Framing Age

Ageing populations have gradually become a major concern in many industrialised countries over the past fifty years, drawing the attention of both politics and science. The target of a raft of health and social policies, older people are often identified as a specific, and vulnerable, population. At the same time, ageing has become a specialisation in many disciplines – medicine, sociology, psychology, to name but three – and a discipline of its own: gerontology.

This book questions the framing of old age by focusing on the relationships between policy making and the production of knowledge. The first part explores how the meeting of scientific expertise and the politics of old age anchors the construction of both individual and collective relationships to the future. Part II brings to light the many ways in which issues relating to ageing can be instrumentalised and ideologised in several public debate arenas. Part III argues that scientific knowledge itself composes with objectivity, bringing ideologies of its own to the table, and looks at how this impacts discourse about ageing. In the final part, the contributors discuss how the frames can themselves be experienced at different levels of the division of labour, whether it is by people who work on them (legislators or scientists), by people working with them (professional carers) or by older people themselves.

Unpacking the political and moral dimensions of scientific research on ageing, this cutting-edge volume brings together a range of multidisciplinary, European perspectives, and will be of use to all those interested in old age and the social sciences.

Iris Loffeier is a permanent Research Fellow in Sociology at HESAV (Haute École de Santé Vaud), Lausanne, Switzerland.

Benoît Majerus is an Associate Professor at the University of Luxembourg, Luxembourg.

Thibauld Moulaert is Associate Professor at the Université de Grenoble-Alpes, France.

Routledge Studies in the Sociology of Health and Illness

For a full list of titles in this series, please visit www.routledge.com.

Framing Age

Contested Knowledge in Science
and Politics

**Edited by Iris Loffeier, Benoît
Majerus and Thibauld Moulaert**

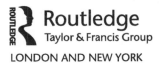

Routledge
Taylor & Francis Group

LONDON AND NEW YORK

First published 2017
by Routledge

2 Park Square, Milton Park, Abingdon, Oxfordshire OX14 4RN
52 Vanderbilt Avenue, New York, NY 10017

*Routledge is an imprint of the Taylor & Francis Group,
an informa business*

First issued in paperback 2019

British Library Cataloguing-in-Publication Data
A catalogue record for this book is available from the British
Library

Library of Congress Cataloging-in-Publication Data
Names: Loffeier, Iris, 1983- editor. | Majerus, Benoãit, editor. |
Moulaert, Thibauld, editor.
Title: Framing age: contested knowledge in science and politics /
edited by Iris Loffeier, Benoãit Majerus and Thibauld Moulaert.
Other titles: Routledge studies in the sociology of health and illness.
Description: Abingdon, Oxon; New York, NY: Routledge, 2017. |
Series: Routledge studies in the sociology of health and illness |
Includes bibliographical references and index.
Identifiers: LCCN 2016055455
Subjects: | MESH: Aged | Sociological Factors | Public Policy |
Aging | Europe Classification: LCC RA418 | NLM WT 30 |
DDC 362.1—dc23
LC record available at https://lccn.loc.gov/2016055455

ISBN: 978-1-138-68383-9 (hbk)
ISBN: 978-0-367-34922-6 (pbk)

Typeset in Times New Roman
by codeMantra

Contents

List of figures and tables

Figures

Tables

Acknowledgements

This book takes its origin in an international conference organised in March 2015 in Luxembourg by the Framing Age (FRAMAG) research team. Johanna Tietje, Sophie Richelle and Manon Pinatel gave a lot to the organisation and we want to thank them in the first place. Many additional people at the University of Luxembourg worked tirelessly to pull the two-day conference together. We especially appreciated the organisational talents of Jolanda Brands, and want to thank her as well as all the conference participants for their contribution to the debates.

We owe to the Luxembourgish Fonds National de la Recherche the possibility of both our team work and the conference. They have been generous supporters for more than three years through the funding scheme CORE, allowing us to experience ideal academic research. We also want to thank Dieter Ferring and his research unit Integrative Research Unit on Social and Individual Development (INSIDE) who helped us finance this event along with a distant, critical but favourable support. We address our many thanks to the History Institute under the direction of Michel Margue and the research unit Identités, Politiques, Sociétés, Espaces (IPSE) under the direction of Christian Schulze for their generous grants.

Stephen Katz, in addition to be a key inspirator and reference had the kindness and generosity to encourage us in the early stages of this book project. His endorsement has been crucial for our whole enterprise, and we are very grateful to him. Grace McInnes and Louisa Vahtrick were then the first at Routledge to make us move forward, and they were followed by Shannon Kneis and Lianne Sherlock on the long road of assembling, editing and finally publishing what once where conference talks. We are very obliged to them and to everyone working at the editing process for making this tangible.

Additionally, we want to address the contributors to this volume with our profound gratitude, as we have been tremendously demanding to them. We much appriciated their patience and enthusiasm to the final stages of this project. Meeting them and having the chance to exchange with such great researchers has been an immense pleasure to the three of us throughout the last two years. Last but not least, Juliette Rogers should be praised for her fantastic language and translating skills, and her prodigious editing contribution to this volume. She relentlessly pushed all of us to reformulate, clarify and strengthen our ideas, far past her due time. We wish to thank her in particular for her amazing work and help.

Iris Loffeier, Benoît Majerus and
Thibauld Moulaert

Introduction

Contested knowledge of ageing. Stepping out to frame the larger picture

*Iris Loffeier, Benoît Majerus
and Thibauld Moulaert*

Since the mid-twentieth century the ageing population has gradually become a major political and scientific concern in most industrialised countries. Politically, welfare states' social and health policies target specific segments of the population such as 'elderly people', people with loss of autonomy, 'seniors' or older workers. At the same time, ageing has become a specialisation in many academic disciplines – medicine, sociology and psychology prominent among them – and it may yet become a specialised subfield in gerontology. From the perspective of knowledge studies, ageing provides a compelling case study in the 'regionalisation of knowledge' (Bernstein, 2000, p. 9): an area ('region') of knowledge that gathers discourses from many horizons and various disciplines. The contours of ageing as a region of knowledge were more or less defined over a century ago, alongside the invention of the terms gerontology (coined in 1903 by Elie Metchnikoff) and geriatrics, although the boundaries,[1] forms, and contents of knowledge production are still in flux today. This book's focus is investigating such a region not as a natural or given phenomenon, but rather as a space of contested knowledge production. It seeks to empirically question scientific, political and everyday framings of age by focusing on the relationships between the production of knowledge, its uses in policy making and daily experience, and the social actors who take part in such dialectics.

What boundaries does knowledge impose around age and ageing as public issues? How do older people and age-policy experts experience those boundaries? How does the focus on old age 'other' older adults? How is this otherness defined? What are the effects of such schemes of knowledge? What is at stake in the production of age-related frames, including those the social sciences help build? On what foundations are some of these boundaries based? Which debates do they feed and perpetuate? What do references to science mean, in practical terms? This volume sets out to answer these questions by bringing together research from Belgium, France, Germany, Luxembourg, Norway, Spain, Sweden and Switzerland. Contributing historians, sociologists, anthropologists and philosophers all focus on the core empirical elements that are at issue when the topic of ageing is addressed, including the contributions scientific discourses make to frame-building. Twelve original chapters based on field or archival research offer insight into perceptions of ageing by showing what is highlighted and obscured by frames of ageing, and how such frames are (re)produced in a variety of ways and countries, at different scales of observation, and in a variety of discourses.

The book has three objectives. First, its focus arose from the observation of a double gap in social science research on ageing. For one thing, there is a dearth of research questioning the construction of a region of knowledge of ageing, and little recent work has unpacked its political and moral dimensions and impacts. As the example of 'alarmist demography', the concomitant fear of a 'decline' in population (Katz, 1992), and many chapters in this book demonstrate, the moral content of knowledge and discourses on ageing needs to be assessed. For another thing, research has largely ignored political, media and common uses of scientific knowledge, and has tended to analyse such uses more as coherent objects than polyphonic discourse (Ducrot, 1984). Media and political discourses on ageing are fuelled by the legitimacy of scientific discourse, while scientific discourses and research trends are partly shaped by public funding. Approaching the subject from different social sciences and countries, this volume intends to show that interactions between knowledge production and age policies are, among other things, strongly expressed through 'moral entrepreneurship' (Becker, 1966) and are built through direct and indirect exchanges between science and policy.

The second aim of this book is to expand the international perspective of ageing studies by acknowledging and moving past the Anglophone narrative in the field. Such a 'predominantly Anglo-American (UK–USA–Canada) emphasis' has already been identified in certain texts (Nikander, 2009, p. 650), but rarely remedied (Lamb, 2015). The ageing-studies literature about the United States is unquestionably rich, but too often conclusions for the US are transposed unchanged into European contexts, regardless of its very different chronologies and actors. The case of pension systems exemplifies such differences. The diversity of European welfare states involving numerous players – be it states as such or various semi-public institutions created after 1945, such as social security in France or the so-called 'Nordic model' – necessarily leads to structurally different settings and paths, as Esping-Andersen archetypically presented in *The Three Worlds of Welfare Capitalism* (1990).[2] A comparative and transnational approach makes it possible to elaborate an understanding of Europeanisation processes and highlight national and local differences. In this sense, bringing together researchers from various parts of Europe and assembling works from several language areas of the continent – although also 'overwhelmingly Western' (Troyanski, 2016, p. xv) in both global and European terms – seemed to be a reasonable first step towards meeting this international challenge. The result already makes valuable contributions without overly blurring specificities of time and space. (Re)introducing European voices from a variety of countries and language areas will hopefully open the way for other epistemologies and scientific communities to join the reflexive debate.[3]

Third, this book can be understood as an epistemological attempt to situate knowledge of ageing. It is not part of what could be called ageing studies, but it does engage with it in many respects. But before developing this third aim any further, we should first give an overview of the central debates in the region of knowledge in which we as editors situate this volume.

Who talks about ageing?

A central but implicit issue in ageing research has been defining which disciplines are most legitimate for exploring the topic. Competing disciplines and specialists have been claiming to be the legitimate authority to 'talk about' ageing throughout the twentieth century and into the twenty-first. The medical and social sciences were probably the first sources of conflicting claims to being the legitimate voice of age studies. The medicalisation of ageing (Le Bihan & Mallon, 2014), which is one of the dominant critical master narratives of the twentieth century, appears to be part of the wider phenomenon of 'scientification of the social' (Raphael, 1996) in which social problems, formerly understood as political, come to be seen as scientific issues instead. Social scientists have accused the biological/medical lens of perceiving ageing as a process of senescence of the 'aged body' (Katz, 1996). That said, the medicalisation of ageing seems like a distinctly social-science discourse, therefore attesting to their early presence in the region of knowledge. In other words, the social sciences played a meaningful role in the struggle over age studies, having interests and 'ways of knowing' (Pickstone, 2001) of their own to defend, although their participation was uneven over time and from place to place.

Social sciences at the heart of the knowledge-region of ageing

While North American social scientists' claims on ageing emerged in the 1930s (Achenbaum, 1995) and more broadly during the Great Depression (Park, 2009), the starting point of such a struggle in France can be traced to the 1960s (Feller, 2005, p. 13) and 1970s, the period of the first oil crisis and strong attacks upon the welfare state (Rosanvallon, 1981). In Belgium, the call to study the social dimension of senescence beyond its medical aspects was made at the First Conference of the International Association of Gerontology, held in Liège in July 1950.[4]

Within the social sciences, both sociology of ageing in continental Europe (Hummel *et al.*, 2014; Van Dyk, 2015) and Anglo-American critical gerontology have taken a markedly ambivalent stand, positioning themselves simultaneously as active partners in the region of knowledge (notably by participating in defining and evaluating policies on ageing) and as external and critical observers of this process. This tension between theory and practice seems to remain intractable and has led to the formula that there are two types of sociologist (Katz, 2014), the supposedly 'purist' academic/ theoretical sociologist and the more result-oriented 'applied' sociologist. Their respective accusations of lacking proper scientific objectives and holding forth without empirical knowledge pressure everyone in the field to take sides.[5]

More broadly, other social science disciplines also claim the right to legitimately work on the topic, and perhaps with less disarray than in sociology. For instance, in France (and elsewhere, see Katz, 1992; Mottu-Weber, 1994) demography was a key player in getting old age labelled as a public problem, and it made several claims to ownership. Such claims occurred at different periods in different places, consequently affecting power relations between scientific disciplines within each country. From its inception in 1945 through the 1950s, the French Institut National d'Études Démographiques (National Institute of Demographic Studies, INED) was virtually the idealtype of the nascent 'expertise' paradigm of the second half of the twentieth century (Delmas, 2011). INED asserted a scientific rationale to argue for the depolitisation of major socio-economic questions, without denying science the ability to intervene in policy. As Paul Paillat, a demographer working for INED, wrote in 1960 in *Population*, INED's journal: 'Our only aim is to supply rational policy with basic data' (p. 10). INED was nevertheless quite successful at taking control of age, because it was INED that framed the paradigms presented by the French Laroque Report. Published in 1962, it was the work of an official commission charged with exploring the issue of ageing in France. To this day, it is widely referred to as the first and foremost political attempt to assess ageing and define it with precision. In Germany, however, demography was partially discredited for the role population studies had played in National Socialism, and national leaders of the second half of the twentieth century could not approach anything resembling population control until the 1980s at the earliest (Overath, 2011).[6] Instead, social psychology took a very early interest in ageing issues in Germany, as evidenced by an early longitudinal study started in Bonn in the 1960s, the Bonner Gerontologische Längsschnittstudie (Gerontological longitudinal study from Bonn, BOLSA). One of the founding participants in the BOLSA study, psychologist Ursula Lehr, became a member of the German Parliament and served as federal Minister for the Family from 1989 to 1990.[7] In the social sciences, psycho-gerontological approaches gradually but unquestionably came to dominate the region.

These examples, further compounded by inclusion of economists' analyses of retirement, make it untenable to think that the social sciences were absent from the process of defining ageing: they have been central actors. Social science disciplines have been involved in the process of building, confirming and legitimating the category of old age. But the 'human sciences'[8] have played only a minor role, and are clearly latecomers to the vast field of ageing studies.

Contrasted disciplinary and epistemological traditions at stake

The major reason for this lesser engagement in the French and German human sciences is the prominence of the notion of social class in sociology and history since the 1960s, so the notions of age or generations did not resonate as paradigms (Mallon *et al.*, 2014, p. 12). This is notably evident in French sociological production of the second half of the twentieth century, in which, for instance, the schools of neither Pierre Bourdieu nor Alain Touraine produced major research on ageing,[9] with the noticeable exception of the works of Anne-Marie Guillemard. She is the only disciple of Alain Touraine – and was the only French sociologist for several decades – who showed a continued interest for the topic since her major seminal book, *La retraite: une mort sociale*, in 1972 and her later work on French public policy's role in producing ageing (Guillemard, 1980). Similar to Anglo-American gerontology's growing interest in actors and their experience beyond the analysis of structures and their effects (Phillipson, 1998), a new generation of sociologists has only slowly emerged since the 1990s. They have been showing less interest in the social production of ageing by public policy and more attention to the micro-production and experiences of ageing, through attention to the role of the couple during retirement (Caradec, 1996) or interactionist study of the experience of living in retirement homes (Mallon, 2004). Regardless, there are still no sociological journals devoted to ageing as an issue in France or Germany, although sociologists have been quite present as authors and board members of the French journals *Gérontologie et société* and *Retraite et Société*, and the German journals *Zeitschrift für Gerontologie und Geriatrie*. This is in stark contrast to publications focusing on identity markers such as class, gender and even other generational categories, such as youth.

The same can be said for history. The notion of generation was absent from historiography for quite some time. Starting in the 1970s, as social history developed in Europe, age slowly appeared as a category, first for youth (Heilbronner, 2008) and then old age. It was the dominant demography that initially got historians interested in generations, which they mainly used to reconstruct a demographic history of old age going back to the sixteenth century, where systematically structured archival records were available. Parallel to this interest, often contextualised in a long-term perspective, some historians focused on the more recent period, especially the last third of the nineteenth century and the first third of the twentieth century. They reconstructed the gradual development of the welfare state, paying particular attention to the expansion of pension systems, among other things. Generally speaking, this historiography painted a rather grim picture of what modernisation did to old age, a view that has been nuanced in the last 15 to 20 years. The cultural turn that also influenced historiography questioned the narrative of the 'golden age', showing that the introduction of class, race and gender into analyses of old age revealed that the once seemingly homogeneous group of older people had in fact always been highly heterogeneous (Thane, 2003, p. 93; Blessing, 2010; Kampf, 2015). To this day, the historiography of ageing remains very fragmented and marginal within historical scholarship (Kampf, 2015).[10] Although there was a sudden fancy for the topic in the 1980s and 1990s that made it seem that the history of ageing might be a whole new domain for historical research (Mottu-Weber, 1994), such interest appears to have been short lived. Although there were a handful of such researchers in each country in the 2010s, it seems rather unrealistic to talk of 'humanistic gerontology'. Other than sociology, the human sciences of history and anthropology[11] thus far do not seem to have been able to establish an age-specific subfield or develop a common vocabulary through interdisciplinary journals or organisations.

Beyond the involvement of particular disciplines, research has focused on different interests over time and in different places. In Anglo-American critical gerontology, social policies and welfare (among other concepts) have been explored and built using 'moral economy', as seen in works of Phillipson (1982) and Walker (1981) in the United Kingdom, Estes (1979) and Minkler and Estes (1991) in the United States, and Myles (1984) in Canada.[12] This literature's general argument is that older people are excluded from social life and marginalised as a consequence of capitalism and its regulation. This 'political economy' perspective was joined by other emerging fields of knowledge like 'human gerontology' (Gubrium, 1993) and 'cultural studies' (Featherstone & Hepworth, 1989, 1990; Cole, 1992; Blaikie, 1999) to form 'critical gerontology'. Devoting more space to the agency of older adults and exploration of the effects of ageing's cultural dimensions from a historical perspective, these approaches are attentive to discourses, images and popular culture, and are particularly sensitive to diversity, paradoxes and individualism, opening new avenues for research. Inspired by Habermas and other scholars, attention to praxis (Moody, 1988, 1993) and the relationship between science and action (Dannefer *et al.*, 2008) has opened additional approaches[13] to this eclectic field of research. This eclecticism is visible in the dedicated *Journal of Aging Studies*. It has been also at the centre of reflection about the constitution of proper regions of research, whether it be gerontology itself (Achenbaum, 1995; Katz, 1996; Park, 2009) or sub- and side-categories such as critical gerontology or the more recent cultural gerontology.

Attempts to structure the field and recent claims to legitimacy

The structuring of this eclectic field is strongly connected to claims over what 'good' research on ageing should be. Such claims were one of the organising principles of the aforementioned literature about ageing, and they primarily appear in the debate over naming sub-disciplines that accompanies such work. Choice of the labels that the region of knowledge and its sub-fields should bear is connected to contrasting definitions of what 'ways of knowing' (Pickstone, 2001) and research communities they embrace.

Gerontology? While numerous publications have wondered if it should be considered an actual discipline (see, for example, Levine, 1981; Lowenstein, 2004) and related to 'the need for theory' (Biggs *et al.*, 2003) or perhaps be thought of as a profession instead (Hirschfield & Peterson, 1982), its diversity in methods and communities has been repeatedly put into question. Social gerontology? Critical gerontology? Cultural gerontology?[14] In the social sciences, the structure of interdisciplinary sub-categories of ageing is one of many sites of contested knowledge production. While Anglo-American social scientists have appropriated (and modified) the category of gerontology with the addition of qualifying prefixes, the Francophone social sciences (Moulaert, 2012) have almost completely rejected this label. This difference is also found in the degrees offered by university-level social science programmes: for instance, while David A. Peterson states that Master's degrees in gerontology are very common and similar in the United States (Peterson, 1984), Françoise Leborgne-Uguen and Simone Pennec (2012) show that in France, unlike Quebec and Brasil, ageing studies degree programmes make no reference to gerontology in either their names or curricula, and choose to refer to a variety of classic academic disciplines instead.

There are also differences among countries in the ways in which categories of knowledge are divided that can be seen as temporary outcomes of struggles over legitimacy. This essentially means that similar discourses, understood as belonging to different categories of knowledge, do not represent the same contexts, voices or degree of legitimacy, and so they cannot be assumed to convey identical contents and conceptions. Let alone the epistemological distance revealed in the uses and status of the work of certain theorists (especially Foucault), cultural studies, and 'French Theory' in diverse scientific communities on both sides of the Atlantic (Cusset, 2003) – and thus presumably around the world – despite the seeming similarity of references and associated vocabulary. This might nuance Troyanski's statement on the worldwide scientific uniformity of the region of ageing studies: 'It almost doesn't matter where the research is being done. The models are international. (…) [S]cholarly frameworks are globalized, and often the terms of the debate have their origins in the West' (Troyanski, 2016, p. 124). Even 'in the West', knowledges of ageing develop at different paces and with disparate contents. This is especially evident concerning language areas, but also occurs within national borders and communities (including scientific communities), as many chapters of this book illustrate.

Stepping out of ageing studies: A proposal for another structure of knowledge, non-regional and multi-disciplinary

This book brings together researchers whose practices are grounded in different but complementary disciplines. The wide-ranging chapters and disciplines each contribute pieces to an empirically grounded puzzle, respecting their classic disciplinary standards while stepping in some way out of ageing studies. The guiding hypothesis is that ageing studies, as a region of knowledge, should first be thought of as a subject for analysis before being taken as an object to be defined. This makes it possible to focus on the forms, contents, structures and uses of knowledge, creating the potential for new knowledge on ageing that might not require new subdivisions of knowledge, further facilitated by at least temporarily stepping out of such a region of knowledge. This is not, however, to deny the value of ageing-studies publications that will be widely cited: the specificities of ageing must be studied and the relationship between action and knowledge taken into account. Our initiative is simply different in some respects, and hopefully complementary to ageing studies. In reference to critical gerontology's own original self-critique (Katz, 1996), we are gambling on the heuristics of researchers of different disciplines and topics joining forces. For one thing, we believe ageing studies benefits from the standard tools of anthropology, history, sociology and philosophy, not to mention their divisions of labour and the dialogue between them. Additionally, in contrast with 'critical-', 'social-' and 'cultural'-gerontology, providing an arena for dialogue for researchers who are not exclusively specialised in ageing opens the way for a novel grasp of its specificities while making a serious effort to answer the call for 'undisciplining old age' (Katz, 1996). We want to emphasise the fact that specialising research exclusively on ageing runs the risk of making ageing appear distinctive as a result of the division of labour in the field of knowledge production, rather than due to its actual specificities. Epistemologically, a specialised region of knowledge presupposes the phenomenon's specificities and takes them for granted. Methodologically, social studies of ageing are in most cases based on empirical enquiry conducted exclusively with older people, although comparative methods and tools are necessary to provide the basis for demonstrating specificities. Such choices limit the phenomenon to a pre-defined segment of the population, confirming epistemological specificities with methodologically induced ones. This is why we were particularly attentive to boundaries, to such an extent that the notion structures the book.

   This book is organised in four parts, each addressing the social challenges associated with the boundaries of age as a region. Part I is devoted to demonstrating that the frame of old age fundamentally delimits the projected futures of societies as well as individuals. It probes what lies at the heart of the framing of ageing: agency over the future. Part II shows how framings of old age define and delimit groups and communities, fixing certain categories of otherness from numerous possibilities; 'older people' is the obvious one, but national and 'cultural' communities are also in play. In other words, Part II is about how the boundaries between categories unite and separate, defining multiple kinds of insiders and outsiders. Part III gets to the ties between 'the political' and science, assessing how their social foundations work together, from collaborative exchange through points of tension. It focuses on the bridges and connections between each side of a boundary, in this case between science and 'the political'. Finally, Part IV stresses the actual actions that can appropriate and modify boundaries, how such boundaries are adjusted and experienced by actors at different levels. Like Part I, this last section starts with a chapter providing a macro-level analysis, then shifts to the meso-level, and concludes with insights on the micro-level.

Part I: The future at the heart of the region of ageing

Part I sheds light on how the intersection of expert knowledge and old-age policy influences the construction of both individual and collective relationships to future. Each in its own way, the three chapters illustrate that trying to glimpse and rationalise the future using simplified and recontextualised scientific discourses contributes to the construction of ageing as a public, political and individual problem. The section starts by setting the scene, introducing the frequent site where science and policy first encounter each other in the realm of ageing: demography, which is called upon even more than usual to shape the debate by bringing numbers to the table. Reinhard Messerschmidt (Chapter 1) radically unpacks the choices behind demographic projections and dissemination to analyse how they interact with media discourses. He shows how the media's recontextualisation of demographic discourses on ageing ultimately results in reducing it to the depiction of a distressing future. His conclusion illustrates how difficult it is for demography to present more nuanced proposals that would or could be widely circulated. At an intermediary level bridging society and the individual, Cécile Collinet and Matthieu Delalandre (Chapter 2) explore the ways in which prevention discourses relate individual life planning to the future of society in the promotion of physical activities for the not-yet-elderly. Their contribution painstakingly documents how national, European and international plans for prevention policy evoke complex scientific knowledge to further justify governance according to anticipated future trends. They show how such complexity is nonetheless simplified, as probabilistic relations become causal relations and uncertainty is transformed into strong statements. At the micro-level, Mark Schweda and Larissa Pfaller (Chapter 3) shed light on the entanglement of 'regimes of truth' and 'regimes of hope' in their description of how people use expert knowledge in anti-ageing medicine. Although expert knowledge tends to govern the relationship between the present and future under a regime of certainty, they show that even the most enthusiastic users of anti-ageing medicine accept the unknown space between their present lifestyle and the future to which it might lead. Rather than purely acritical belief, they observe and identify a series of connected and nuanced positions – with more subtlety than media and policies – that show how the future is actually something individuals also work on.

Part II: Defining boundaries, defining insiders and outsiders

Part II brings to light the many ways in which the category 'old age' defines communities and groups, not only within its boundaries but also beyond the targeted public. Its three chapters are informative on the ways this category can be instrumentalised and used ideologically as a rhetorical strategy in several arenas. Authors reveal how dwelling on supposed elderly misery (be it social, biological or both) paves the way for 'moral entrepreneurs' (Becker, 1966) and targeted ideologies that paradoxically weaken social bonds. Magnus Nilsson (Chapter 4) examines uses of the stereotype of the deserving old person as an ideological tool in nationalist discourse in several discursive arenas in Sweden (but with clear resonance for other European countries). Study of such discourses allowed him to clearly outline how nationalism can articulate with the welfare of older people, implicitly casting some kinds of people outside the borders of admitted European political communities. This not only occurs in public debate but also at the very heart of scientific concepts like the 'moral economy of ageing' (Kohli, 1991). Nilsson exposes the ideological character of the category of old age that defines both the people it refers to and 'the community, as such'. Alexandre Lambelet (Chapter 5), in his study of public discussion of sexual and suicide assistance in Switzerland, shows how labelling people as old and elderly also specifies activities. He analyses how the definition of 'the elderly' reframes what individuals do, adapting the terms of the debate to perceived needs and rights of older people that are inspired by particularly populist and miserabilist interpretations. Finally, Richard C. Keller (Chapter 6) continues these reflections in his analysis of 'the *canicule*' in France, the 2003 heat wave that lead to staggering death rates of elderly people, and the political shock wave that followed. He found that an increasingly strident discourse gradually framed the elderly of France as a population at the limits of citizenship and a burden for an emerging postindustrial nation. He notably shows how considering the aged body through a biological lens can justify exclusion of the 'frail' elderly from the social contract when their death, illnesses, difficulties or loneliness are understood as normal.

Part III: Bridges between science and policy

In Part III, three contributions further deepen this approach, showing that scientific knowledge itself is a compromise with objectivity and has ideologies of its own. The authors open the knowledge production field to prove that neither scientists nor their output are free from particular interests, ideologies or rhetoric. Beyond ideology, those chapters' depictions unveil the actual scientific activities that contribute to shaping frames of ageing, a scientific undertaking that is strongly connected to social work and evolving 'realities' of how knowledge of the elderly is partly produced for policy making. Pursuing the archaeology of knowledge, Nicole Kramer (Chapter 7) explores gender and ageing issues by tracing the connections between elder care policies, scientific discourses and feminist claims. Using archival materials to track their historical contexts in careful detail, she provides clear insight on colluding or opposing interests that paradoxically appeared in discourses of similar content. Her analysis also documents how these different social arenas legitimise one another and how they are simultaneously mutually beneficial and competing in a struggle for legitimacy. Antía Pérez-Caramés (Chapter 8) unpacks the situation in Galicia – also known as the 'oldest region of Spain' – to stress the overlap of demographic knowledge and political orientations in relation to media discourses. Relations between 'alarmist demographers', the press and policy makers are revealing of how pro-natalist solutions become consensus and are promoted with minimal discussion despite the fact that they represent a complete political reversal. Her contribution also illustrates how alarmist demographic knowledge circulates between national borders, from France to Spain. Nicolas Belorgey (Chapter 9) presents the current instrument for assessing dependency in France (the AGGIR scale) resulting from geriatric medicine's political and strategic struggle for greater control over a period of over 20 years. Dissecting the AGGIR scale's internal operation and historical implementation, he shows that inventing the measurement process was not only about knowledge production on the part of geriatricians, but also about taking real political action and securing control over the domain for their profession.

Part IV: Experiencing, playing with, shifting boundaries

Frames are not only built, they are also experienced. Authors in Part IV illustrate how frames can be experienced at different levels of the division of labour, whether by people who build them (legislators and scientists), people using them (professional caregivers) or 'elderly people' themselves. Lucie Lechevalier Hurard and Benoît Eyraud (Chapter 10), examining the issues raised by the limitation of freedom of movement in elder care, portray the long-lasting challenges in setting the perimeters defining a category of elderly people to be specifically protected by law. They show that there is still no consensus over elderly people as a group in civil law, as the ideal balance between protection and stigmatisation remains elusive or even impossible. They demonstrate how boundary-making nonetheless had a pivotal moment in the 2000s concerning elderly people with Alzheimer's disease or dementia. Without a firm legal consensus on the elderly in civil law, specific soft law has been providing the only possible answer by setting boundaries within the category instead. This chapter illustrates how difficult the issue of boundaries has been for those in charge of formally delimiting them. Although the category of elderly people seems to be self-evident and well established, this chapter shows how wide the actual gap is between representations of old age and how it is institutionalised in law. Jingyue Xing and Solène Billaud (Chapter 11) present how colleagues from two distinct professional backgrounds in France (nursing and social work) build their own shared expertise and approach to autonomy assessment. They describe how they manipulate apparently rigid frames when evaluating the needs of elderly people living at home. Their meso-level findings serve as a call for greater attention to the role of intermediate professions – street-level bureaucrats – in charge of public policies. Last, Aske Juul Lassen (Chapter 12) provides a more micro-level analysis with the observation of specific situations and very usefully enhances the definition of the concept of 'technologies'. He explores elderly people's leisure activities through the frame of active ageing policies, revealing how far they are from expert definitions. Some older billiards players do not see themselves as active agers, despite the fact that their practices unexpectedly fall into the institutional frame of active ageing, the existence of which they acknowledge and work to transform. The three last chapters seem to be a final reminder that a specific kind of social activity always accompanies frames: play with the very boundaries they impose.

Notes

1 We also use Basil Bernstein's metaphor of the boundary, which relates to classification. Classification is the very activity that creates categories, categories of knowledge among them. Boundaries separate categories from one another (as 'insulation', in Bernstein's terms) and are maintained, reinforced or weakened by power relations and struggles – that is, by their social basis (Bernstein, 2000, p. 99). In this sense, regions are a type of category of knowledge, as are academic disciplines, and boundaries are what separate, for instance, sociology from psychology, 'the elderly' from 'young people', etc.

2 His model was also critically revised to include Southern European welfare states (Ferrera, 1996) and take better account of gender issues (Lewis, 1992). From a similar international perspective, Guillemard (2010) shows how the place of older people in employment (at work, retired or going into early retirement) varied according to the welfare state, relations between the parties involved and cultures of ageing.

3 Publishing such work in English is part of a more general position on research and its language of expression. As continental European researchers, we argue that there is need for national-language-based scientific publishing. But we also strongly advocate for the sharing of local ways of practising research and locally situated results in English to contribute to global heuristics.

4 Reports of the first international conference on gerontology, Liège, 10–12 July 1950, *Revue médicale de Liège*, V(20); http://digitalassets.lib.berkeley.edu/irle/ucb/text/lb001454.pdf, accessed 26 December 2016.

5 So far very few scholars have attempted to bridge the alleged 'gap'. Such distinctions also exist in other disciplines, such as among geriatricians; see Belorgey's chapter in this volume.

6 A feature that links Germany and Spain (see Messerschmidt & Pérez-Caramés in this volume).

7 For further reading: Birren, James E., and J.J.F. Schroots. 'The History of Geropsychology'. In *Handbook of the Psychology of Aging*, edited by James E. Birren and K.W. Schaie, 5th ed., 3–28. San Diego: Academia Press, 2001; and Birren, J.E., and J.J.F. Schroots, eds. *A History of Geropsychology in Autobiography*. Washington: American Psychological Association, 2000.

8 A term in common use in Europe referring to disciplines addressing the biological, social and cultural aspects of human existence, including sociology, anthropology, history and philosophy.
9 Rémi Lenoir, a disciple of Pierre Bourdieu, briefly worked on the topic at the end of the 1970s before changing orientation.
10 In contrast to youth studies, which even has its own journal in France: *Revue d'histoire de l'enfance 'irrégulière' (Journal of the History of 'Irregular' Childhood)*.
11 This despite the creation of an international Association for Anthropology and Gerontology in 1978, and the recognition of ageing as 'an explicit topic of anthropological research' in the 1970s (Degnen, 2015, p. 106).
12 Anne-Marie Guillemard's work could also be considered close to such a perspective, despite being more concerned with the sociology of public ageing-related policies rather than social gerontology.
13 This specific effort to connect research and action also motivated Phillipson and Walker's original call for 'critical gerontology' removed from the 'mainstream' (1987).
14 The example of the recent handbook on the subject of 'cultural gerontology' (Twigg & Martin, 2015a, 2015b), embracing broad fields of knowledge from the social sciences and humanities, can be read as a new attempt to impose a categorical structure on a field of knowledge, with a claim of legitimacy as its starting point.

References

Achenbaum W. Andrew (1995), *Crossing Frontiers: Gerontology Emerges as a Science*. Cambridge, New York, Cambridge University Press.
Becker Howard (1966), *Social Problems: A Modern Approach*. New York, Wiley.
Bernstein Basil (2000), *Pedagogy, Symbolic Control and Identity. Theory, Research, Critique*. Oxford, Rowman & Littlefield Publishers [1996].
Biggs Simon, Lowenstein Ariela & Jon Hendricks (eds) (2003), *The Need for Theory*. Amityville, NY, Baywood.
Blaikie Andrew (1999), *Ageing and Popular Culture*. Cambridge, Cambridge University Press.
Blessing Bettina (2010), 'Die Geschichte des Alters in der Moderne: Stand der deutschen Forschung', *Medizin, Gesellschaft und Geschichte*, Vol. 29, pp. 123–150.
Caradec Vincent (1996), *Le couple à l'heure de la retraite*. Rennes, Presses Universitaires de Rennes.
Cole Thomas (1992), *The Journey of Life: A Cultural History of Aging in America*. New York, Cambridge University Press.
Cusset François (2003), *French Theory: Foucault, Derrida, Deleuze & Cie et les mutations de la vie intellectuelle aux États-Unis*. Paris, La Découverte.
Dannefer Dale, Stein Paul, Siders Rebecca & Robin Shura Patterson (2008), 'Is That All There Is? The Concept of Care and the Dialectic of Critique', *Journal of Aging Studies*, Vol. 22, no. 2, pp. 101–108.
Degnen Cathrine (2015), 'Ethnographies of ageing'. In Twigg Julia and Wendy Martin, *Routledge Handbook of Cultural Gerontology*. Oxford and New York, Routledge, pp. 106–112.
Delmas Corinne (2011), *Sociologie politique de l'expertise*. Paris, La Découverte.
Ducrot Oswald (1984), *Le dire et le dit*. Paris, Les éditions de Minuit.
Esping-Andersen Gøsta (1990), *The Three Worlds of Welfare Capitalism*. Cambridge, Polity Press.

Estes Caroll (1979), *The Aging Enterprise. A Critical Examination of Social Policies and Services for the Aged*. San Francisco, Jossey-Bass.

Estes Carroll, Biggs Simon & Chris Phillipson (2003), *Social Theory, Social Policy and Ageing: A Critical Introduction*. London, Open University Press.

Featherstone Mike & Mike Hepworth (1989), 'Ageing and Old Age: Reflections on the Postmodern Lifecourse'. In Bytheway Bill, Kiel Teresa, Allatt Patricia and Allan Bryman (eds), *Becoming and Being Old*. London, Sage, pp. 143–157.

Featherstone Mike & Mike Hepworth (1990), 'Images of Ageing'. In Featherstone Mike and Andrew Wernick (eds), *Images of Ageing*. London, Routledge, pp. 29–48.

Feller Elise (2005), *Histoire de la vieillesse en France 1900–1960. Du vieillard au retraité*, Paris, Éditions Seli Arslan.

Ferrera Maurizio (1996), 'The "Southern Model" of Welfare in Social Europe', *Journal of European Social Policy*, Vol. 6, no. 1, pp. 17–37.

Gubrium Jaber F. (1993), *Speaking of Life: Horizons of Meaning for Nursing Home Residents*. New York, Walther de Gruyter.

Guillemard Anne-Marie (1972), *La Retraite: une mort sociale. Sociologie des conduites en situation de retraite*. Paris/La Haye, Mouton.

Guillemard Anne-Marie (1980), *La vieillesse et l'État*. Paris, Presses Universitaires de France.

Guillemard Anne-Marie (1986), *Le Déclin du social: Formation et crise des politiques de la vieillesse*. Paris, Presses Universitaires de France.

Guillemard Anne-Marie (2010), *Les défis du vieillissement. Âge, emploi, retraite. Perspectives internationales*. Paris, Armand Colin.

Heilbronner Oded (2008), 'From a Culture for Youth to a Culture of Youth: Recent Trends in the Historiography of Western Youth Cultures, *Contemporary European History*, Vol. 17, no. 04, pp. 575–591.

Hirschfield Ira S. & David A. Peterson (1982), 'The Professionalization of Gerontology', *The Gerontologist*, Vol. 22, no. 2, pp. 215–220.

Hummel Cornelia, Mallon Isabelle & Vincent Caradec (eds.) (2014), *Vieillesses et vieillissements: regards sociologiques*. Rennes, Presses Universitaires de Rennes.

Kampf Antje (2015), 'Historians of Ageing and the "Cultural Turn"'. In Twigg Julia and Wendy Martin (eds.), *Routledge Handbook of Cultural Gerontology*. Oxford and New York, Routledge, pp. 45–52.

Katz Stephen (1992), 'Alarmist Demography: Power, Knowledge, and the Elderly Population', *Journal of Aging Studies*, Vol. 3, no. 6, pp. 203–225.

Katz Stephen (1996), *Disciplining Old Age: The Formation of Gerontological Knowledge*. Charlottesville, VA and London, University Press of Virginia.

Katz Stephen (2003), 'Critical Gerontology Theory: Intellectual Fieldwork and the Nomadic Life of Ideas'. In Biggs Simon, Lowenstein Ariela and Jon Hendricks (eds), *The Need for Theory*. Amityville, NY, Baywood, pp. 15–31.

Katz Stephen (2014), 'What Is Age Studies?', *Age Culture Humanities*, no. 1, http://ageculturehumanities.org/WP/what-is-age-studies/, accessed 20 December 2016.

Kohli Martin (1991), 'Retirement and the Moral Economy: An Historical Interpretation of the German Case'. In Minkler Meredith and Caroll L. Estes (eds), *Critical Perspectives on Aging: The Political and Moral Economy of Growing Old*. Amityville, NY, Baywood.

Lamb Sarah (2015), 'Beyond the View of the West. Ageing and Anthropology'. In Twigg Julia and Wendy Martin (ed.), *Routledge Handbook of Cultural Gerontology*. Oxford and New York, Routledge, pp. 37–44.

Le Bihan Blanche & Isabelle Mallon (eds) (2014) 'La médicalisation de la vieillesse, enjeux et ambivalences', *Retraite et Société*, Vol. 67, no. 1.

Leborgne-Uguen Françoise & Simone Pennec (2012), 'Réflexions à partir d'une expérience universitaire de formations en sciences sociales dans le domaine du vieillissement', *Gérontologie et société*, Vol. 3, no. 142, pp. 57–80.

Lechevalier Hurard Lucie (2015), 'Être présent auprès des absents. Ethnographie de la spécialisation des pratiques professionnelles autour de la maladie d'Alzheimer en établissement d'hébergement pour personnes âgées'. *Thèse pour le grade de docteur en sociologie*, Paris 13 Nord.

Levine Martin (1981), 'Guest Editorial: Does Gerontology Exist?', *The Gerontologist*, 1981, Vol. 21, no. 1, pp. 2–3.

Lewis Jane (1992), 'Gender and the Development of Welfare Regimes', *Journal of European Social Policy*, Vol. 2, no. 3, pp. 159–173.

Lowenstein Ariela (2004), 'Gerontology Coming Of Age: The Transformation Of Social Gerontology into a Distinct Academic Discipline', *Educational Gerontology*, Vol. 30, no. 2, pp. 129–141.

Mallon Isabelle (2004), *Vivre En Maison de Retraite. Le Dernier Chez-Soi*. Rennes, Presses universitaires de Rennes, coll. Le sens social.

Mallon, Isabelle, Cornelia Hummel, et Vincent Caradec. 2014. Vieillesses et vieillissements: les enjeux d'un ouvrage. In *Vieillesses et vieillissements: regards sociologiques*, édité par Cornelia Hummel, Isabelle Mallon, et Vincent Caradec, 9–19. Rennes: PUR.

Metchnikoff Élie (1903), *Études sur la nature humaine: essai de philosophie optimiste*. Paris, Masson.

Minkler Meredith & Caroll L. Estes (eds.) (1991), *Critical Perspectives on Aging: The Political and Moral Economy of Growing Old*. Amityville, NY, Baywood.

Moody Harry R. (1988), 'Toward a Critical Gerontology: The Contribution of the Humanities to Theories of Aging'. In Birren James E., Bengtson Vern L., and Donna E. Deutchman (eds), *Emergent Theories of Aging*. New York, Springer, pp. 19–40.

Moody Harry R. (1993), 'Overview: What Is Critical Gerontology and Why Is It Important?'. In Cole Thomas, Achenbaum Andrew W., Jakobi Patricia L. and Robert Kastenbaum (eds), *Voices and Visions of Aging: Toward a Critical Gerontology*. New York, Springer, pp. xv–xli.

Mottu-Weber Liliane (1994), 'Être vieux à Genève sous l'ancien régime'. In Heller Geneviève (ed.), *Le Poids des ans. Une histoire de la vieillesse en Suisse Romande*. Lausanne, SHSR & Éditions d'en bas, pp. 47–66.

Moulaert Thibauld (2012), 'Pourquoi les francophones préfèrent-ils la sociologie du vieillissement à la gérontologie critique?', *Gérontologie et Société*, Vol. 142, No. 3, pp. 81–99.

Myles John (1984), *Old Age and the Welfare State: The Political Economy of Public Pensions*. Boston, MA, Little Brown.

Nikander Pirjo (2009), 'Walking the Talk: Becoming One's Own Data as Critical Scholar', *Review Essay, Ageing & Society*, Vol. 29, No. 4, pp. 649–651.

Overath Petra (ed.) (2011), *Die vergangene Zukunft Europas: Bevölkerungsforschung und -prognosen im 20. und 21. Jahrhundert*. Köln, Böhlau.

Paillat Paul (1960), Les moyens d'existence des personnes âgées: le schéma démo-économique', *Population*, Vol. 15, no. 1, p. 10.

Park Hyung Wook (2009), 'Refiguring Old Age: Shaping Scientific Research on Senescence, 1900–1960', *Phd Dissertation*, University of Minnesota.

Peterson David A. (1984), 'Are Master's Degrees in Gerontology Comparable?', *The Gerontologist*, Vol. 24, no. 6, pp. 646–651.

Phillipson Chris (1982), *Capitalism and the Construction of Old Age*. London, MacMillan.

Phillipson Chris (1998), *Reconstructing Old Age: New Agendas in Social Theory and Practice*. London, Sage Publications.

Phillipson Chris & Alan Walker (1987), 'The Case for a Critical Gerontology'. In Di Gregorio Silvana (ed.), *Social Gerontology: New Directions*. London, Croom Helm, pp. 1–15.

Pickstone John V. (2001), *Ways of Knowing: A New History of Science, Technology, and Medicine*. Chicago, University of Chicago Press.

Raphael Lutz (1996), 'Die Verwissenschaftlichung des Sozialen als methodische und konzeptionelle Herausforderung für eine Sozialgeschichte des 20. Jahrhunderts', *Geschichte und Gesellschaft*, Vol. 22, no. 2, pp. 165–193.

Rosanvallon Pierre (1981), *La Crise de l'État-Providence*. Paris, Seuil.

Thane Pat (2003), 'Social Histories of Old Age and Aging', *Journal of Social History*, Vol. 37, no. 1, pp. 93–111.

Troyanski David G. (2016), *Aging in World History*. Routledge, New York.

Twigg Julia & Wendy Martin (2015a), 'The Challenge of Cultural Gerontology', *The Gerontologist*, Vol. 55, no. 3, p. 353–359.

Twigg Julia & Wendy Martin (eds) (2015b), *Routledge Handbook of Cultural Gerontology*, Oxford and New York, Routledge.

Van Dyk Silke (2015), *Soziologie des Alters*. Bielefeld, Transcript Verlag.

Walker Alan (1981), 'Towards a Political Economy of Old Age', *Ageing & Society*, Vol. 1, No, 1, pp. 73–94.

Part I

Future at the heart of the ageing region

1 Demographic change as dystopia

Contemporary German discourses on ageing, between science and politics

Reinhard Messerschmidt

Embedded in a long tradition of demographic dystopias, which Spanish demographer Andreu Domingo (2008) examined in the popular literature of the last two centuries, contemporary discourses of demographic change raise a variety of questions. Over 20 years ago, gerontologist Stephen Katz stated that 'popular and professional discourses which currently accentuate the demographic features of aging populations are characterized by their alarmism' and named this phenomenon 'alarmist demography' (1992, p. 204). He situated such alarmism in governmental narratives on the aged sub-population and its collective dependency, where popular media and think tanks 'depict the elderly emptying the coffers of the welfare state and creating a tax burden beyond the means of the labour force to support', giving the appearance that 'the growing aging population is threatening to create an economic crisis with profound consequences for healthcare systems, social security programmes, industrial and intergenerational relations' (ibid., pp. 203–204). This chapter will resituate in the present what he could see so clearly in the past.[1] Demographic change, typically understood as the ageing of the population (Schimany, 2003) with respect to its subsequent shrinkage (Kaufmann, 2005), has become commonplace in German social-science and mass-media discourse since the turn of the millennium. Although the 'fear of population decline' ebbed and flowed over the past century, according to Teitelbaum and Winter (1985, p. 1), 'depending both upon demographic realities and perceptions of the links between population change and economic, social, and political power', the 'flow' of contemporary discourses should be understood in the context of strategies of governmentality addressing individual and population ageing. In fact, the current flow can be interpreted as resulting from the prevailing economization of the social (Bröckling, 2007) and embedded in specific programmes of governmentality, such as the growing entrepreneurship of the self(s), which can no longer expect social care from the state. Declarations that social security systems are endangered and consequently need to be increasingly privatized are legitimized by demographic claims to knowledge of the future, which we will refer to as 'future knowledge' (Hartmann & Vogel, 2010). This can be interpreted as being part of contemporary 'neosocial governmentality'

(Lessenich, 2008) or the 'neosocial market economy' (Vogelmann, 2012). As this chapter will show, privatization of benefits (for insurance companies, the financial market, and the 'silver economy' driven by the rising consumption by older people and for age-specific needs) contrasts with the socialization of costs (e.g. prolonged working life/later retirement, 'active' and productive ageing, direct or indirect cuts in social insurance). Nevertheless, governmental programmes and associated governments of the self are not necessarily successful (Bröckling *et al.*, 2010), because individuals can always partially or entirely reject the related discourses.[2]

This chapter's main objective is to reveal the order of demographic future knowledge and its discursive depth structures (Diaz-Bone, 2013), in the sense of underlying orders of thought and communicational power (Reichertz, 2015). Foucault's manifold legacy (Messerschmidt, 2016) allows examination of its conditions of possibility. The chapter thus analyses both of the discursive fields that provide the fundamentals of a specific contemporary governmentality of demographic change. The first section, concerning the fabrication of demographic future knowledge, focuses on the underlying 'rationality' consisting of key categories, measures (e.g. fertility rates or dependency ratios), and population projections in the scientific field, and the following section empirically situates 'garbled demography' (Teitelbaum, 2004) in the present by describing discursive regularities in 3810 German media texts dating from 2000 to 2013. The final section will connect these discursive fields to 'demographization' (Barlösius, 2007, 2010) and outline a specific governmentality of demographic change.

The order of demographic future knowledge

Foucauldian analysis of the discourse of demographic change starts with its underlying epistemological orders, in sense of rules or, as he called it, the 'system of formation' (1972, p. 43), a thought system containing categories, measures and concepts that serve as conditions for the related statements' existence. Before any assumptions can be asserted about the demographic future, it is necessary to know the present. Already at this stage, scientific discourse contains a variety of observable problems that will be summarized in what follows. Despite all possible ruptures, demographic thought has a central regularity: a territorially defined population and its dynamics. Defining a population involves both the inclusion and exclusion of people. The latter is closely tied to the concept of nation-state and reflected in the genealogically problematic concept of 'Volk' as 'community of descent' in Germany (Brubaker, 1990, p. 396, Overath & Schmidt, 2003; see also Nilssen's chapter in this volume for a Swedish perspective), in its implicit or even explicit form (Etzemüller, 2007, p. 145). Meanwhile, a minority of German demographers have demonstrated the constructivist character of the concept of 'population' (Mackensen *et al.*, 2009). A population is constructed insofar as it depends on borders drawn in relation to the historical development of the nation-state and political decisions (Etzemüller, 2008, p. 203).

At first glance, the resulting distinction between national citizens and 'others' resulting from such boundaries appears obvious, but the issue becomes problematic with further reflection. The approximate estimates of 'illegal' migration (for lack of data) are but one of the problems. This distinction is still visible (and quite questionable) when demographic models exclude the German-citizen children of immigrants and continue to assume that there are two separate sub-populations (Bohk, 2012), one allegedly 'autochthonous' and another that will never lose the 'migrant-background' label. The key demographic concept of population is neither neutral nor natural. There are currently only two published monographs dealing with German 'population discourse' (Hummel, 2000; Etzemüller, 2007), both of which conceptualizing it as a substantially monolithic discourse that can be traced back to the emergence of demography in the late eighteenth century. These publications unquestionably contribute to a better understanding of the history of contemporary demographic discourse, whereas this chapter devotes more attention to discourses of demographic change in the present. The sociologist Diana Hummel (2000, p. 15) identified demography as a genuine 'political science' and pointed out that 'population' was clearly already a political concept starting with the emergence of the study of demography as the explanation and prognostication of population dynamics for political regulation purposes. Her detailed and demographically informed analysis has great historical depth, starting with the emergence of demography in the late eighteenth century, but ends exactly at the moment when discourses of demographic change become widespread in the German public via the mass media. For this reason, the analysis presented in this chapter covers the years 2000 to 2013. Furthermore, Michel Foucault's later works (2007, 2008, 2010, 2011) were not yet available when Hummel wrote her monograph.

Demographic processes are primarily visible through numbers, which demographers produce, calculate and interpret. Etzemüller's position (2008, p. 210), that 'the discourse works only through its visualization, because demographic processes as such are invisible' lacks additional focus on the underlying epistemic regularities concerning the measurement of these processes. Nevertheless, visualization plays a crucial role in framing media reception: although demographic discourses cannot be entirely reduced to visualization, graphs do in some ways produce stronger statements compared to tables or sentence form. This is caused by a 'symbolic surplus', as Eva Barlösius termed it in her critique of the 'demographization of the social' (2007, p. 17), characterized by graphs that evoke one specific interpretation of the consequences (2010, p. 232). Population pyramids, popularized by Friedrich Burgdörfer in 1932 (Etzemüller, 2007, p. 85) and still used for describing a population's changing age structure, already present a strongly normative framework for interpretation. The visual scheme – from the age-structure 'pyramid' of circa 1900 to the 'urn' of 2050 – is indeed a classic feature of 'apocalyptic' population discourses. Technically, this scheme is rooted in an 'ideal' total fertility rate (TFR) of 2.1 children per woman, the so-called replacement fertility rate for a stationary population.

Implicitly embedded interpretation is rarely as obvious as in this case, however. Looking at a recent press release from the German Federal Statistical Office (Destatis) presenting the future of the German population over the next 50 years reveals many interesting details. In the German versions[3] (e.g. Destatis, 2015a), the subtitle reads 'coordinated pre-calculation of the population' instead of speaking of coordinated population projection. This slight difference reflects the notable tension with Destatis' deterministic population projections (see Figure 1.1). Comparison to a probabilistic projection by the Vienna Institute of Demography (VID, see Figure 1.2), which is also scenario-based but includes uncertainty in the visualization, makes the main difference in the power of each statement visible.

The Destatis graph only shows the outcome of two 'moderate' scenarios that clearly indicate a decline, whereas the VID projection shows a possible range of outcomes under the given premises with different probabilities. In absolute numbers,[4] there is no significant difference between the results of Destatis' upper limit scenario and the median of the VID projection. However, the graph from Destatis lacks information that is provided in the VID graph, and the scales of the axes are strikingly different. While the x-axis shows a lengthy historical time horizon before the projection period starts, the y-axis has an unusual gap between 0 and 60. The consequence of both modifications is a more dramatic (visual) decline, resulting in the first graph containing a more 'newsworthy' statement. If we treat each population projection graph as a discourse, namely a 'group of statements that belong to a single system of formation' (Foucault 1972, p. 107), the task

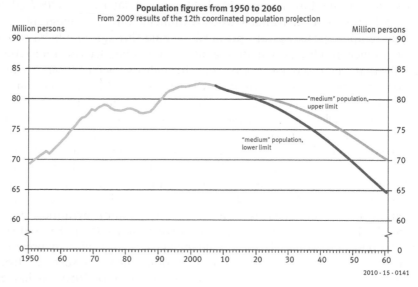

Figure 1.1 A deterministic population projection. Source: Destatis, 2009.

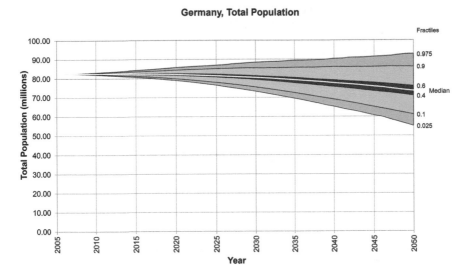

Figure 1.2 A probabilistic population projection. Source: Scherbov *et al.*, 2008.

is to analyse the system of formation of each one. Although the premises of both graphs are comparable, the conclusions to which they allude are fundamentally different. Both projections refer to the same measures and produce a very similar range of results (at least as numerically[5] represented in tables), but they differ strongly in visualization, especially where considerations of uncertainty are concerned. Population projections can only be as good as the underlying assumptions about the future development of fertility, mortality and migration. Destatis uses twelve scenarios combined with three additional 'model-calculations', but most of these scenarios are excluded in Figure 1.1. Their underlying assumptions are described in tables in the appendix, without results or visualization (2009, pp. 36–41); the results of these scenarios can only be downloaded separately as an Excel spreadsheet. If we compare these assumptions with indicators' past trajectories, all scenarios have an artificially static character in common, so the difference between a scenario and 'model-calculation' seems to vanish.

The TFR (see Figure 1.3) has obviously declined since the 1960s, in both parts of Germany. Although the declining trend is well documented for the past, experts designing scenarios are confronted with Hume's problem of induction (a.k.a. 'Russell's inductivist turkey'[6]): why should the trend continue? Even assuming that it does, the three stable scenarios offered by Destatis' experts are still epistemologically questionable, especially regarding limitations of the TFR metric described later in this chapter. The premises become even more problematic if we look at net migration

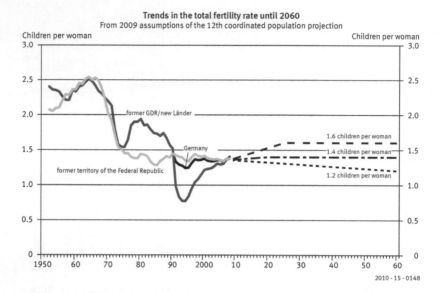

Figure 1.3 Trends in the total fertility rate until 2060. Source: Destatis, 2009.

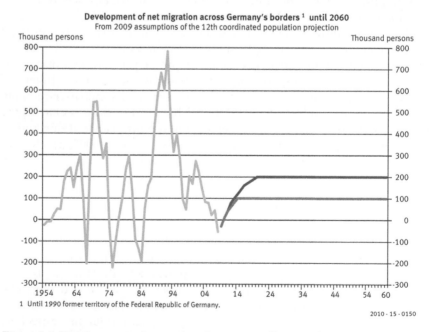

Figure 1.4 Development of net migration across Germany's borders until 2060.
        Source: Destatis, 2009.

(see Figure 1.4). The only two options included in Destatis' projections are either 100,000 or 200,000 persons per year. But these numbers had already been noticeably surpassed by 2011 (Destatis, 2012), and in 2012 net migration was nearly twice as high as the higher scenario, with 394,900 people (Destatis, 2013). This is not a case of an unexpected 'black swan',[7] however, since migration is well known as an unpredictable factor that is highly dependent on political decisions.

Both examples illustrate that the results of population projections are highly dependent on underlying assumptions of fertility, mortality and migration. Among those, only mortality trends seem to be relatively certain. As to the TFR, or more exactly 'period TFR', abbreviated PTFR), the problem is more complex than induction. Tomáš Sobotka and Wolfgang Lutz have recently emphasized that:

> a strong case for stopping the use of the period TFR as a one-fits-all [sic] fertility indicator which is currently common practice. ... demographers who still choose to use the period TFR should stop referring to it as the 'mean number of children per woman', which it evidently is not.
>
> (2011, p. 655–656)

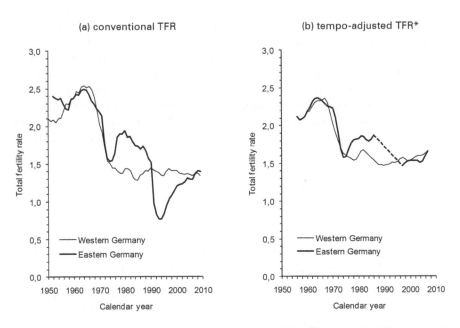

Figure 1.5 Conventional and tempo-adjusted total fertility rates in Western and Eastern Germany, 1950–2010. Source: Luy and Pötzsch, 2010, p. 622.

Destatis uses this same problematic description on the y-axis of its diagram. Moreover, the conventional PTFR is distorted by tempo effects (Bongaarts & Feeney, 1998) from birth timing and the exclusion of future births by women who have not yet completed their reproductive phase. There are approaches to estimating a tempo-adjusted TFR that try to compensate for underestimation (see Figure 1.5), but the 'real' cohort TFR (CTFR) is available only for cohorts that have completed their reproductive phase.

Sobotka and Lutz (2011, p. 638) are critical of the fact that 'in the public discourse relatively few references are made to cohort fertility as the adequate measure of fertility or to other indicators of period fertility that may better reflect changes in fertility trends'. They moreover emphasize that there is hardly any public discussion of these issues. Both conclude that '[t]he choice of the most appropriate indicator must depend on the question asked' (2011, p. 656). Scientifically this conclusion seems almost trivial, but the complexity of demographic measures seems to be a strong obstacle for journalistic mediation of this issue.[8]

The same could be said about the dependency ratio,[9] which is an age-based construction with considerable influence over the projected consequences of demographic change, especially where social insurance is concerned. The conventional dependency ratio is the ratio of the 'dependent' sub-population (typically calculated as the number of people aged 65+) divided by the number of people of working age (15 or 20 to 64). Sanderson and Scherbov's (2010, p. 1287) critique points out that, '[w]hen using indicators that assume fixed chronological ages, it is implicitly assumed that there will be no progress in important factors such as remaining life expectancies and in disability rates'. Consequently, they present a prospective old-age dependency ratio (POADR) using an age forecasting measure that would reduce the projected increase for 2050 by one-third, whereas a disability-adjusted dependency ratio leads to a reduction by more than two-thirds (see Table 1.1). The 'drama' of demographic change loses its alleged justifications and becomes much less dramatic when these possible alternatives are added on to all the uncertainties and limitations presented earlier.

Although critical analysis of demographic measures and their construction does provide more deeply considered perspectives, the process should still not be understood as realistic: some measures may be suited to specific contexts, but they are still researcher-created constructs that may be more or less close to demographic 'reality', especially that of the future. Measures can only be evaluated in retrospect, as shown earlier with the TFR. Such reflexivity is understood according to Pierre Bourdieu's position,

> that the scientific struggle is arbitrated by reference to the constructed 'real'. In the social sciences, the 'real' is indeed external to and independent of knowledge, but it is itself a social construction, a product of past struggles which, at least in this respect, remains at stake in present struggles. ... Social science is, then, a social construction

of a social construction. ... Reflexivity is ... the only way out of the contradiction which consists in demanding a relativizing critique and relativism for the other sciences, while remaining attached to a realist epistemology.

(2004, p. 88)

Furthermore, Alain Desrosières discussed the problem of tension between realism and conventionalism specifically regarding the criteria for quality in official statistics and concluded that differentiation based on structuralism-inspired compromise solutions[10] can help people to 'understand the often obscure debates and controversies triggered by statistical arguments, both in the public arena and in the social sciences' (2009, p. 321). With respect to central demographic concepts, such a debate would only be obscure if consequential reflection upon the boundaries of this construction is neglected. This differentiation is compatible with the epistemological position that Ian Hacking (2002) described as 'dialectical realism'. It accommodates the specific character of demographic (future) constructs as discursive games of truth intertwined with power relations, avoiding the trap of epistemic relativism. As we have seen, central concepts of the demographic 'formal core' (Hummel, 2000, p. 229) like population, age and other measures are misinterpreted as 'objective' facts by some demographers and most

Table 1.1 Different types of dependency ratios by Sanderson and Scherbov

OADR (Old-age dependency ratio)

	2005–10	*2025–30*	*2045–50*
Germany	0.33	0.48	0.63
increase	–	0.15	0.30
%	–	45.45	90.91

POADR (Prospective OADR)

	2005–10	*2025–30*	*2045–50*
Germany	0.21	0.25	0.34
increase	–	0.04	0.13
%	–	19.05	61.90

ADDR (Adult disability dependency ratio)

	2005–10	*2025–30*	*2045–50*
Germany	0.12	0.13	0.15
increase	–	0.01	0.03
%	–	8.33	25.00

Source: Sanderson and Scherbov (2010); the author's calculations for the percentage of increase. Shows lower figures for POADR and even lower figures for adult disability dependency ratio (ADDR).

journalists. This is the main cause of what is at best reductionist, but often false, mediation of demographic knowledge in public discourse: in other words, 'garbled demography', which will be illustrated below with analysis of the media corpus.

Garbled Demography? Demographic change in German mass media, 2000 to 2013

Michael S. Teitelbaum explains the oversimplification and problematic reduction of complexity as resulting from 'fundamental cultural differences between demographers and journalists, and an equally large divergence in the incentive structures faced by professionals in these two domains' (2004, p. 317). In addition to the misinterpretation of projections as forecasts, he criticizes journalists' attraction to long projection intervals, given the uncertainty of projections over time. Consequently, demographers aiming for public impact tend to produce simplified press releases or finding summaries, fully aware of the journalistic expectations:

> In part the fault may lie with sometimes imprecise prose in demo-graphic reports, as when 'projections' and 'forecasts' are confused with each other, or when the future tense form 'will' is used rather than the conditional 'would' in describing the quantitative outputs of such projections. In part we may fairly attach responsibility to public relations or public information staff, who are motivated to craft pithy sentences for press releases that will capture the attention of busy journalists. In part the error lies with journalists, who focus on long-term projections because they can produce major demographic changes, but interpret them as 'forecasts.' Finally, politicians and activists have been known to take hypothetical demographic scenarios as 'recommendations' if these serve their purposes.
>
> (Teitelbaum, 2004, p. 325)

Although this is a convincing description of elements limiting discourse where the functional logics of the press and media are concerned, the problem of demographic power/knowledge seems to be more complex, as the following overview of the analysis of the mass-media discourse illustrates.

The corpus of media materials for public discourse analysis was compiled using the online archives of leading German newspapers and magazines and Nexis.[11] It consists of 3810 articles covering the 14-year period from 2000[12] to 2013, in which the number of articles increases steadily except for 2007 and 2008, and after 2011 due to the closure of the *Financial Times Deutschland* (see Figure 1.6).

Although as a practical matter it is illusory and unrealistic to think that a corpus can be complete, the selection of sources was intended to be as complete as possible. Quantity matters in corpus construction only insofar

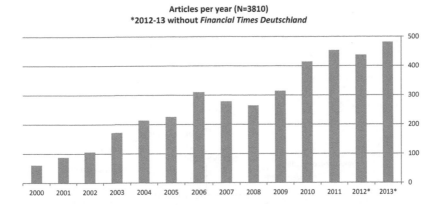

Figure 1.6 Overview of articles over time.

as the risk of excluding important elements must be minimized. The corpus was formed according to the following selection criteria: digital availability over the entire period, representation of the entire political spectrum, and presence of specific arguments regarding demographic change. One possible bias is the combination of search keywords and categories, which were tested in various combinations before downloading the articles in order to obtain as many articles matching the criteria as possible.

The analysis itself focuses primarily on qualitative aspects, although code frequencies in the annotation process were also quantified. In this mixed-method 'transfer design' (Kuckartz, 2014, p. 87), code frequencies are only used to describe the internal relationships of discursive regularities. The resulting numbers can be interpreted as power vectors in the discourse that correlate with the possible impact of certain statements or data sources and agents. Moreover, their distribution indicates how demographic knowledge is used in the mass media. The corresponding regularities in fact result from scientists, journalists, politicians and other experts' practices that both affect the discourse, and are affected by it. Figure 1.7 shows the main categories of the system of more than 39,000 codes, which correspond to the main lines of argumentation.

We begin with a look at the references to demographic knowledge in Figure 1.8.

The most commonly appearing 'input' categories, such as (over-)ageing, shrinking and low fertility, show a declining trend over the analysis period. The same is observed for references to population projections, although the decrease is less pronounced due to their key role. Codes that appeared less frequently, such as internal migration, do not follow this trend and tend to remain relatively stable at a lower impact level. After several years of repetition, the main categories seem to have become increasingly commonsense. This corresponds to the concurrent growing tendency for 'namedropping',

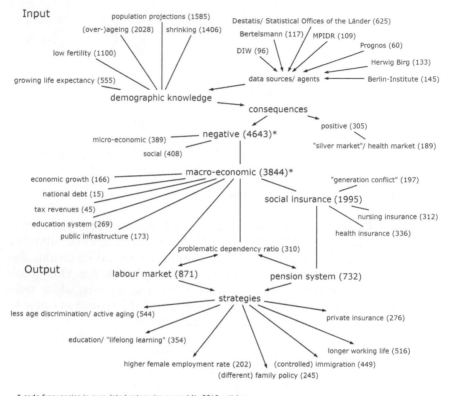

Figure 1.7 MAXMaps visualization of the code system (main elements).

where demographic change, ageing society and the like are mentioned without any further development of the underlying demographic concepts (see Figure 1.9).

More telling patterns can be observed in Figure 1.10, which takes a closer look at data sources and agents.

First, governmental data sources remain continually present at a high level. In particular, the graph representing Destatis shows the impact of the 'coordinated population projections' of 2003, 2006 and 2009. Second, the graph for individuals and networks shows a peak in the beginning, followed by a strong decline. Herwig Birg, who publically expressed his political views on population agency in the press and two monographs (2001, 2005) heads the list of experts on Destatis' population projection scenarios (Destatis, 2009, p. 10) and is at the vanguard. The Rürup Commission has a comparable role

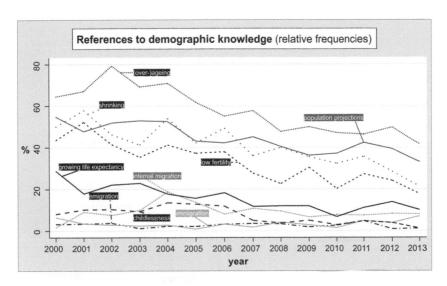

Figure 1.8 Percentages of articles each year referring to demographic knowledge.

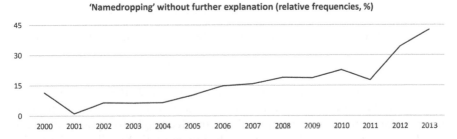

Figure 1.9 'Namedropping' on demographic or population change/development (percentage of articles per year).

as a key player in the partial privatization of the German pension system. As Birg and the Commission lose visibility, think tanks and lobby organizations take over. The most present is the Berlin-Institut für Bevölkerung und Entwicklung (Berlin Institute for Population and Development),[13] which regularly links population projections to regional rankings of future demographic competitiveness on a numerical scale represented by corresponding red or green coloured areas on a visualization map. These rankings apply a Spencerian social Darwinism to regional disparities, and naturalize the Matthew effect[14] regarding the support of economically successful regions with population increase and the corresponding abandonment of deindustrialized and/or shrinking population areas. This rationality, with alleged scientific justification, results in articles with headlines such as 'Germany

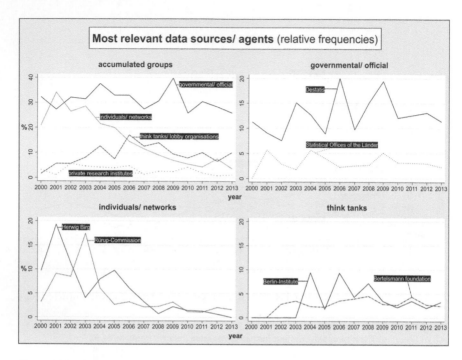

Figure 1.10 Percentages of annual articles referring to groups of data sources or agents over time.

2014: Humans Go, Wolves Come' (*Financial Times Deutschland*, 18 August 2004). The Berlin Institute continuously tried to crush any remaining solidarity relating to the constitutionally guaranteed right to equality of living conditions in Germany. Its implicit solution, suitable for all social and demographic problems, seems to be competition and the marketization of its every aspect. Various other lobby organizations and think tanks addressed other topics, e.g.:

1   The Initiative Neue Soziale Marktwirtschaft (New Social Market Economy Initiative) and the related Institut der deutschen Wirtschaft Köln (Cologne Institute for Economic Research),[15] which focus primarily on social policy and the labour market (in favour of the latter).
2   The powerful Bertelsmann Stiftung (Bertelsmann Foundation), which promotes new public management (in demographic as well as other contexts) on all governmental levels from municipalities up to the federal government, through tools such as a web-portal named 'Wegweiser Kommune' (Signpost Municipality)[16] containing nine so-called 'demography-types' with different action strategies.

3   The Deutsches Institut für Altersvorsorge (German Institute for Retirement Provisions)[17] and the former Institut für Wirtschaft und Gesellschaft (Institute for Economy and Society, IWG), which advocate for privatization of the pension system justified by future demographic developments.

These examples are only the tip of the iceberg (see Messerschmidt 2014 for a complete list, and the forthcoming monograph for detailed information); in fact lobbying's influence on mass-media discourse is massive. The code frequencies of both the Berlin Institute and the Bertelsmann Foundation are higher than those of the Max-Planck-Institut für demografische Forschung (Max Planck Institute for Demographic Research, MPIDR,[18] see Figure 1.7), which is the most relevant public research centre. These dynamics' traces are visible in the codes for negative consequences of demographic change (see Figure 1.11). They represent future problems or challenges that correspond to the solution strategies being promoted for individuals and society at large (see Figure 1.12).

Although addressing social insurance is a stable element in both of Figures 1.11 and 1.12, all related lines peak between 2000 and 2003, which corresponds to the peak of 'individual/network' influence during the same period found in Figure 1.10. A strong decline follows, and both topical discursive strands become more diversified, corresponding to the growing influence of think tanks and lobby organizations. In this diversification process, discursive strands aiming to mobilize aged people in particular become more relevant. After reforms of the pension system that lead to massive pension cuts and partial privatization to meet the demands of insurance

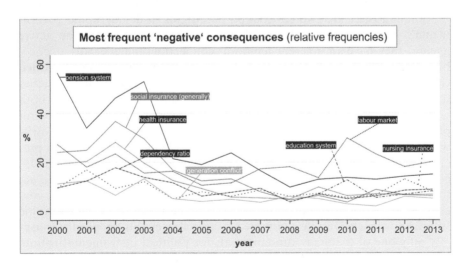

Figure 1.11 Most frequently appearing 'negative' consequences of demographic change over time (percentages of annual articles).

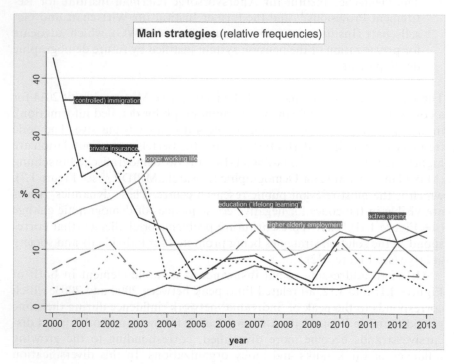

Figure 1.12 Selected solution strategies over time (percentages of annual articles).

companies and the financial markets, 'active ageing' becomes a dominant element of the public discourse (Van Dyk *et al.*, 2013; Denninger *et al.*, 2014).

Although there are two co-existing paradigms of demographic governmentality, one focusing on the social security system and the other on 'active ageing', they have an inherent temporal connection: the allegedly science-based raising of the retirement age and prolongation of employment opened the discursive space to an increased mobilization of potential productivity and growth at the cost of previously 'unproductive' retirement. In both governmentality paradigms, normative discourses become 'true' by dint of repetition, backed with claimed scientific objectivity. This only works when closely connected to power relations (see Figure 1.10), or more precisely with a growing communicative power in discourse (Reichertz, 2015) corresponding to the wide-ranging efforts of various data sources and actors, be they governmental or private. Over the entire analysed period, governmental and official data sources provide the majority of demographic future knowledge. Despite a notable bias (see above), this knowledge is usually only one of the many fundamentals for political instrumentalization. While in the first years there is a strong observable influence of individuals and networks supporting pension reforms, think tanks also show a growing influence corresponding to economic interests, which are connected to governmental programmes of a neoliberal, or more precisely neosocial, character. With this terminology, Stephan Lessenich (2008, summarized below in the apt words of Vogelmann) argues that the term 'neoliberal':

> might disguise rather than reveal what is happening today, because neo-liberalism is a political rationality trying to govern without making recourse to the 'trans-actional' reality called society, whereas today's governmental practices make up and rely on a new form of 'the social': the neosocial.
>
> (Vogelmann, 2012, p. 16)

On the one hand, the state rejects its former responsibility in the domain of social policy in favour of private insurance and assets on the financial or real estate markets. On the other hand, there is a rising quotient of governmentality of the self that fills the gap. It corresponds to the allegedly permanent, creative, flexible, self-responsible, risk-conscious and consumer-oriented model of entrepreneurship of the self (Bröckling, 2007), but manifesting in new domains, such as lifelong learning to stay available to the job market for as long as possible, longer working lives and productive mobilization after the age of retirement.

Although language is not the main focus of a Foucauldian discourse analysis of statement systems, it plays an important role in the dramatization process, especially for the first demographic governmentality paradigm. There are generally three main commonalities in alarmist demography language use. The most frequent code, 'dramatic' or 'drastic' development(s), shows a strong peak in the beginning followed by a strong decline in 2006, when the first few critical articles were published (see Figure 1.13):

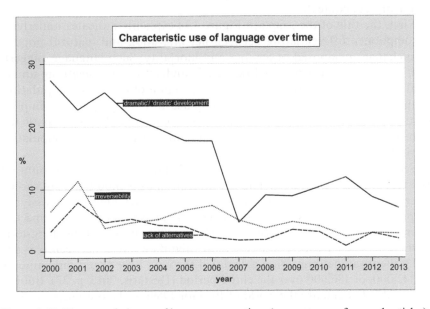

Figure 1.13 Characteristic use of language over time (percentages of annual articles).

The appearance of critical articles cannot be taken as an indicator of a general shift in the mass-media discourse. Although there are a few critically reflexive articles, the vast majority still fits Katz's description of 'alarmist demography'. A 'new culture of change' (Schwentker & Vaupel, 2011, p. 3) towards a post-alarmist demography seems to emerge in the scientific discourse, but it is still far from holding a hegemonic position and continues to lack appropriate transfer into the mass media.

Demographization as ahistorical ontology of the present

Foucault, when explaining his conception of an ontology of the present, wondered, 'What is the present reality? ... What is the present field of possible experiences?' (2010, p. 20). This is a noticeably broader approach than Ian Hacking's reception of Foucault's early works would have it, where he historicized conceptual analysis as 'analysis of words in their sites' (2002, p. 24). Although it has changed slightly over time concerning recent consequences and strategies and in some details with respect to modifying population projections, the contemporary demographic ontology of the present is a relatively stable discourse due to the solidity of its 'formal core' and related orders of (future) knowledge (see above). In particular, Destatis' most recent population projections (2015) show an ahistorical understanding of migration processes, which are obviously of great importance in a period of globalization and the current 'refugee crisis'. Although this context is not directly relevant to the scope of the analysis of media texts from the 2000–2013 period, reflection on some crucial elements of the recent projection is necessary to relate critique of the underlying narrow demographic 'formal core' to the present context.

First, the title of the graph in Figure 1.14 explicitly indicates underlying assumptions, differentiating between net migration and 'natural population change', composed of fertility and mortality. Such language suggests that migration across national borders is understood as something unnatural, introducing exclusion into the construction of a national population. Although this terminology is commonplace in demography, the implicit distinction is even more problematic when compounded by systematic underestimation of net migration in the assumptions going into population projections.

Second, these assumptions have been debatably adjusted to account for the recent past (see above). The net migration of 500,000 in 2014 should decrease 'step-wise' to 100,000 or 200,000 by 2020, the same figures assigned to previous projection's assumptions. The discursive rationality behind this is an ahistorical form of 'normalism' (Link, 2006) based on the 'long-term average' of seven decades: despite several 'migration waves' between 1954 and 2013, the mean net migration calculated through 1989 would only amount to 142,000, or 186,000 over the entire period (Destatis, 2015, p. 37). But is it reasonable to compare the world of 1954 (or 1989) to the present, especially

Natural population change and net migration
From 2014, results of the 13th coordinated population projection

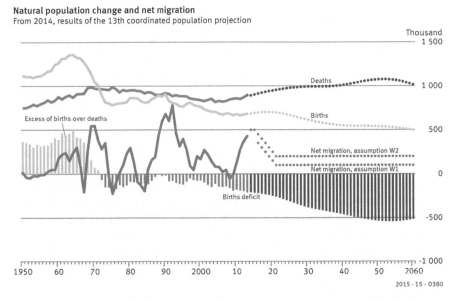

Figure 1.14 Migration assumptions of the most recent German population projection.
   Source: Destatis, 2015.

in the field of migration? Such an abstract numerical conception of the trajectories of demographic indicators seems to be blind to history and the obvious fact that today's world has changed substantially in terms of globalization and migration flows.

'Demography Drives Your Future' – the current slogan of Europe's leading demographic research institute network[19] – seems highly plausible. Given this rising (bio)political volatility, Foucault's keywords 'security, territory, and population' (2007), originally referring to the emergence of population statistics in the late eighteenth century, are still central issues, but need to be resituated in the context of population ageing and shrinking. Internal security has always been the focus of anti-immigration political positions and this discursive strand is doubtlessly on the rise since early 2016. A second major discursive strand, the territorial integrity of (German) national/state and European Union borders, is also being renegotiated, even by political parties having held different positions in the past. Even prior to the onset of the European 'refugee crisis', the assumptions of the 'financial crisis' period reflected either a positivist ivory tower perspective or a problematic and implicitly normative perspective encompassing 'Fortress Europe' and the contemporary resurgence of nationalisms. Although Destatis' explanations tend to favour the first strand, the possible discursive connection with the latter leaves room for political instrumentalization. Numerically,

Destatis divides 'source countries' into two categories, the first consisting of aged populations from southern or eastern Europe, 'which mostly produce so-called work-migration', and the second consisting of younger populations from Afghanistan, Iraq and Syria, which are 'characterized by asylum-seekers' (Destatis, 2015, p. 38). According to Destatis, in 10 to 20 years the first category would have fewer people in migration-active ages, so local demand for employees would rise. There would be more advantages to the second migration category if there were no substantial changes in local conditions. Additionally, there would be potential for migration from Africa and Asia. These factors alone are already in notable tension with the projection's migration assumptions. Furthermore, Destatis does not address the possibility that the complex and hard to predict 'crises' facing Europe today could also require fundamental changes in immigration and integration policies. Foucauldian discourse analysis is inadequate for discerning whether this omission might be related to the fact that Herwig Birg, the individual with the greatest discursive communication power (Reichertz 2015, see Figure 1.10), is listed as supporting experts thanked in the acknowledgements of Destatis' most recent population projection (2015, 11), as in earlier press releases.

Birg recently (2015) published a new 'demographic prognosis' whose title translates to 'The ageing republic and the failure of policy', and his scientific and mass-media publications unstintingly argue for 'generation replacement' via in-country births instead of immigration. The same argumentation exists in an older prototypical example of alarmist demography in present German discourse of demographic change. The most influential German tabloid, *BILD*, printed the following text on 15 March 2006, with the headline 'Experts Are Warning: We Germans Will Die Out in 12 Generations!' According to 'Germany's Most Famous Population Scientist Prof. Herwig Birg':

> In 2100 the number of Germans have will shrunk to 46 million, in 2300 we will be ... shortly before extinction ... This demographic change will pursue us over many generations ... Because the unborn cannot beget children. Germans must be aware that political promises – secure pensions, secure future – are worthless.

Alarmist statements like these are found often in the analysed media corpus – and a high percentage of them refer to or are written by Herwig Birg, who, since retiring from university professorship in 2004, has been working in 'research, consultancy, and presentations' for 'the economy, organizations, and public clients' according to his website.[20] Regardless of Birg's empirically unclear motives and at best implied nationalist/conservative statements in his media discourse, Destatis' most recent and preceding population projections show strong indications of demographization in relation to the demographic 'formal core' and its underlying assumptions. According to

Barlösius' critique (2010, p. 232), demographization consists of three specific elements that are 'characteristic of the present debate about demographic change': First, visualizations suggest (or allege) unambiguity in the assumption that the future can be extracted from the past and present, and already include a specific interpretation of the consequences of demographic change. Second, the graphic representations embody a fundamental change of the perspective: 'instead of society, there is more talk of population; instead of social change, there is more talk of demographic change', especially regarding future social and economic sustainability. Third, demographic representations are technocratically constructed, consequently implying which actions are necessary and which governmental interventions will succeed in realizing the planned future. Analysis of demographic future knowledge and its underlying orders of knowledge in media discourse from 2000 to 2013 flesh out the picture of garbled demography as a meaning-reducing apparatus. The two discursive fields are reciprocally intertwined: the epistemic rules of formation already show a noticeable bias rather than their proclaimed scientific objectivity.

Concluding remarks

As this chapter has demonstrated, demographic future knowledge is based on categories and measures that are researcher-made constructs, and their demographic 'reality' is as problematic for demographers as it is epistemologically questionable when alarmist consequences and implicit political positions are concerned. This bias is massively radicalized in the mass-media discourse described above, which would not exist without specific demographic future knowledge discourses. Various 'experts' and think tanks serving the interests of the financial and insurance industries play a crucial role in the radicalization process. As this chapter has emphasized, both discursive systems are governed by the persistent fundamental rule of a logic of '*ceteris paribus*', the 'irritating assumption that only one parameter will change, but everything else will remain constant' (Schwentker & Vaupel, 2011, p.5). This premise opens the way for the reductionist demographization of the social future in favour of neosocial market logics that are promoted as if there were no alternative.

Consequently, alternative solutions to supposedly demographic problems remain unexplored because demographic change is usually offered as the explanation for such problems, even those arising from non-demographic causes that might actually be more influential than demographic ones. A potentially endless list of critical questions could be asked and discussed, scientifically as well as politically, but given the limited length of this chapter, it will end with only three: First, to what extent is demographic future knowledge empirically grounded regarding anticipated population ageing and shrinking, and how strongly politically charged is this order of knowledge? Second, is there a scientific answer to the question of the best design for social insurance, especially the pension system, or are there only political positions hidden behind allegedly scientific 'answers'? Third, to what extent do we deal with problems of an ageing society, on topics such as pensions, the labour market, or the real estate market? Hegemonic narratives turn out be less convincing, or even misguiding, when examined in detail and in the context of alternative explanations such as the financial crisis, tax policy, rising social inequality, lobby interests, urbanization and regional disparities, and other social, political and economic realities. Although this chapter covered some such aspects, a full range of scientific and society-wide debates, currently only existing in the margins, are needed to establish a post-alarmist view of ageing in both fields.

Notes

1 Parts of this analysis have been published in Messerschmidt 2014 and 2016, with different emphases, from earlier stages of research.
2 To examine the extent of their 'success', qualitative interviews can provide supplemental insights that surpass the scope of the Foucauldian toolbox. For German 'active ageing' discourses, see Denninger *et al.* (2014). For an analysis of 'active ageing' through everyday practices in Danish senior centres, see Lassen, this volume.
3 Titles and citations from sources in German are the author's translations.
4 According to Destatis (2009, p. 46), the population in 2050 would amount 73.61 million for the upper limit (and 69.41 million lower limit) as compared to a median of 73.44 million in the VID projection (Scherbov *et al.* 2008, p. 40).
5 Destatis' minimum amounts 64.37 million in 2050 (Model-calculation with zero net migration), whereas the maximum amounts 82.58 million (Model-calculation with TFR=2.1), as compared to a range from 61.08 to 86.09 million for the 80 per cent prediction interval of the VID projection.
6 According to Alan Francis Chalmers (1999, p. 45), Bertrand Russell was referring to David Hume's problem of induction (Hume, 1896), concerning the epistemological risk of using inductive reasoning to interpret single events into a general statement. He raises the problem with the story of an 'inductivist turkey' who observed friendly humans feeding him every day at 9 a.m. and generalized this experience – until Christmas morning.
7 Nassim N. Taleb (2007) situated Karl Popper's 'black swan' example (2002, p. 378) in context of the financial crisis; Popper originally expressed his scepticism of inductive reasoning (as in footnote 6) as follows: 'no matter how many instances of white swans we may have observed, this does not justify the conclusion that all swans are white'.
8 Journalists are not the only ones to experience this obstacle. Generally, non-experts struggle for an appropriate understanding of such data, which affects all readers of 'garbled demography' in the press, be they scholars in other disciplines or interested citizens.
9 See also Belorgey's chapter in this volume on the social construction of dependency in France.
10 'Several compromise solutions are available to ease this tension. They rely on the principle of separating the signifier (the measurement) and the signified (the object to be measured), while linking them by means of varied correspondence terms' (Desrosières 2009, p. 321). Desrosières already raised the problem more than a decade earlier in his monograph *The Politics of Large Numbers* (1998, pp. 1) because 'it is difficult to think simultaneously that the objects being measured really do exist, and that this is only a convention'.

11 www.nexis.com (formerly LexisNexis, accessed 1 October 2016) offers a commercial press database, which, despite excluding some articles by freelancers, is relatively useful for the construction of press text corpora.
12 The decision to start of analysis in 2000 was based on the sufficient number of articles appearing in the corpus that year, unlike previous years.
13 www.berlin-institut.org, accessed 1 October 2016.
14 Briefly, this is accumulated (dis)advantage, which Robert K. Merton (1968) developed in the context of scientific reward systems but which is easily transferable as a fundamental principle of capitalist societies, where the rich get richer and the poor get poorer (e.g. Piketty 2014).
15 Initiative Neue Soziale Marktwirtschaft, www.insm.de; Institut der deutschen Wirtschaft Köln, www.iwkoeln.de, accessed 1 October 2016.
16 www.wegweiser-kommune.de, accessed 1 October 2016.
17 www.dia-vorsorge.de, accessed 1 October 2016.
18 www.demogr.mpg/de, accessed 1 October 2016.
19 www.population-europe.eu, accessed 1 October 2016.
20 www.herwig-birg.de/, accessed 1 October 2016.

References

Barlösius Eva (2007), 'Demographisierung des Gesellschaftlichen. Zur Bedeutung der Repräsentationspraxis'. In Barlösius Eva & Daniela Schiek (eds.), *Demographisierung des Gesellschaftlichen. Analysen und Debatten zur demographischen Zukunft Deutschlands*. Wiesbaden, VS, pp. 9–36.

Barlösius Eva (2010), 'Bilder des demografischen Wandels'. In Hartmann Heinrich & Jakob Vogel (eds.), *Zukunftswissen. Prognosen in Wirtschaft, Politik und Gesellschaft seit 1900*. Frankfurt and New York, Campus, pp. 231–248.

Birg Herwig (2015), *Die alternde Republik und das Versagen der Politik*. Münster, Lit.

Bohk Christina (2012), *Ein probabilistisches Bevölkerungsprognosemodell. Entwicklung und Anwendung für Deutschland*. Wiesbaden, Springer VS.

Bongaarts John & Griffith Feeney (1998), 'On the Quantum and Tempo of Fertility', *Population and Development Review*, 24 (2), pp. 271–291.

Bourdieu Pierre (2004), *Science of Science and Reflexivity*. Translated by Richard Nice. Chicago, University of Chicago Press.

Bröckling Ulrich (2007), *Das unternehmerische Selbst. Soziologie einer Subjektivierungsform*. Frankfurt am Main, Suhrkamp.

Bröckling Ulrich, Krasmann Susanne & Thomas Lemke (2010), *Governmentality. Current Issues and Future Challenges*. New York, Routledge.

Brubaker Rogers (1990), 'Immigration, Citizenship, and the Nation State in France and Germany: A Comparative Historical Analysis', *International Sociology*, 5 (4), pp. 379–407.

Chalmers Alan Francis (1999), *What Is This Thing Called Science?* Third edition. Queensland, University of Queensland Press.

Denninger Tina, van Dyk Silke, Lessenich Stephan & Anna Richter (2014), *Leben im Ruhestand. Zur Neuverhandlung des Alters in der Aktivgesellschaft*. Bielefeld, transcript.

Desrosières Alain (1998), *The Politics of Large Numbers: A History of Statistical Reasoning*. Cambridge, Mass, Harvard University Press.

Desrosières Alain (2009), 'How To Be Real and Conventional: A Discussion of the Quality Criteria of Official Statistics', *Minerva*, 47 (3), pp. 307–322.

Diaz-Bone Rainer (2013), 'Sozio-Episteme und Sozio-Kognition. Epistemologische Zugänge zum Verhältnis von Diskurs und Wissen'. In Viehöver Willy, Keller Reiner & Werner Schneider (eds.), *Diskurs – Sprache – Wissen*. Wiesbaden, Springer VS, pp. 79–96.

Destatis (2009), *Germany's Population by 2060. Results of the 12th Coordinated Population Projection*. Wiesbaden, Statistisches Bundesamt, www.destatis.de/EN/Publications/Specialized/Population/GermanyPopulation2060.pdf?—blob= publicationFile (Accessed 5 January 2014).

Destatis (2012), *Press Release 255 / 2012–07-25. Germany's Population Increasing in 2011 for the First Time Since 2002*. Wiesbaden, Statistisches Bundesamt, www. destatis.de/EN/PressServices/Press/pr/2012/07/PE12_ 255_12411.html (Accessed 5 January 2014).

Destatis (2013), *Press Release 354 / 2013–10-22. Number of Foreigners in the Central Register Increases 4.1% in 2012*. Wiesbaden, Statistisches Bundesamt, www. destatis.de/EN/PressServices/Press/pr/2013/10/PE13_ 354_12521.html (Accessed 5 January 2014).

Destatis (2015), *Germany's Population by 2060 - Results of the 13th Coordinated Population Projection*. Wiesbaden, Statistisches Bundesamt, www.destatis.de/EN/Publications/Specialized/Population/GermanyPopulation2060_5124206159004. pdf?__blob=publicationFile (Accessed 15 February 2016).

Destatis (2015a), *Bevölkerung Deutschlands bis 2060. 13. Koordinierte Bevölkerungsvorausberechnung*. Wiesbaden, Statistisches Bundesamt, www.destatis.de/DE/PresseService/Presse/Pressekonferenzen/2015/bevoelkerung/Pressebroschuere_Bevoelk2060.pdf?__blob=publicationFile (Accessed 24 July 2015).

Domingo Andreu (2008), '"Demodystopias": Prospects of Demographic Hell', *Population and Development Review*, 34 (4), pp. 725–745.

Etzemüller Thomas (2007), *Ein ewigwährender Untergang. Der apokalyptische Bevölkerungsdiskurs des 20. Jahrhunderts*. Bielefeld, transcript.

Etzemüller Thomas (2008), '"Dreißig Jahre nach zwölf?" Der apokalyptische Bevölkerungsdiskurs im 20. Jahrhundert'. In Nagel Alexander-Kenneth, Schipper Bernd U. & Ansgar Weymann (eds.), *Apokalypse. Zur Soziologie und Geschichte religiöser Krisenrhetorik*. Frankfurt am Main and New York, Campus, pp. 197–216.

Foucault Michel (1972), *The Archaeology of Knowledge and The Discourse on Language*. New York, Pantheon Books.

Foucault Michel (2007), *Security, Territory and Population (Lectures at the Collège De France 1977–78)*. Ed. by Michel Senellart. Basingstoke, Palgrave Macmillan.

Foucault Michel (2008), *The Birth of Biopolitics (Lectures at the Collège De France, 1978–1979)*. Ed. by Michel Senellart. Basingstoke, Palgrave Macmillan.

Foucault Michel (2010), *The Government of Self and Others (Lectures at the Collège De France, 1982–1983)*. Ed. by Frédéric Gros. Basingstoke, Palgrave Macmillan.

Foucault Michel (2011), *The Courage of the Truth (The Government of Self and Others II: Lectures at the Collège de France, 1983–1984)*. Ed. by Frédéric Gros. Basingstoke, Palgrave Macmillan.

Hacking Ian (2002), *Historical Ontology*. Cambridge, Mass, Harvard University Press.

Hartmann Heinrich & Jakob Vogel (eds.) (2010), *Zukunftswissen. Prognosen in Wirtschaft, Politik und Gesellschaft seit 1900*. Frankfurt and New York, Campus.

Hume David (1896), *A Treatise of Human Nature*. Reprinted from the Original Edition in three volumes and edited, with an analytical index, by L.A. Selby-Bigge, M.A. Oxford, Clarendon Press [1739].

Hummel Diana (2000), *Der Bevölkerungsdiskurs*. Opladen, Leske & Budrich.

Katz Stephen (1992), 'Alarmist Demography: Power, Knowledge, and the Elderly Population', *Journal of Aging Studies*, 6 (3), pp. 203–225.

Kuckartz Udo (2014), *Mixed Methods*. Wiesbaden, Springer VS.

Lessenich Stephan (2008), *Die Neuerfindung des Sozialen. Der Sozialstaat im flexiblen Kapitalismus*. Bielefeld, transcript.

Link Jürgen (2006), *Versuch über den Normalismus. Wie Normalität produziert wird*. Göttingen, Vandenhoeck & Ruprecht.

Luy Marc & Olga Pötzsch (2010), 'Estimates of the Tempo-adjusted Total Fertility Rate in Western and Eastern Germany, 1955–2008', *Comparative Population Studies – Zeitschrift für Bevölkerungswissenschaft*, 35 (3), pp. 605–636.

Mackensen Rainer, Reulecke Jürgen & Josef Ehmer (eds.) (2009), *Ursprünge, Arten und Folgen des Konstrukts 'Bevölkerung' vor, im und nach dem 'Dritten Reich'*. Wiesbaden, VS.

Merton Robert (1968), 'The Matthew Effect in Science', *Science*, 159 (3810), pp. 56–63.

Messerschmidt Reinhard (2014), '"Garbled Demography" or "Demographisation of the Social"'? A Foucauldian Discourse Analysis of German Demographic Change at the Beginning of the 21st Century', *Historical Social Research*, 39, H.1, pp. 299–335.

Messerschmidt Reinhard (2016), 'Revealing the Governmentality of Demographic Change in Germany with the Discourse-analytical "Toolbox" of Foucault'. In McIlvenny Paul, Zhukova Klausen Julia & Laura Bang Lindegaard (eds.), *New Perspectives on Discourse and Governmentality*. Amsterdam, John Benjamins, pp. 353–386.

Overath Petra & Schmidt Daniel (eds.) (2003), *Volks-(An)Ordnung. Einschließen, ausschließen, einteilen, aufteilen!* Leipzig, Leipziger Universitätsverlag.

Piketty Thomas (2014), *Capital in the Twenty-First Century*. Translated by Arthur Goldhammer. Cambridge, Mass., Harvard University Press.

Popper Karl (2002), *The Logic of Scientific Discovery*. London and New York, Routledge Classics.

Reichertz Jo (2015), 'Wie erlangt man im Diskurs Kommunikationsmacht?', *Journal for Discourse Studies*, 3(3), pp. 258–272.

Sanderson Warren C. & Sergei Scherbov (2010), 'Remeasuring Aging', *Science*, 329 (5997), pp. 1287–1288.

Scherbov Sergei, Mamolo Marija & Wolfgang Lutz (2008), *Probabilistic Population Projections for the 27 EU Member States Based on Eurostat Assumptions*. Vienna, Vienna Institute of Demography, www.oeaw.ac.at/vid/download/edrp_2_08.pdf (Accessed 5 January 2014).

Schimany Peter (2003), *Die Alterung der Gesellschaft. Ursachen und Folgen des demographischen Umbruchs*. Frankfurt am Main, Campus.

Schwentker Björn & James W. Vaupel (2011), 'Eine neue Kultur des Wandels', *ApuZ. Aus Politik und Zeitgeschichte*, 10–11, pp. 3–10.

Sobotka Tomáš & Wolfgang Lutz (2011), 'Misleading Policy Messages Derived from the Period TFR: Should We Stop Using It?', *Comparative Population Studies – Zeitschrift für Bevölkerungswissenschaft*, 35 (3), pp. 637–664.

Taleb Nassim Nicolas (2007), *The Black Swan. The Impact of the Highly Improbable*. New York, Random House.

Teitelbaum Michael S. (2004), 'The Media Marketplace for Garbled Demography', *Population and Development Review*, 30 (2), pp. 317–327.

Teitelbaum Michael S. & Jay M.Winter (1985), *The Fear of Population Decline*. Orlando, Academic Press.

Van Dyk Silke, Lessenich Stephan, Denninger Tina & Anna Richter (2013), 'The Many Meanings of "Active Ageing". Confronting Public Discourse with Older People's Stories', *Recherches Sociologiques et Anthropologiques*, 44 (1), pp. 97–115.

Vogelmann Frieder (2012), 'Neosocial Market Economy', *Foucault Studies*, 14, pp. 115–137.

2 Recommendations concerning the use of physical exercise to improve the wellbeing of older people in France

Cécile Collinet and Matthieu Delalandre

The concept of wellbeing first appeared in preventive policies on ageing in the second half of the twentieth century. The ability to remain active was progressively depicted as the condition of this wellbeing, making 'active ageing' (Moulaert & Viriot Durandal, 2013) an ideal model for ageing successfully. This model interlinks three main aspects: social participation, health, safety.

The Madrid international plan of action on ageing adopted in 2002 by the United Nations Organization (UNO) recommended that its member states give priority 'to improving health and wellbeing in ageing' (UNO, 2002, p. 15). The WHO (World Health Organization) specified in its international plan *Active Ageing: A Policy Framework* (2002) that the need was to 'ensure the wellbeing of older people' (p. 4), and that active ageing 'enables older people to manage their potential of physical, social and mental wellbeing throughout their life' (p. 12). The correlation between activity and wellbeing was thus reaffirmed in the European Healthy Ageing programme initiated in 2003 and including the WHO as a partner: 'We find higher levels of wellbeing and physical ability in active people' (p. 17). In addition, the promotion of ageing has taken different forms: if the WHO and the UNO emphasized a holistic approach on individual lifestyles, on the European level the central aspect was more a question of the socio-professional integration of older people (Lassen & Moreira, 2014).

International studies and recommendations found an echo in the French preventive policies from the early 2000s. In fact, if the 1962 Laroque report (Laroque, 1962), marking the acknowledgement of the first French public policies on preventive ageing (in France public action is often organized by commissioning programmes and documented reports from experts), mentions eight times the notion of wellbeing without seriously developing it, the notion of subjective wellbeing was not further researched until it appeared in the *Ageing Well National Plan 2007–2009* (Ministry of Health and Solidarity, Ministry of Social Security, Older People, Disabled People and Families, Ministry of Youth, Sports and Community Organisations, 2007). This plan was particularly important in the setting up of prevention policies on ageing. The importance given to wellbeing can again be found in the report by Dr Ladoucette (Ladoucette, 2011), commissioned by the Ministry of Labour, Work and Health, centring on the links between wellbeing and mental health.

The suggestions in the different French and international plans consisted in an interlinking between a state of health and wellbeing, its measurement through various means, and recommendations to accomplish this. These were articulated round a preventive tripod (Aquino, 2009) that included directives on nutrition, physical exercise and the cultivation of social connections. Establishing this corpus of knowledge, along with an epistemic community (Haas, 1992) supporting it, contributed in modelling an image of ageing. The texts of major international organizations came from the convening of experts and the establishment of a corpus of scientific knowledge (Viriot Durandal & Moulaert, 2014), and justified the case of active ageing as a model of ideal ageing. In this way, scientific expertise took part in the production of a norm (Trépos, 1996): *Active ageing* and its underlying idea of wellbeing ('ageing well' in France) were in fact a combination of scientific, political and ethical considerations, and therefore necessarily normative (Stenner *et al.*, 2011).

In the field of science, the studies were equivocal and finally led to prescriptive usable principles that were intended to be easily assimilated by the targeted public. Even so, the mobilization of scientific knowledge in the international plans and reports and their relay at the French level was carried out in a reduced way. The diversity of research, its complexity or divergence, was often levelled out. This study shows that the heterogeneity of scientific literature tended to decrease producing a simple causal link between doing physical activities and wellbeing. This knowledge led to a set of usable practical directives along with norms adopted in France by the concept of *ageing well* (and is consistent with the holistic view of *active ageing* developed by the WHO). These formed a frame of reference (Jobert & Muller, 1987; Muller, 1990) and were at the core of different texts guiding preventive policies on ageing. This frame of reference is analysed here through three of its constituent dimensions: the norms it conveys (corresponding to criteria for ageing well), algorithms (causal relations between recommendations and health and economic consequences) and depictions (of successful ageing).

A great deal of sociological research has already been carried out on the physical activity of older people (quantitative surveys: Burlot & Lefèvre, 2009; Crosnier, 2005; Truchot, 2002; qualitative surveys: Feillet, 1996, 2006; Feillet & Roncin, 2006; Hénaff-Pineau, 2008, 2009; Tulle, 2008). These studies focus on showing the nature of physical activities practised by older people, the history of this practice or even their attitude towards the body. By contrast, analysis of texts at different levels of public action through the triple focus of physical activity, wellbeing and scientific directives has not been carried out (in his thesis Hénaff-Pineau refers to texts without doing a systematic analysis); this is our aim here. The difficulty in mobilizing scientific knowledge in the directives linked to ageing well is particularly interesting in the case of physical activities. They are one of the prescribed recommendations regularly cited in political texts and have led to abundant scientific literature on the subject of their impact on health.

This work is supported by the analysis of a corpus of texts composed of various international and French national reports and preventive plans on ageing published since the 1960s. The corpus was made up through a progressive inventory. We selected the texts on the national level (From the Laroque report in 1962 to the Ageing Well Plan 2007–2009 and the Ladoucette report in 2011) and international level (notably the UNO, the WHO, the Organization for Economic Co-operation and Development and the European Union) cited in literature (Lassen & Moreira, 2014; Viriot Durandal & Moulaert, 2014). We collected original texts. After an extensive reading, we isolated the passages concerning wellbeing on the one hand, and physical activities on the other to produce a more precise analysis. We also took into account other official guidelines (addressing the question of the physical activity of older people) identifying those seeming to indicate significant changes in the depiction of ageing and in the courses of action considered (Raymond & Grenier, 2013). More recently, from the 2000s, our focus on the use of physical activities for prevention led us to include, at the French national level, programmes specific to physical activities or those linked to nutrition. Most of the texts were available on Internet; certain previous ones (for example the Laroque report in France) were consulted in the library. In all, the corpus is composed of nearly 40 texts.

Alongside this corpus of 'institutional' texts, another contains 20 scientific papers addressing the question of the links between wellbeing and physical activity of older people collected from literature reviews; next to existing review (like the one made by the National Institute for Health and Medical Research or INSERM: Institut National de la Santé et de la Recherche Médicale, 2008), we searched for a series of keywords in the *PubMed* database (principally, the following key words were used: physical activity, ageing, older adults, wellbeing, wellness). We began with literature reviews and then enlarged the corpus by examining the texts cited in these reviews. Then we started comparing the 'scientific corpus' back with the 'institutional' corpus.

Our chapter is structured in three phases. After highlighting the importance of physical activities in national and international texts dedicated to preventive ageing, we examine the scientific debates concerning the role of physical activity on wellbeing to show how a usable frame of reference has been established.

Preventive ageing, wellbeing and physical and sports activities in international and French national programmes

The idea of a positive impact of physical activity on the health and wellbeing of older people is supported in the texts of the major international bodies on the subject. It was not always the central element of preventive ageing in all the texts, as other factors appeared, for instance professional environment, or physical and social lifestyle (here the *Global Age-friendly Cities Guide*, published by the WHO in 2007 can be cited). However, physical activity is very present in several major texts published by the WHO or the European Union and, when mentioned, its positive effects are firmly asserted.

For example, the guidelines published by the WHO in 2002 for the second world assembly on ageing, developed the notion of active ageing in great detail and stated that 'Participation in regular, moderate physical activity can delay functional decline. It can reduce the onset of chronic disease in both healthy and chronically ill older people' (p. 23). In addition it was specified that, in terms of political intervention, information campaigns culturally compatible with the target population should be carried out, access to physical and sports activities should be made easier, and that the public and professionals should be made aware of the importance of remaining active during ageing (WHO 2002, p. 48).

Some texts approached the effects of physical and sports activities in a more multi-factorial way. Doing physical activities could have effects on different levels: psychological (on mental health), social and physiological. The document published under the title *Healthy Ageing: A Challenge for Europe* indicates that: 'For example physical activity is often practised together with other people and hence also affects the social determinants' (Berenson, 2007, p. 23). The following is stated further on in the text: 'Other evidence shows the mental health benefits of physical activity' (p. 78). The document reports the results set out in various articles along these lines and includes the recommendations formulated some years before by the American College of Sports Medicine (ACSM). These were very often repeated in the texts studied: 'Moderate physical activity on three-to-five occasions per week with a duration of 30–60 minutes seems to be effective in reducing blood pressure' (p. 99). If the idea of wellbeing and quality of life was introduced in advance and presented as being correlated to doing physical activity, only one study assessing wellbeing and its parameters was actually cited: 'and older people who are physically active report higher levels of wellbeing and physical function than the less active do' (Spirduso & Cronin, 2001). Other studies reflect a more exclusively somatic notion of health. It should be noted that few texts cite the studies on which they are based.

The need for regular physical exercise to improve the health and wellbeing of senior citizens was also accepted and set up on a national level in France. Several official guidelines on French health promotion policies highlighted the importance of practising physical activity and its beneficial impact on health and wellbeing. The National Ageing Well Plan for 2007–2009 mentions that 'clinical data showing the positive and long-term effects of physical activity on health has been available for a long time.

Physical activity improves health and wellbeing' (p. 11). Here the authority of scientific clinical knowledge was called on to justify the need to promote physical activity among senior citizens through different measures: creation of a reference guide, support for sports federations, improvement of training for professionals, assessment of physical capabilities of senior citizens and publicity campaigns. In the Nutrition and Health National Programme (PNNS) 2011–2015, certain measures aim to promote physical activity among specific groups, notably among older people (Ministry of Labour, Work and Health, 2011). The PNNS, structured on a 5-year programme basis, links nutrition with the promotion of physical activity. The strategic axis of the three succeeding PNNS (2001–2006, 2007–2010, 2011–2015) were directed towards communication, information, education, improvement of the physical and nutritional environment in relation to the recommendations concerning physical activities. The promotion of physical and sports activity was to be done through

> the creation and distribution of a directory of sports associations offering activities for people over 50; the development of the offer of physical activities in institutional establishments for dependant older people (EHPAD: Établissement d'Hébergement pour Personnes Âgées Dépendantes) and in retirement homes and residences for older people; the synchronization of fall prevention programmes.
>
> (Ministry of Labour, Work and Health, 2011, p. 28)

These recommendations can also be found in the Aquino report:[1] 'Regular practise of moderate physical activity contributes to healthy ageing and improves the functional state of frail, or becoming frail, older people' (Aquino, 2013, p. 61). In the different texts, the link between physical activity and wellbeing is asserted and justifies a set of measures aiming to promote physical and sports activities. The underlying intention was that if studies show a correlation between the levels of wellbeing and physical activity, encouragement of the population to do physical activity would increase the level of individual wellbeing. The link between physical activity and wellbeing is often described as causal and correlated. However, correlation does not mean causes. From this standpoint, the way in which scientific results on the subject were used contributed in stressing the need for a norm of wellbeing: doing regular, moderate physical activity became essential for those wanting to remain in good health and maintain their wellbeing. Here our findings agree with those of Hénaff-Pinault (2008, 2009) concerning medical prescriptions for physical and sports activities.

Scientific knowledge under debate

Although the link between physical activity and wellbeing is confirmed in policy guidelines, it remains under discussion in scientific literature.

Nuanced scientific results

While recognizing the research carried out, it should be noted that scientific literature was more nuanced on the subject than the political texts promoting wellbeing. Effectively, many studies tend to show the existence of a correlation between the assessment of wellbeing and regular physical activity, whether with older people, children, teenagers or young adults (Krawczynski & Oszewski, 2000). Different indicators for measuring wellbeing support these conclusions: depression, hypochondria, feeling of 'purpose in life', anxiety, etc. (Ibid.; Fukukawa *et al.*, 2004; INSERM, 2008). However, the question was not an issue of total consensus and there are diverging or at least nuanced results. For example, for Fukukawa *et al.* (2004), the effects of physical activity on wellbeing depend on the age of the subject. The effects were more significant for those aged 65 to 79 years old than for the youngest adults. Whereas for Netz and his colleagues (2005), the effects diminish with age and the wellbeing of those over 76 years old raises other issues than physical activity. Finally, for some, the source of wellbeing was not physical activity itself but rather the associated psychological factors: positive attitude of onlookers, breaking free from negative thoughts, new learning and encounters (Lawlor & Hopker, 2001).

The causal link discussion

It is also important to underline that the demonstration of a correlation does not mean there is a direct, univocal causal link. If certain studies lean towards a causal link between physical activity and wellbeing, this deduction is far from reaching a consensus and even raises doubts and uncertainties not visible in the international and national reports and texts. For a certain number of authors the causal link made between physical activity and wellbeing of older people was not obvious (e.g. Scully *et al.*, 1998; Penedo & Dahn, 2005). These claim that although a correlation between physical exercise and psychological wellbeing had been observed, there was little experimental proof to support the thesis of a direct causal link between physical exercise and wellbeing of older people. Furthermore, several researchers highlight methodological limitations (for example Lotan *et al.*, 2005); according to them, they could not allow a conclusion to be reached that by doing more physical activity, a so-called inactive older person would improve his/her level of wellbeing.

Doubts concerning the establishing of recommendations on physical activity

Despite reference to studies that led to results in favour of a correlation or causal link between physical activity and wellbeing, it remains difficult to convert research results into precise practical recommendations on the kind of physical exercise to carry out. The literature review conducted by Scully *et al.* (1998) is very instructive in this respect. For the authors, strong evidence shows the somatic effects of physical exercise. By contrast, little evidence demonstrates the effects on psychological wellbeing and therefore does not allow the production of precise recommendations concerning physical exercise. The authors cite many studies. For example, McAuley (1994) identified a correlation between physical exercise and several dimensions of wellbeing but was unable to formulate practical recommendations indicating the kind of exercise that would be beneficial in a particular situation (strength-building, endurance, etc.). In a more specific way, Scully *et al.* (1998) were interested in different dimensions of wellbeing: anxiety, depression, etc. and came to virtually the same conclusions each time (INSERM cites this literature review several times in their report, in 2008, on the effects of physical activity on health).

The scientific literature analysed demonstrates a positive effect of exercise on the level of anxiety, though the kind of exercise practised does not appear to have an effect on the results. The impact study on depression gives the same results, as does the study concerning the link between physical exercise and self-esteem. The authors tried to investigate the links between the various kinds of activity and different dimensions of self-esteem (perceived competency in sport, perception of the physical self, etc.), but the literature did not reveal which kind of exercise was most effective on a particular dimension of self-esteem. In their conclusion, the authors regretted that precise recommendations concerning physical activities could not be drawn from this research and asserted that future research should be directed towards this point in particular (Scully *et al.*, 1998). More recent studies on the links between physical activity and psychological wellness are not more precise, physical exercise is usually understood in a general way, without really differentiating the kind of exercises carried out (for example Klusmann *et al.*, 2012).

The texts from national and international institutions depict a consensual and homogeneous corpus of knowledge, though this was not the case. If physical activity was generally considered as beneficial for somatic health parameters, the correlation between the practise of physical activities and wellbeing was less consensual. The existence of divergent results needing to be qualified could in fact be observed. Furthermore, the reports and plans studied highlight a simple causal link between physical activities and wellbeing, whereas scientific literature on the subject is more measured. Lastly, the certainty in the formulation of recommendations usually reproduced a 'general' set of standards for everyone in an equal way: moderate physical activity should be practised almost daily. However their establishment did not identify with the different studies although the recommendations themselves were simple and functional.

The modelling of a usable frame of reference

With the support of scientific knowledge, the different texts modelled a set of recommendations in coordination with standards and representations to form what French public action experts call a 'frame of reference' (Jobert & Muller, 1987; Muller, 1990). This was at the core of preventive policies on ageing and was used to guide them. More precisely, this frame of reference contributed to the structuring of *values* and *norms* (criteria for ageing well), mobilized *algorithms* (causal relations between recommendations and economic and health consequences) and produced *depictions* (of successful ageing). The interlinking of these levels can be found in the referred texts.[2]

Causal relations between recommendations and consequences on health can be observed. They already existed, even if in very general, in the Laroque report, 1962:

> Without a doubt a diet deficient in proteins, a prolonged imbalance between intellectual and physical activities, living and working conditions inappropriate to the biological and psychological capabilities of the individual, lack of psychological preparation for retirement and growing old, accelerate for many adults the process of ageing.
>
> (Laroque, 1962, p. 110)

The recommendations became progressively more precise in the texts from 1990–2000 both in France and internationally:

> Adults aged 65 years and above should do at least 150 minutes of moderate-intensity aerobic physical activity throughout the week, or do at least 75 minutes of vigorous-intensity aerobic physical activity throughout the week, or an equivalent combination of moderate- and vigorous-intensity activity... . Aerobic activity should be performed in bouts of at least 10 minutes duration... . Adults of this age group with poor mobility should perform physical activity to enhance balance and prevent falls on 3 or more days per week.
>
> (WHO, 2010, p. 8)

In France for example the National Prevention Plan through Physical and Sports Activity (PNAPS: Plan National de Prévention par l'Activité Physique ou Sportive, Ministry of Labour, Work and Health, 2008) recommended that assessments on physical abilities should be carried out. Programmes implemented by specialized sports federations were cited, as well as examples and guiding principles for training, taken from documents in use in other countries (e.g. Canada). For example, to develop the aerobic endurance of older people considered as 'frail' (this category gathers those who are neither 'independent' nor 'dependent') 20 minutes of continued activity was recommended three times a week, at a low or medium intensity, however it was specified that 'these exercises should be carried out after those that develop strength-endurance and balance' (Ministry of Labour, Work and Health, 2008, p. 121).

The recommendations progressively took the form of operational procedures. On an international level and in many French texts (for example the National Plan on Ageing Well) the recommendations were rooted in the slogan: 'a brisk walk of at least thirty minutes per day'. Thirty minutes of moderate physical activity per day first appeared in 1995 in conjunction with the ACSM, the CDC (Centers for Disease Control and Prevention), the WHO and the IFSM (International Federation of Sports Medicine). This maxim was present in most of the texts that followed.

More precisely the prevention agencies as well as the texts and reports provide additional information. In France, the French Agency for Food and Health Safety (AFSSA: Agence Française de Sécurité Sanitaire des Aliments), under the authority of the Ministry of Health, published a practical guide giving simple instructions for the practise of physical activity: 'The equivalent of at least thirty minutes of brisk walking per day', 'Integrate in everyday life any form of physical activity (walking, cycling, gardening...) and sports activities (gymnastics, yoga, swimming...)', 'To be beneficial, do physical activity by periods of at least ten minutes' (AFSSA, 2008, pp. 4–5). Three profiles were established, not in terms of age group but in categories of sports people concerned. The people schematized in the first category were in the 'I'm very active' and 'I do sport' stages. For this group advice on nutrition and medical appointments was given. The second category referred to the 'I'm not very active' and 'I don't like sport' profile. Here the recommendations advised walking and taking advantage of certain opportunities in everyday life to 'move', such as using the stairs instead of the lift, doing odd jobs, gardening, doing the housework or going dancing. Two double pages were dedicated to people who did not like sport. Finally the people corresponding to the profile: 'I would like to do a physical or sports activity again' were advised to start slowly, and to adapt their diet and many examples of activities were given. In the same spirit the *Reference Frame of Good Practices* published by the National Institute for Prevention and Health Education (INPES: Institut National de Prévention et d'Education pour la Santé), proposed a *Practical Guide in 11 Recipes and 10 Physical Exercises* (INPES, 2012).

These directives were linked to values and norms (which are closely interlinked) corresponding to criteria for ageing well that refer to three central notions: autonomy (in opposition to dependency), activity in the sense here of social dynamism and responsibility (autonomy and responsibility are important values and define norms of activity). In France, autonomy was therefore at the core of the Aquino report (2013); the main challenge was to preserve it. To achieve this, physical activity was a central element: 'six kinds of key strategies are recognized as efficient in international literature to promote the health of independent people of 55 years old and over living at home' (p. 16). Physical activity (exercises for endurance, muscle-training, maintaining balance and suppleness) is therefore listed before information/ communication, education of the group, telephone follow-up, assessment of individual needs and environmental risks, home visits. Here it is worth noting that reference to international literature is considered as an authoritative argument to justify a set of recommendations.

It was emphasized that older people could maintain their social dynamism if they remained physically active. The AFSSA specified the importance of 'eating better' and 'exercising daily' to succeed in 'simply "Ageing Well"', while continuing to live according to your wishes' (AFSSA, 2008, p. 2) and the *Passport to Active Retirement* (Published in 2007 by the Ministry of Social Security, Older People, Disabled People and Families) originally proposed as part of the Ageing Well Plan included information on health, personal assistance and voluntary work. This document has been available from pension offices since 2007. It defends the idea that retirement is an active time of life as it enables people to take up an activity again, take the time to look after themselves, share their experience by doing voluntary work because support and services on offer allow more time for others: 'It's the time to take up gymnastics, gardening, swimming or walking...' (p. 6).

The basic idea throughout these recommendations is activity. Being active became essential and the incentives to get moving were many: older people, seniors should not just be pensioners content to wait

> resting till the end of their lives, but be people taking part ...in social life. ... Retirement should not be a bleak period before death or a repetitive life in 'idleness', disconnected from other younger people, but a new, enthusiastic period of life, during which we keep learning while continuing to teach and pass on our experience.
>
> (Bsc & Rey, 1998, p. 211)

But as Lamb clearly shows, the emphasis on positivity and individual autonomy can be very *disturbing* for older people and could make them feel guilty (Lamb, 2014). This individual autonomy and responsibility resulted not so much from a direct moralizing discourse than from the knowledgeable statements. Finally, the normative aspect of the frame of reference was hidden behind the recourse to bio-medical knowledge.

Finally, a depiction of 'ageing well' puts individual empowerment at the heart of the procedures. Wellbeing depends on capability and the notion of empowerment became central. This concept of ageing joined the idea of 'promoting health' highlighted since the Ottawa Charter (WHO, 1986) and was based on two main elements: communities must create favourable environments for individuals (WHO, 2007), and reciprocally individuals must develop skills and behaviours guaranteeing their own health. In other words, health and wellbeing thus relied as much on individual responsibility as on external factors:

> Active ageing policies and programmes recognize the need to encourage and balance personal responsibility (self-care), age-friendly environments and intergenerational solidarity. Individuals and families need to plan and prepare for older age, and make personal efforts to adopt positive personal health practices at all stages of life. At the same time supportive environments are required to 'make the healthy choices the easy choices.'
>
> (WHO, 2002, p. 17)

(For an account of personal 'active ageing' in everyday use in daycentres, see Lassen's chapter here).

Accepting responsibility was rooted in the knowledge on links between lifestyles and foreseeable consequences (like tobacco or alcohol abuse, and inactivity) and on a body of knowledge both scientific and popular through media campaigns on prevention or specialist press. This knowledge refers first to the link established between physical activity and health (modelled as seen earlier in a simple and causal way) and then to the simple practical instructions. For example, walking for 30 minutes per day or the more recent 10,000 steps, launched by Hatano (1993) from Japan, contribute to a combination of duration and number of steps.

The depiction of 'ageing well' in the texts studied was that of a prepared and well thought out process. They refer to a person actively involved in social sphere, living life to the full and who looks after themselves; this person feels a responsibility for its future state of health, knowing that the community will later take care of him/her in one way or another. In effect, the individual develops its activity aware of the dangers and anticipates the consequences of their behaviour (Genard, 2007; see Schweda & Pfaller in this volume) for a discussion of usual experience of anti-ageing products and services in Germany). People are now required to manage themselves, be subjects of their own lives, be responsible for themselves and the community. Wellbeing is an individual and subjective factor and its requirement has become an element of public health.

Conclusion

We showed that the notion of wellbeing first appeared in preventive policies on ageing during the second half of the twentieth century. French texts followed international recommendations which establish a simple causal link between physical activity and wellbeing of individuals, whereas scientific literature on the subject is more careful.

The different plans and official guidelines of French national and international policies in favour of ageing well bring to light the notion of activity, with a view to empowerment. Certain authors consider that this focalization causes anxiety in older people (Lamb, 2014), and that it can lead to a form of self-blame (Billé and Martz, 2010). In exchange for the support given by the community, older people should remain physically and socially active: a prerequisite of good health and wellbeing. The notion of empowerment is transferred from a collective and individual responsibility to an individual one (even though this responsibility remains flexible). Promoting active ageing (internationally) or ageing well (in France) was interpreted by highlighting good practices, by the instruction to be physically active, and justified by recourse to a body of scientific knowledge. In this way, the empowerment of individuals resulted not so much from a direct moralizing discourse than from the knowledgeable statements enabling people to anticipate the consequences of their lifestyle. Finally, it was an evidence that the normative aspect of the frame of reference for public policies was both masked and justified by the recourse to scientific and/or medical knowledge. This observation completes the studies of other authors who have worked on different sources (for example Laliberte Rudman, 2006).

However, without falling into a radical relativism, it is worth noting that science can be seen in this study as an authority, used as a tool to justify a certain normative idea of what ageing should be like. The case for recommendations concerning physical activity is from this viewpoint characteristic: the effects of physical activity on biological health parameters are certainly widely agreed but the links between physical activity and wellbeing are far from having just a causal, direct and unquestionable relationship, as also observed by Tulle (2008) through his study of scientific literature. As can be seen in other fields of public action, the opinion of scientific experts (even reported) was considered as authoritative (Roy, 2001), whereas in fact scientific texts are heterogeneous, steeped in reservations and uncertainty.

Notes

1 Three reports on ageing were published in 2013 (Aquino, 2013; Rivière, 2013, Pinville, 2013).
2 We have chosen to start from the algorithms which are recurrent in the corpus to go to depictions, values and norms.

References

AFSSA (2008), *Le guide nutrition à partir de 55 ans*. Paris.
Aquino Jean-Pierre (2009), 'Prévention en gérontologie et plan national "Bien vieillir"'. In Bourdillon François, *Traité de prévention*. Paris, Flammarion, pp. 298–306.
Aquino Jean-Pierre (2013), *Anticiper pour une autonomie préservée: Un enjeu de société*. Paris, Rapport du comité 'Avancée en âge, prévention et qualité de vie'.
Berenson Karin (2007), *Healthy Ageing. A Challenge for Europe*. Stockholm, Swedish National Institute of Public Health.
Billé Michel & Didier Martz (2010), *La Tyrannie du Bien vieillir*. Paris, Le Bord de l'eau.

Bosc Yves & Jean-François Rey (1998), 'Vieillissement et mauvais vieillissement', *Prévenir*, no. 35, pp. 207–211.

Burlot Fabrice & Brice Lefèvre (2009), 'Les pratiques physiques des seniors', *Retraite et société*, Vol. 58, no. 2, pp. 133–158.

Crosnier Dominique (2005), 'Les activités physiques et sportives des seniors'. In Muller Lara, *La pratique des activités physiques et sportives en France*, Paris, Ministère de la Jeunesse, des Sports et de la Vie associative et INSEP, pp. 81–98.

Feillet Raymonde (1996), *Représentations du vieillissement et attitudes des retraités et des jeunes en situation de confrontation sur le terrain sportif.* Thèse de doctorat en sciences humaines, Université Paris V.

Feillet Raymonde (2006), *Corps, Vieillissement et identité: Entre préservation et présentation de soi. Place des activités physiques et sportives.* Toulouse, Érès.

Feillet Raymonde & Charles Roncin (2006), *Souci du corps, sport et vieillissement.* Paris, Érès.

Fukukawa Yasuyuki, Nakashima Chiori, Tsuboi Satomi, Kozakai Rumi, Doyo Wataru, Niino Naoakira, Ando Fujiko & Hiroshi Shimokata (2004), 'Age differences in the effect of physical activity on depressive symptoms', *Psychology and Aging*, Vol. 19, no. 2, pp. 346–351.

Genard Jean-Louis (2007), 'Capacités et capacitation: Une nouvelle orientation des politiques publiques'. In Cantelli, Fabrizio & Jean-Louis Genard, *Action Publique et Subjectivité. Droit et Société*, no. 46, Paris, Librairie Générale de Droit et de Jurisprudence, pp. 41–64.

Haas Peter M. (1992), 'Introduction: Epistemic communities and international policy coordination', *International Organization*, Vol. 46, no. 1, pp. 1–35.

Hatano Yoshiro (1993), 'Use of the pedometer for promoting daily walking exercise', *International Council for Health, Physical Education, and Recreation*, Vol. 29, pp. 4–8.

Hénaff-Pineau Pia-Caroline (2008), *Pratiques physiques des seniors et vieillissement: Entre raison et passion. Analyse sociologique de la transformation des pratiques avec l'avancée en âge.* Thèse de doctorat en sciences du sport, de la motricité et du mouvement humain, Université Paris-Sud 11.

Hénaff-Pineau Pia-Caroline (2009), 'Vieillissement et pratiques sportives: Entre modération et intensification', *Lien social et politiques*, no. 62, pp. 71–83.

INPES (2012), *Guide pratique en 11 recettes et 10 exercices physiques.* Paris.

INSERM (2008), *Activité physique. Contextes et effets sur la santé.* Paris, INSERM.

Jobert Bruno & Pierre Muller (1987), *L'État en action. Politiques publiques et corporatismes.* Paris, PUF.

Klusmann Verena, Evers Andrea, Schwarzer Ralph & Isabella Heuser (2012), 'Views on aging and emotional benefits of physical activity: Effects of an exercise intervention in older women', *Psychology of Sport and Exercise*, Vol. 13, no. 2, pp. 236–242.

Krawczynski Marcin & Henryk Olszewski (2000), 'Psychological well-being associated with a physical activity programme for persons over 60 years old', *Psychology of Sport and Exercise*, Vol. 1, no.1, pp. 57–63.

Ladoucette (de) Olivier (2011), 'Bien-être et santé mentale: Des atouts indispensables pour bien vieillir', *Rapport remis au Ministère du travail, de l'emploi et de la santé*, Paris.

Laliberte Rudman Debbie (2006), 'Shaping the active, autonomous and responsible modern retiree: An analysis of discursive technologies and their links with neo-liberal political rationality', *Ageing & Society*, Vol. 26, no. 2, pp. 181–201.

Lamb Sarah (2014), 'Permanent personhood or meaningful decline? Toward a critical anthropology of successful aging', *Journal of Aging Studies*, Vol. 29, pp. 41–52.

Laroque Pierre (1962), *Politique de la vieillesse. Rapport de la Commission d'étude des problèmes de la vieillesse.* Paris, La documentation française.

Lassen Aske Juul & Tiago Moreira (2014), 'Unmaking old age: Political and cognitive formats of active ageing', *Journal of Aging Studies*, Vol. 30, no.1, pp. 33–46.

Lawlor Debbie A. & Stephen W. Hopker (2001), 'The effectiveness of exercise as an intervention in the management of depression: Systematic review and meta-regression analysis of randomised controlled trials', *British Medical Journal*, Vol. 322, no. 7289, pp. 763–767.

Lotan Meir, Merrick Joav & Eli Carmeli (2005), 'A review of physical activity and well-being', *International Journal of Adolescent Medicine and Health*, Vol. 17, no. 1, pp. 23–31.

McAuley, Edward (1994), 'Physical activity and psychosocial outcomes'. In Bouchard Claude, Shephard Roy J. and Thomas Stephens, *Physical Activity, Fitness, and Health.* Champaign, Human Kinetics, pp. 551–568.

Ministry of Health and Solidarity, Ministry of Social Security, Older People, Disabled People and Families, Ministry of Youth, Sports and Community Organisations (2007), *Plan national 'Bien viellir' 2007–2009.* Paris.

Ministry of Labour, Work and Health (2008), *Plan national de prévention par l'activité physique ou sportive.* Paris.

Ministry of Labour, Work and Health (2011), *Plan National Nutrition Santé 2011–2015.*

Ministry of Social Security, Older People, Disabled People and Families (2007), *Passeport pour une retraite active.* Paris.

Moulaert Thibauld & Jean-Philippe Viriot Durandal (2013), 'Production et rapport aux normes contemporaines du vieillir. Le vieillissement décliné', *Recherches sociologiques et anthropologiques*, Vol. 44, no. 1, pp. 1–156.

Muller Pierre (1990), *Les politiques publiques.* Paris, PUF.

Muller Pierre (2000), 'L'analyse cognitive des politiques publiques: Vers une sociologie politique de l'action publique', *Revue française de science politique*, Vol. 50, no. 2, pp. 189–207.

Netz Yael, Wu Meng-Jia, Becker Betsy Jane & Gershon Tenenbaum (2005), 'Physical activity and psychological well- being in advanced age: A meta-analysis of intervention studies', *Psychology and Aging*, Vol. 20, no. 2, pp. 272–284.

Penedo Frank J. & Jason R. Dahn (2005), 'Exercise and well-being: A review of mental and physical health benefits associated with physical activity', *Current Opinion Psychiatry*, Vol. 18, no. 2, pp. 189–193.

Pinville Martine (2013), *Relever le défi politique de l'avancée en âge. Perspectives internationales*, Rapport remis au premier ministre, Paris.

Raymond Émilie & Amanda Grenier (2013), 'The rhetoric of participation in policy discourse: Toward a new form of exclusion for seniors with a disability?', *The Canadian Journal of Aging*, Vol. 32, no. 2, pp. 117–129.

Rivière Daniel (2013), *Dispositif d'activités physiques et sportives en directions des âgés*, Rapport remis aux ministres, Ministère des affaires sociales et de la santé, Paris.

Roy Alexis (2001), *Les experts face au risque. Le cas des plantes transgéniques.* Paris, PUF.

Scully Deirdre, Kremer John, Meade Mary M., Graham Roger & Katrin Dudgeon (1998), 'Physical exercise and psychological well-being: A critical review', *British Journal of Sports Medicine*, Vol. 32, no. 2, pp. 111–120.

Spirduso Waneen W. & Leilani D. Cronin (2001), 'Exercise dose-response effects on quality of life and independent living in older adults', *Medicine and Science in Sports and Exercise*, Vol. 33, no. 6S, pp. S598–S608.

Stenner Paul, McFarquhar Tara & Ann Bowling (2011), 'Older people and "active ageing": Subjective aspects of ageing actively', *Journal of Health Psychology*, Vol. 16, no. 3, pp. 467–477.

Trépos Jean-Yves (1996), *Sociologie de l'expertise*. Paris, PUF.

Truchot Guy (2002), 'Les seniors'. In Mignon Patrick & Guy Truchot, *Les pratiques sportives en France*. Enquête 2000, Paris, Ministère des Sports et INSEP, pp. 41–46.

Tulle Emmanuelle (2008), 'Acting your age? Sports science and the ageing body', *Journal of Aging Studies*, Vol. 22, no. 4, pp. 340–347.

UNO (2002), *Rapport de la Deuxième Assemblée Mondiale sur le Vieillissement*. Madrid 8–12 Avril 2002, New York, Nations Unies.

Viriot Durandal Jean-Philippe & Thibauld Moulaert (2014), 'Le "vieillissement actif" comme référentiel international d'action publique: Acteurs et contraintes', *Socio-logos. Revue de l'association française de sociologie [En ligne]*, no. 9. URL: http://socio-logos.revues.org/2814, accessed 31 January 2017.

WHO (1986), *Promotion de la Santé*. Charte d'Ottawa, Ottawa, WHO.

WHO (2002), *Active Ageing: A Policy Framework*. Geneva, WHO.

WHO (2007), *Global Age-friendly Cities Guide*. Geneva, WHO.

WHO (2010), *Global Recommendations on Physical Activity for Health*. Geneva, WHO.

3 'Regimes of hope' in planning later life

Medical optimism in the field of anti-ageing medicine

Mark Schweda and Larissa Pfaller

In 1996, the American osteopaths Ronald Klatz and Robert Goldman, founders of the American Academy of Anti-Ageing Medicine (A4M), declared that 'the future of anti-aging medicine promises the elimination of the disability, deformity, pain, disease, suffering and sorrow of old age' ([1996] 2003, p. 13). 'In a few decades', they predicted, 'the traditional enfeebled, ailing elderly person will be but a grotesque memory of a barbaric past' (ibid., p. 13). Merely 10 years later, the British self-proclaimed biogerontologist Aubrey de Grey even speculated that 'the first person to live to 1000 might be 60 already' (2004). Today, we have almost gotten used to the prevalence of boastful anti-ageing advertisements like the following:

> The future of multivitamins is radically different – and radically better – than anyone ever thought possible. Moreover, it's here now. New science has profoundly expanded our understanding of what's possible in human wellness and anti-ageing. For instance, scientists now believe that if you live to the year 2050, you may not have to get any older.
>
> (Super Nutrition, 2013)

These examples of contemporary anti-ageing discourse attest to the '(bio) medicalization of ageing' – the fact that medicine has become one of the major forces defining the nature of ageing and old age and shaping the everyday life of older people in modern societies (Estes & Binney, 1989; Kaufman *et al.*, 2004). They furthermore illustrate that a considerable portion of the underlying scientific claims and their corresponding anti-ageing medical practices refer primarily to the future: professional discourse involves audacious forecasts and promises about future biomedical developments, expressing remarkable confidence and optimism in scientific progress and technical feasibility. At the same time, the actual interventions anti-ageing professionals offer often depend on identifying individual risk factors for potential ailments to develop preventive strategies for later life and manage a future medical fate. Specifically, the German Society of Anti-Ageing-Medicine (Deutsche Gesellschaft für Prävention und Anti-Aging Medizin, GSAAM) has adopted a policy of framing old age as a decisive risk factor for diseases and public health burdens, with anti-ageing medicine as a strategy for calculating and countering medical risks (Spindler, 2014). By turning ageing into an individual and societal project, anti-ageing essentially involves gambling on the future and the anticipated developments and outcomes of present endeavours. Similar trends in other fields of biomedicine and the life sciences (such as human genetics, stem cell research, reproductive medicine and oncology) have been described in terms of a general shift away from 'regimes of truth' towards 'regimes of hope' (Brown, 2005; Moreira & Palladino, 2005): Instead of 'truth' in the traditional sense of a verifiable correspondence with currently known facts, scientific claims are increasingly concerned with the evocation of elusive future possibilities and the potential of current research approaches and technological perspectives.

Against this background, we investigate the extent to which anti-ageing can be described in terms of 'regimes of hope', discussing the implications for lay persons and users of anti-ageing products and services and highlighting potentially problematic consequences. To do so, we combine an exploration of the professional discourse of anti-ageing medicine in Germany (from interviews with experts, websites and conventions of the GSAAM) with the qualitative content analysis of narrative interviews and focus groups conducted with users of anti-ageing products and services in Germany (96 participants altogether). The aim is to analyse and compare how perceptions of and attitudes towards the future and future health in anti-ageing medical expert discourse are taken up, modified, and problematized in everyday practices. We focus on an attitude we term 'medical optimism', since it is primarily concerned with the problem of raising and maintaining hope in the face of an uncertain future. As our findings will show, the regimes of hope promoted by anti-ageing discourses open spaces for manifold ways of individual self-conception and self-reassurance, but at the same time also create specific moral conflicts and dilemmas for those concerned.

Background: 'Regimes of hope' in anti-ageing medicine

Anti-ageing medicine describes itself as a discrete discipline implementing medical and biogerontological methods and findings for the early diagnosis, prevention, treatment, and/or reversal of age-related changes, disorders and diseases (A4M, 2015). It promises using medical insights and technologies to fight the visual signs and symptoms of ageing, prevent or repair functional ailments and diseases of old age, and prolong the healthspan, average life expectancy or even maximum lifespan in humans. In addition, 'anti-ageing' is also used as a label for a wide range of commercial health, beauty, care, and wellness products and treatments. There have been attempts to establish alternative terms such as 'pro-age', 'reverse-ageing', 'down-ageing' and 'rejuvenation', but 'anti-ageing' is still powerful as a professional guiding concept, popular buzzword and commercial marketing label. It has inspired a dynamic social movement and a broad and expanding industry, but is also subject to controversy in discussions of medical risk, individual suitability and social consequences (Mykytyn, 2006a, 2006b).

The neologism 'anti-ageing medicine' was coined with the founding of the A4M in the United States in the early 1990s. Ever since, the organization has been dedicated to the development and promotion of medical treatments for ageing and its symptoms and effects. Its mission is the 'advancement of technology to detect, prevent, and treat ageing related disease and to promote research into methods to retard and optimize the human ageing process' (A4M, 2015). Today, the A4M comprises over 26,000 members from 120 countries, among them many physicians and researchers as well as political stakeholders (ibid.). From its beginnings, anti-ageing medicine has been at the centre of highly controversial ethical and political debates (Post & Binstock, 2004). In 2002, a number of prominent American gerontologists and geriatricians waged a 'war' on the new self-declared 'profession' and dismissed its promises as baseless and its practices as amounting to commercial quackery that could sometimes be dangerous (Vincent, 2003). The 'anti-ageing' boom has nonetheless continued, transcending the medical sphere and developing into a broad patient/practitioner movement (Mykytyn, 2006b). Anti-ageing organizations were subsequently established in many other parts of the world, especially Australia, Asia and Europe, and they often specifically adapted general medical orientations and objectives into definitions that suit their national contexts.

This is particularly evident with regard to the development of the anti-ageing discourse in Germany. While American anti-ageing medicine is mainly influenced by the A4M, which defines ageing as a treatable biomolecular 'meta-disease', the GSAAM, founded in 1999, formulated a more preventive approach targeting ageing not so much as a disease but rather 'as the major risk factor for widespread diseases and diseases of civilization' (GSAAM, 2015, authors' translation). This shift of emphasis has led the GSAAM to split from the American umbrella organization and its war on ageing as a disease, and to the emergence of a specifically German interpretation of anti-ageing in terms of responsible prediction and prevention to control the risky nature of ageing and old age (Spindler, 2014). Another specificity of the German situation is that the healthcare system is public and based on the idea of solidarity, thus implying that contributors to German public health insurance are responsible for each other. While failure to sustain good health in old age may be considered simple bad luck or inadequate personal foresight in a heavily individualized private system such as that found in the United States, in the German socio-political context ageing also becomes a matter of moral responsibility towards other community members. In contrast to medically necessary treatments, the cost of anti-ageing products and services is not usually covered by German health insurance providers. Anti-ageing thus seems to be something 'special' and rather 'questionable', since health insurance is thought to only accept paying for effective medical treatments (Schweda *et al.*, 2011).

Current approaches to anti-ageing include a wide range of different medical (and para- or pseudo-medical) products and practices (for an overview, see Stuckelberger, 2008). According to their main objectives, three main categories can be distinguished. The *first category* of interventions are aimed at limiting aesthetic signs of ageing, and mostly involve cosmetic treatments of the skin such as Botox or filler injections (e.g. hyaluronic acid, collagen, body fat) to lessen wrinkles, laser therapy or chemical peeling to reduce age spots, or surgical interventions such as facelifts to tighten the skin. Furthermore, special 'anti-ageing' clinics or spas offer 'holistic' approaches involving body care, dietary regimens and lifestyle programmes for a youthful and attractive appearance. Beyond the medical field, 'anti-ageing' is also used as a label for a wide range of common beauty products and services such as face creams, shampoos, dietary supplements, and specific massages and exercises. The *second category* of anti-ageing measures comprises attempts to prevent or remedy functional failure, ailments, and diseases associated with old age. They include various pharmaceutical interventions (e.g. hormone replacement therapies using human growth hormone (HGH) or dehydroepiandrosterone (DHEA) to sustain muscle mass and bone density, statin or chelation therapy to prevent arteriosclerosis or cancer, or Viagra™ to correct erectile dysfunction). In addition, preventive strategies are recommended to facilitate healthy ageing, maintain fitness and capabilities, and keep the body in youthful condition. This mainly includes lifestyle changes like particular exercises, healthy diets and nutrition, mental fitness programs, regular medical check-ups, and avoiding alcohol consumption, smoking and excess weight. A *third category* consists of even more ambitious approaches directly aimed at extending lifespan: prolonging individual life expectancy as well as the human biological lifespan. There are high expectations of caloric restriction (CR), a dietary regimen based on low calorie intake to decelerate biological ageing. Pharmaceutical interventions like hormone replacement therapy (e.g. melatonin, oestrogen and testosterone) and dietary supplements (vitamins, antioxidants, functional foods) are also used for this purpose. Beyond that, 'transhumanist' visions of radical life extension or even biological immortality focus on methods for slowing, stopping or reversing senescence. They are inspired by biological research targeting the shortening of telomeres, the release of free radicals as a by-product of mitochondrial energy metabolism, and cell processes like apoptosis, and they promote the prospect that regenerative medicine or gene therapies might extend the maximum human lifespan far beyond the limit of 120 years.

Despite the great variety of their aims and methods, all anti-ageing projects and practices seem to have one thing in common: they are primarily directed towards the future. Even a Botox treatment is supposed to bring about longer-lasting effects than mere cosmetics. The future perspective seems obvious where preventive interventions are concerned: dietary regimes, exercises and preventive treatments are intended to decrease health risks and improve chances of staying healthy and fit in later life. (Radical) life extension ultimately promises to expand the future horizon of our whole existence beyond all customary temporal measures. Anti-ageing discourse in general frequently speaks of science and technology in terms of progress and interprets them through their historical development in order to stress the breadth of future possibilities. This also explains the prominence (and concurrent blurring) of traditional categories from the philosophy of history, such as 'conservative' or 'progressive', in this context (Horrobin, 2006; Vincent, 2009).

In this strong orientation towards the future, anti-ageing seems to correspond to a more general trend in domains of biomedicine and life sciences including stem cell research, reproductive medicine and oncology. Indeed, recent developments in all these fields have been described in terms of a general shift away from 'regimes of truth' to 'regimes of hope' (Moreira & Palladino, 2005; Petersen & Wilkinson, 2015). In this regard, the status and legitimacy of science and technology are no longer primarily based on their ultimate authority in the prosaic field of objective factual knowledge, methodologically controlled 'evidence-based' claims, and exact, precisely calculated chances and risks. Instead, they increasingly adopt a future-oriented, emotionally charged discourse of open possibilities, excited anticipation and unlimited hope (Brown, 2005, 2006). It seems as though the very uncertainties and imponderables of the corresponding scientific hypotheses and biomedical strategies in fact make them a perfect screen for the projection of prospective desires, aspirations, and plans (ibid.). In a detailed account, Adams *et al.* highlight five distinctive dimensions of this general development: (a) *injunction* as the moral responsibility to anticipate the future and deal with its uncertainties, (b) *abduction* as a way of deriving plans and strategies for an uncertain future from rather fragmentary empirical knowledge, (c) *optimization* as the interminable task of pursuing and achieving the best possible future results, (d) *preparation* as the readiness to prepare in the present for potential future scenarios and problems, and (e) *possibility* as the central buzzword for raising and bolstering hope through technoscience (2009, pp. 254–259). As many critics have noted, the resulting lofty discourses on future developments and possibilities are not only exceptionally vague and controversial, but also pervaded by tangible political and economic interests creating problematic 'dynamics of expectation' (Brown, 2003) or a whole 'political economy of hope' (Novas, 2006).

There have been approaches to apply this theoretical framework to the anti-ageing discourse and movement as well. Here, too, uncertainties are no longer framed in terms of epistemic insufficiencies, but rather as opening up a boundless space of chances and possibilities for the future. Hypotheses, predictions and future scenarios are formulated and shape present perspectives and decisions, generating the dynamic of 'hype' or self-fulfilling prophecy (Petersen & Seear, 2009; Mykytyn, 2010a, 2010b). To date, however, most relevant empirical studies focus on professional anti-ageing practitioners

(Mykytyn, 2006b; Flatt *et al.*, 2013; Spindler, 2014). By contrast, little is known about how the actual users of anti-ageing products and services perceive the promotion of these regimes of hope or how they deal with their own hopes and uncertainties regarding the future (Watts-Roy, 2009; Pfaller, 2016).

Sample and methods

In order to examine everyday perceptions of the uncertainties of anti-ageing futures and strategies for addressing them, we analysed 20 narrative in-terviews and 12 moderated focus group discussions of eight to ten partic-ipants conducted with users of anti-ageing medicine in Germany (a total of 96 participants).[1] All interviewees and focus group participants were re-cruited through flyers and advertisements in specific online forums, snow-ball sampling and relevant public events. We aimed for a balance of both age and gender while selecting participants and composing focus groups. The final sample had broad socio-demographic variety, thus allowing us to explore lay perspectives on anti-ageing in Germany across a wide range of individual viewpoints, situations, and backgrounds. The participants' ages ranged from 20 to 85 years, with an average of 56 and a median of 61 years. They represented a great diversity of educational, professional, and socio-economic backgrounds from Western, Eastern, Northern, and Southern regions of Germany, rural as well as urban (for more detailed information, see Schweda and Pfaller, 2014).

The interviews and focus groups took place in different German cities (Erlangen, Göttingen, Berlin, Rostock, Nuremberg, Munich and Leipzig) between 2011 and 2012. The interviews were conducted using an interview guide. Two facilitators moderated the focus groups using a semi-structured list of questions on the importance of anti-ageing, anti-ageing practices, and preventive measures, as well as scenarios on the risks and opportunities of life extension. The interviews and group discussions were recorded and transcribed, then pseudonyms were assigned; only indicators of the speakers' gender (Mr/Ms) and age (in parentheses) were retained.

The material was analysed according to qualitative content analysis (Mayring, 2000) using Atlas.ti® scientific software. The coding process was conducted in two steps: an initial basic coding step to identify main the-matic fields was then followed by a step of in-depth coding to structure the material into finer categories. This method made it possible to group indi-vidual statements into a few prevailing rationales, while at the same time interpreting them as 'documentation' of overarching individual orienta-tions (Bohnsack, 2008). In the following section, we describe some of these lines of thought and general orientations towards anti-ageing medicine that users and interested laypersons bring to the fore in dealing with the expert claims accompanying anti-ageing medicine and the future.

Empirical results: Dealing with hope in the practice of anti-ageing

Our study uncovers a wide range of attitudes towards anti-ageing medicine, from total rejection to active and ardent pursuit and advocacy. In total, four major strategies for dealing with the relevant expert claims and imperatives could be identified: The first can be described as *medical optimism*, since it is based on a strong belief in medical science and technologies and their continual advancements. The second one could be labelled *preventive maximalism*, as it tries to cope with the uncertainty of anti-ageing futures by maximizing preventive efforts. A third strategy pursues *ritualized wellbeing*, focusing more on increasing personal wellness than actual medical effects. The fourth strategy is *considered rejection*, questioning the scientific validity of anti-ageing claims or the relevance of the underlying objectives (for a more detailed description, see Schweda and Pfaller, 2014). Here we will take a closer look at the perspectives and arguments subsumed under the first strategy, *medical optimism*. While all the other strategies are concerned with somehow dealing with an essentially uncertain, unpredictable future, this one is more about the production of certainty. As the findings show, users of anti-ageing measures find different bases for hope, but also point to problematic aspects of unreflective scientific optimism.

Generating optimism

One central element in 'optimistic' users' descriptions of anti-ageing medicine was the value and authority of the scientific knowledge upon which the corresponding interventions are supposedly based. The conviction that 'science will guide the way' was often depicted as an integral part of an autonomous, proactive and rational attitude and lifestyle in opposition to obscurantism, fatalism and superstition. Although scientific knowledge and its resulting technologies are not uncritically accepted, they appear more reliable and viable than any other available orientation system:

> For me, the most important thing is that you yourself decide about your own life. I'm not saying that religion and all that is nonsense, but you have to live your own life and take your fate in your own hands. And the tools for that are technology, medicine, and so on. And that's why I trust in that. Of course, they aren't perfect ... but it's the only thing we have!
>
> (Mr I (32), interview)

An important master narrative in this medical optimism was scientific progress. The users were not merely convinced of the validity of the scientific knowledge used as the basis for anti-ageing interventions thus far. They often also interpreted its evolution in terms of progress and thus formulated extremely optimistic assumptions about its further development. In light of this background conception of scientific progress, some of the users virtually considered themselves as representing an avant-garde, like this married couple:

> Ms O (73): Basically, we are always one step ahead of the general public. ... That's the cutting edge, but one day, everybody will get there. And maybe one day, our friends will have to admit...
> Mr O (73): 'You were right all the time. And we were wrong!'

The avant-garde perspective permeates the whole anti-ageing discourse. Its specific appeal to 'optimistic' users is that it couches the narrative of progress in historical terms in order to explain – and indeed turn the tables on – the discrepancy between their personal belief in anti-ageing medicine and the incomprehension of their social circles. They may feel misunderstood and ridiculed by their families and friends right now, but are actually ahead of their time: their current outsider status is merely due to a backward, underdeveloped state of public awareness. As it becomes better known, scientific truth will ultimately prove them right.

The broad historicizing approach is not only necessary to putting the truth of anti-ageing science into perspective, but its practical usefulness as well. Conviction in medical progress makes it easier to envision and interpret the often modest benefits of anti-ageing interventions as evidence of continuous gradual (or even accelerating) advancement. Thus, a male participant explained his fundamental conviction that

> you can definitely buy time when you behave right and take advantage of the whole range of technological, medical possibilities. And if you are really optimistic, you can assume that research will be much more advanced in 20 years.
>
> (Mr I. (32), interview)

This 'abductive' argument (Adams *et al.*, 2009) connects personal biography and general history while at the same time helping to bridge the gap between the rather modest or even dubious effectiveness of currently available anti-ageing interventions and the bold promises of considerable life extensions in the future. Even though present anti-ageing treatments may appear to be unspectacular, it still seems rational to pursue them in order to gain time. This mirrors a common logic found in professional discourse as well: anti-ageing medicine may not bring about one single, ultimate breakthrough, but it can incrementally buy the time needed to develop increasingly effective interventions in the future. Hence, linear or exponential medical progress is presumed to be a necessary precondition for successful anti-ageing careers.

Varieties of evidence

Interestingly, 'optimistic' anti-ageing users' strong reliance on medical science, technology, and progress does not necessarily have to be based on or explicitly refer to actual scientific evidence, e.g. concrete biogerontological research or biomedical studies. In fact, in our interviews and focus groups, this confidence was rather frequently expressed in terms of a general emotional attitude of trust in scientific expertise, technological effectiveness, and their gradual accumulation and refinement. At times, this attitude was even accompanied by a certain sense of mission, an impulse to defend and promote the blessings of anti-ageing medicine:

> I realized how little regular people know about ageing processes and I was shocked! ... Then I started, you could say, educational work.
>
> (Mr N (72), interview)

Not only is the objective scientific persuasiveness of anti-ageing practices brought to bear in this context, but the inscrutable validity of subjective, often bodily, experience as well. This kind of experience can apparently function as a specific kind of evidence in its own right, perhaps comparable to the particular experiential evidence often stressed by proponents of homeopathy and other alternative treatments:

> Well, I have my own approach ... It's simply a branch that's really hard to prove. ... It's kind of a matter of opinion. Well, in my case, I do find evidence. In my opinion, it has nothing to do with beliefs, because it can be proven, seen, noticed, and sensed in every respect.
>
> (Ms A (29), interview)

At times, this personal belief in the effectiveness of anti-ageing medicine is not only expressed in terms of predictive prognoses regarding future effects, but at the same time also actively and almost ritually actualized and reinforced in the performance of tangible anti-ageing practices. More than a simple matter of objective predictions, efficacy must be actively supported and brought about by maintaining an appropriate spirit and suitable attitudes and practices. Thus, the same female speaker explained that

> when I applied lotion to my skin, I always wished it would make the skin particularly beautiful.
>
> (Ms A (29), interview)

This statement expresses a specific sense of 'preparation' (Adams *et al.*, 2009): the activity of rubbing in a particular anti-ageing lotion is ritually linked to the almost incantatory imagination of and longing for an actual improvement of the skin. In this sense, hope appears as a subjective attitude accompanying 'objective' anti-ageing practices, but in fact also acts as an integral ingredient and a necessary precondition for their success. Such interdependency between personal attitude and therapeutic effect is well known from other fields such as oncology and alternative medicine. Hope is invested in anti-ageing, which at the same time also gets reinforced through it, thus developing the dynamic of a self-fulfilling prophecy.

Hope and disappointment

Their strong trust in science and progress notwithstanding, it would be inaccurate to describe 'optimistic' users as naïve believers blindly following anti-ageing promises and marketing strategies. They frequently describe themselves as mature and responsible citizens who have the competence to assess and apply scientific information, thus being on the same level as the experts. Particularly in the interviews, many participants used dialogue with researchers as a kind of platform for presenting themselves as informed and active users of anti-ageing products and services. They usually spontaneously offered arguments and explanations to lend credibility to their stance. But users of anti-ageing products and practices also problematized unconditional belief in medical knowledge and its progress. One common recurrent objection in the discourse was that this kind of 'blind' trust makes you susceptible to commercial exploitation. Thus, one participant explained that medical health programmes on television are often targeted at consumers, and therefore,

> should of course be treated with a degree of caution. First of all, many things are sponsored by the industry. That is, the industry delivers prepared manuscripts for the program, pays a particular sum, and then the stuff will be broadcast. Regardless of whether it is correct or not. And so, watch out!
>
> (Mr T (63), focus group)

Furthermore, personal experience with the failure of preventive strategies based on medical expert knowledge can destroy 'optimists'' basic trust in science and lead to disillusionment and scepticism regarding the value of scientific expertise, thus opening another perspective on anti-ageing. Hence, an older female participant suffering from hypertension recounted:

> I regularly had check-ups and the doctor always said that my cholesterol level is borderline. It is always borderline. And I always said that I eat healthy food and get exercise and so on. I thought that I would really live to be 100 years old this way. Yes, and suddenly one night, my blood

pressure was 230 and I had to be taken to the hospital in an ambulance. And what had happened? The coronary arteries were 80 to 90 per cent blocked.

(Ms U (75), focus group)

Not only are the possible failures of (preventive) anti-ageing medicine brought into the discourse, but also the possible damages it can cause:

Well, you can really damage a lot with it ... especially with medication or other products where the side effects are unknown. I mean, I don't want to shorten my life through medicine.

(Mr J (41), interview)

Against this backdrop, the validity of the claims of prognostic assumptions – and thus the rationality of 'preparation' and 'optimization' (Adams *et al.*, 2009) – can be radically called into question. This does not necessarily turn anti-ageing users into disoriented people adrift in a nebulous field of imponderable uncertainties. But it does mean that other, more personal resources such as rational risk calculation or subjective emotional certainty have to be mobilized to counterbalance scientific uncertainty:

Of course, it is in your hands ... But you never know how much it actually brings about. ... Just to live maybe a year longer. And you never know if it is actually responsible for that one year.

(Ms T (52), focus group)

These findings ultimately allow us to sketch the distinct profile of 'scientific optimism' by contrasting it with the other strategies found in anti-ageing users' statements (Schweda & Pfaller, 2014). One distinctive feature of the 'optimists' is that their perspective on the science and technology behind anti-ageing is embedded in a general attitude of trust and hope towards the future. While others are concerned with managing doubt, they concentrate on generating certainty. Thus proponents of *preventive maximalism* acknowledge that the causes of age-related diseases remain uncertain and the efficacy of preventive interventions may be dubious, but apply the rationale of Pascal's wager to defend the position that it is nevertheless reasonable to employ anti-ageing strategies – just to be on the safe side, in case they might actually turn out to be effective. And proponents of *ritualized wellbeing* completely disconnect anti-ageing's subjective benefits from the objective validity of its claims; for them, the value of anti-ageing is less in its actual medical effects than in a ritualized practice fostering personal wellness. In contrast, the strategies of *scientific optimism* are all about establishing, investing and managing hope. This hope, however, cannot be equated with a naïve or unreflective attitude. It must rather be seen as an active achievement and a deliberate stance supported by a range of considerations, from scientific assessments to historical interpretations of 'progress' to personal experiences (which can also make it susceptible to doubt and disappointment).

Conclusions: Anti-ageing between truth and hope

It has often been noted that the anti-ageing boom is revealing of broader trends and developments in late modern society. In particular, it seems to simultaneously express, shape and change contemporary conceptions of the life course as well as our images of ageing and old age. Thus, from a Foucauldian perspective, anti-ageing medicine has been described as a symptom of the '(bio)medicalization of ageing', subjecting old age to medical jurisdiction and normalization and transforming its normal features into physiological conditions and its anomalies into pathologies to be medically treated and cured (Mykytyn, 2008; Joyce & Loe, 2010). In a similar vein, the anti-ageing boom has also been criticized as representing new forms of governmentality, power and disciplinary control in the neoliberal age, providing technologies of the self that appear all the more subtle and pervasive as they are constitutive of late modern subjectivity, thus acting themselves as forms of *self*-discipline and *self*-control (Katz, 2000; Cardona, 2008).

Another significant aspect of anti-ageing is that it is caught up in the general focal and rhetorical shift towards the future found in contemporary science communication and governance discourses. In light of increased life expectancy, demographic changes and biotechnological innovations, later life seems to have become a vast screen for projecting future scenarios, provisions and plans involving manifold medical options and strategies (for the role of demographic projections, see Messerschmidt in this volume). Consequently, ageing and old age are beginning to lose the appearance of being a natural process and an unalterable fate (Mykytyn, 2006a, 2010a, 2010b). New diagnostic, therapeutic and preventive measures promote the idea of a self-determined ageing process that is to be planned with prudence, foresight and circumspection. These promises of anti-ageing medicine can create uncertainties, provoke disappointment, and lead to an inadequate 'responsibilization of ageing' (Cardona, 2008) – especially when users only have statistically based probabilistic statements of chances and risk, and no causal knowledge of the mechanisms of ageing and disease. The gap between general predictions based on stratified health data and the inevitably individual situation, lifestyle and future of a particular user opens a vast space of problems and insecurity (ibid.).

The findings of our empirical exploration of 'optimistic' anti-ageing users' perspectives and practices in Germany seem to reflect key aspects of these general theoretical discourses. They exhibit many typical features of the general shift from 'regimes of truth' to 'regimes of hope': the general orientation towards the future; the ideal of a self-determined, rational and well-informed agent autonomously mastering later life and old age; the emphasis on anticipating, assessing and preparing for future developments;

the production of optimism by, for instance, interpreting recent scientific developments in terms of progress and extrapolating them into the future; the reference to a range of evidence, from scientific results to personal experience and ritualized re-enforcement (for a current overview: Petersen & Wilkinson, 2014). All in all, our findings indicate that there is no simple binary choice between regimes of truth and regimes of hope in respective users' views on anti-ageing medicine. Rather, both perspectives are intricately intertwined: truth is invested with hope, while hope is backed by truth. In this sense, the truth about ageing is not presented as a given fact; it becomes dependent on our own interpretations, attitudes and behaviours, and thus indeed 'responsibilized' and moralized. It seems as though the 'optimistic' users themselves play a crucial role in making anti-ageing claims come true by translating and re-enacting certain practices in their everyday lives. At the same time, however, we find that the users' statements never simply echo the hopes and hype articulated in prevalent expert discourses. They actually evaluate the epistemological and moral claims of anti-ageing medicine in the logic of everyday life, relativizing its validity in view of their lifestyles and taking account of their personal, biographical, and bodily experiences and orientations. They accept responsibility for their own health and future lives, but also acknowledge epistemic and normative limits to the legitimacy of 'responsibilization'.

Of course, the specific qualitative design of our study and the composition of the sample have certain limitations that need to be taken into account when interpreting these findings. This contribution in particular focuses on an exploration of 'optimistic' users of anti-ageing medicine in Germany. More systematic empirical research is needed in order to draw a richer and more differentiated picture, especially with regard to other types of users and different national contexts. Our considerations nevertheless correspond to recent research on the agency of patients and users vis-à-vis modern biomedicine. Our study thus confirms that the agency of actors is rooted in their ability to resist or negotiate treatment options (Pound et al., 2005; Holt, 2007; Koenig, 2011). In this respect, our findings also indicate that 'optimistic' use of anti-ageing medicine should not be equated with simple unthinking naïveté. It could in fact be that it is 'more about disillusionment with allopathic medicine than it is about controlling bodily ageing' (Watts-Roy, 2009, p. 434). These results help put oversimplified notions of anti-ageing medicine into perspective. By addressing the 'politics of life itself' (Rose, 2001, 2006), anti-ageing not only produces forms of social control and discipline, but at the same time also creates practices of self-fulfilment and self-care. Thus, the actual use of anti-ageing practices and products is not just a consequence of a unidirectional 'colonization of the life world' through modern biomedicine and its irresistible regimes of hope. By the same token, users are not merely passive recipients subjected to the imperatives of individual and socio-political anticipation, preparation and optimization. They also demonstrate their ability to act by questioning the interpretative authority of modern biomedicine, distancing themselves from expert claims and creating alternative criteria and spaces for critical deliberation on truth and hope, although their concrete strategies may fall short of the heroic stances of fervent 'activism' or straightforward 'resistance'. Sociological and ethical analysis should acknowledge the viability and legitimacy of such strategies. This recognition is not tantamount to an uncritical perspective; on the contrary, it can provide the foundation for an improved and better-targeted form of criticism aimed at concrete problems in handling biomedical futures in specific biographical perspectives and socio-cultural settings.

Note

1 The interviews and group discussions took place under the auspices of the research project 'Biomedical Life Plans for Ageing' funded by the German Federal Ministry of Education and Research (Project No. 01GP1004).

References

Adams Vincanne, Murphy Michelle & Adele E. Clarke (2009), 'Anticipation: Technoscience, Life, Affect, Temporality', *Subjectivity*, 28(1), pp. 246–265.

American Academy for Anti-Ageing Medicine (A4M) (2015), *A4M Overview*, www. a4m.com/about-a4m-overview.html, accessed 6 February 2017.

Bohnsack Ralf (2008), *Rekonstruktive Sozialforschung: Einführung in qualitative Methoden*. Opladen, Verlag Barbara Budrich.

Brown Nik (2003), 'Hope Against Hype – Accountability in Biopasts, Presents and Futures', *Science Studies*, 16(2), pp. 3–21.

Brown Nik (2005), 'Shifting Tenses: Reconnecting Regimes of Truth and Hope', *Configurations*, 13(3), pp. 331–355.

Brown Nik (2006), 'Shifting Tenses – from Regimes of Truth to Regimes of Hope', *Shifting Politics – Politics of Technology – The Times they are A-changin'*, Groningen, April, pp. 21–22.

Cardona Beatriz (2008), '"Healthy Ageing" Policies and Anti-ageing Ideologies and Practices: On the Exercise of Responsibility', *Medicine, Health Care and Philosophy*, 11(4), pp. 475–483.

De Grey Aubrey (2004), 'We Will Be Able to Live to 1000', *BBC News* (3 December), http://news.bbc.co.uk/2/hi/uk/4003063.stm, accessed 6 February 2017.

Estes Carroll L. & Elizabeth A. Binney (1989), 'The Biomedicalization of Ageing: Dangers and Dilemmas', *The Gerontologist*, 29(5), pp. 587–596.

Flatt Michael A., Settersten Richard A., Ponsaran Roselle & Jennifer R. Fishman (2013), 'Are "Anti-ageing Medicine" and "Successful Ageing" Two Sides of the Same Coin? Views of Anti-ageing Practitioners', *The Journals of Gerontology Series B: Psychological Sciences and Social Sciences*, 68(6), pp. 944–955.

German Society of Anti-Ageing Medicine (GSAAM) (2015), *GSAAM – Über uns*, www.gsaam.de/gsaam-ueber-uns.html, accessed 6 February 2017.

Holt Martin (2007), 'Agency and Dependency within Treatment: Drug Treatment Clients Negotiating Methadone and Antidepressants', *Social Science & Medicine* 64(9), pp. 1937–1947.

Horrobin Steven (2006), 'Immortality, Human Nature, the Value of Life and the Value of Life Extension', *Bioethics*, 20(6), pp. 279–292.

Joyce Kelly & Meika Loe (2010), 'A Sociological Approach to Ageing, Technology and Health', *Sociology of Health & Illness*, 32(2), pp. 171–180.

Katz Stephen (2000), 'Busy Bodies: Activity, Ageing, and the Management of Everyday Life', *Journal of Ageing Studies*, 14(2), pp. 135–152.

Kaufman Sharon R., Shim Janet K. & Ann J. Russ (2004), 'Revisiting the Biomedicalization of Ageing: Clinical Trends and Ethical Challenges', *The Gerontologist*, 44(6), pp. 731–738.

Klatz Ronald & Robert Goldman (2003), *The New Anti-ageing-revolution. Stopping the Clock for a Younger, Sexier, Happier You.* North Bergen, Basic Health Publications.

Koenig Christopher J. (2011), 'Patient Resistance as Agency in Treatment Decisions', *Social Science & Medicine*, 72(7), pp. 1105–1114.

Mayring Philipp (2000), 'Qualitative Content Analysis', *Forum Qualitative Sozialforschung/Forum: Qualitative Social Research*, 1(2): Art. 20, http://nbn-resolving. de/urn:nbn:de:0114-fqs0002204, accessed 6 February 2017.

Moreira Tiago & Paolo Palladino (2005), 'Between Truth and Hope: On Parkinson's Disease, Neurotransplantation and the Production of the "Self"', *History of the Human Sciences*, 18(3), pp. 55–82.

Mykytyn Courtney Everts (2006a), 'Anti-ageing Medicine: Predictions, Moral Obligations, and Biomedical Intervention', *Anthropological Quarterly*, 79(1), pp. 5–31.

Mykytyn Courtney Everts (2006b), 'Anti-ageing Medicine: A Patient/Practitioner Movement to Redefine Ageing', *Social Science & Medicine*, 62(3), pp. 643–653.

Mykytyn Courtney Everts (2008), 'Medicalizing the Optimal: Anti-ageing Medicine and the Quandary of Intervention', *Journal of Ageing Studies*, 22(4), pp. 313–321.

Mykytyn Courtney Everts (2010a), 'A History of the Future: The Emergence of Contemporary Anti-ageing Medicine', *Sociology of Health & Illness*, 32(2), pp. 181–196.

Mykytyn Courtney Everts (2010b), 'Analyzing Predictions: An Anthropological View of Anti-ageing Futures'. In Fahy Gregory M., West Michael D., Coles L. Stephen & Steven B. Harris (eds.), *The Future of Ageing*. Dordrecht, Heidelberg, London, New York, Springer Netherlands, pp. 23–38.

Novas Carlos (2006), 'The Political Economy of Hope: Patients' Organizations, Science and Biovalue', *BioSocieties*, 1(03), pp. 289–305.

Petersen Alan & Kate Seear (2009), 'In Search of Immortality: The Political Economy of Anti-ageing Medicine', *Medicine Studies*, 1(3), pp. 267–279.

Petersen Alan & Iain Wilkinson (2014), 'The Sociology of Hope in Contexts of Health, Medicine, and Healthcare', *Health*, 19(2), pp. 113–118.

Pfaller Larissa (2016), *Anti-Ageing als Form der Lebensführung*. Wiesbaden, Springer VS.

Post Stephen G. & Robert H. Binstock (eds.) (2004), *The Fountain of Youth. Cultural, Scientific, and Ethical Perspectives on a Biomedical Goal*. Oxford, New York, Oxford University Press.

Pound Pandora, Britten Nicky, Myfanwy Morgan, Yardley Lucy, Pope Catherine, Daker-White Gavin & Rona Campbell (2005), 'Resisting Medicines: A Synthesis of Qualitative Studies of Medicine Taking', *Social Science & Medicine*, 61(1), pp. 133–155.

Rose Nikolas (2001), 'The Politics of Life Itself', *Theory Culture Society*, 18(6), pp. 1–30.

Rose Nikolas (2006), *Politics of Life Itself: Biomedicine, Power and Subjectivity in the Twenty-first Century*. Princeton, Princeton University Press.

Schweda Mark, Herrmann Beate & Georg Marckmann (2011), 'Anti-Ageing-Medizin in der gesetzlichen Krankenversicherung? Sozialrechtliche Entscheidungspraxis und gerechtigkeitsethische Reflexion'. In Maio Giovanni (ed.), *Altwerden ohne alt zu sein. Ethische Grenzen der Anti-Ageing-Medizin*. Freiburg i. Br., Karl Alber, pp. 172–193.

Schweda Mark & Larissa Pfaller (2014), 'Colonization of Later Life? Laypersons' and Users' Agency Regarding Anti-ageing Medicine in Germany', *Social Science & Medicine*, 118, pp. 159–165.

Spindler Mone (2014), *Altern Ja-Aber Gesundes Altern: Die Neubegründung der Anti-Ageing-Medizin in Deutschland*. Wiesbaden, Springer VS.

Stuckelberger Astrid (2008), *Anti-ageing Medicine: Myths and Chances*. Zürich, Hochschulverlag.

Super Nutrition Inc. (2013), *10 Years Younger: Anti-Ageing Vitamins Start Now*. www.super-nutritionusa.com/.

Vincent John A. (2009), 'Ageing, Anti-ageing, and Anti-anti-ageing: Who are the Progressives in the Debate on the Future of Human Biological Ageing?', *Medicine Studies*, 1(3), pp. 197–208.

Vincent John A. (2003), 'What is at Stake in the 'War on Anti-ageing Medicine'?', *Ageing and Society*, 23(5), pp. 675–684.

Watts-Roy Diane M. (2009), 'A Protest Vote? Users of Anti-ageing Medicine Talk Back', *Health Sociology Review*, 18(4), pp. 434–445.

Part II
Defining boundaries, defining insiders and outsiders

4 Nationalism and the moral economy of ageing

Magnus Nilsson

The notion of a 'moral economy of ageing' has been developed as a way to understand the moral precepts that underpin support for the care and welfare of older people in society (Kohli 1991, Svallfors 2008). In gerontology the notion of moral economy has mainly been seen as a function of relations between younger and older members of society, or in other words as an intergenerational contract based on serial reciprocity of the transfer of resources across generations (Minkler & Cole 1992). The notion of a moral economy was partly developed in response to the deficiencies of rational-choice theories, since self-interest alone could not explain the role of norms and morality among motivations for the transfer of resources between groups in a society (Mau 2003). The idea of a moral economy of ageing is based upon a view that normative ideas of reciprocity, justice and obligations influence the way people understand their rights and responsibilities as members of a political community. Additionally, rights and responsibilities concerning public welfare programmes are largely mediated by the notion of deservingness (Collins 1965, Will 1993, Jönson & Nilsson 2007, Slothuus 2007, Crepaz 2008, Petersen *et al.* 2010). Thus, as Sloothus writes, '[c]itizens' willingness to support welfare policies depends to a considerable extent on their perception of the deservingness of welfare recipients' (2007: 327). In line with the moral economy of ageing as a generational contract, the predominant narrative that legitimizes the strong support for welfare and the deservingness of older people in Sweden – as well as in many other countries – is a moral commitment that is justified with reference to prior contributions to society (Anderson 1993, Vincent *et al.* 2001). As van Oorschot writes,

> the neediness of elderly people is rarely doubted, they are seen as a category of people who have delivered their contribution to society, and they are seen as belonging to "us", since they are our parents and grandparents and we ourselves will eventually become pensioners.
>
> (2006: 39 fn 4).

Threats to the moral economy of ageing, and hence to the welfare of older citizens, have mainly been conceived in terms of distrust in public institutions' effectiveness in providing security in old age and the consequences of an ageing population (Moody 2009, Komp & Tilburg 2010, Svallfors 2012). But the risk that has by far gained the greatest interest among scholars is that of generational conflict in discussions about the 'ageing of society' (Higgs & Gilleard 2010).

Even though the moral economy approach is an improvement on rational-choice theories (c.f. Mau 2003, Goerres & Tepe 2010), some aspects need to be problematized so that a fuller understanding of older people's status in the moral economy of the welfare state may emerge. The way in which deservingness is associated with certain social categories or groups depends on how their situation and characteristics are framed. Particular catego-ries are seen as 'deserving' because relations between those categories and society (where relations of obligation and reciprocity are played out) have been actively articulated. Thus, as Will (1993) indicates, deservingness is dependent on the way that claims are embedded in a narrative context, and this holds for older people as well, as we saw in van Oorschot's earlier quote describing older people as 'belonging to "us"'. An analysis of this narrative including older people in a 'we', a political community, is nonetheless largely absent in the literature on support for the welfare of older people and the constitution of the moral economy of ageing. The political community is instead seen as a neutral context. This understanding of the moral economy of ageing neglects the importance of the articulation of political community as well as how it actively contributes to the construction of the category of older people and its relations to other groups, categories and institutions. In this chapter I will discuss and illustrate how conceptions of the welfare of older people are contingent on the articulation of the political commu-nity, and how notions of 'society' and 'the nation' are central to the moral economy of ageing in a setting characterized by competing notions of what constitutes *the* political community.

The chapter is based on a study of how the welfare of older people in Sweden is articulated in relation to the nation-state. Central to the study's analytical strategy is analysis of actors' discourse on the far right of the political spectrum, since they tend to show strong interest in the welfare of older people and use this to problematize what is taken for granted in main-stream public discourse. Data for this analysis comes from a wide range of sources, including news media, official documents, events for older people and social media discussions.

I will start by explaining my position on the notion of political commu-nity, which lays the groundwork for the discussion that follows.

The contested nature of the political community

The concept of political community is central to understanding attitudes towards the welfare state and the moral economy of old age. Paradoxically, the literature on the moral economy of ageing largely takes the definition of a political community and how it is configured for granted, with no further discussion. Even in social science in general, the political community is generally equated with the country, society or State under study, and the members of the political community are assumed to be the citizens of that entity (Calhoun 1999, Elliott & Turner 2012). As Elliott and Turner (2012: ix) write, this is based on an assumption that 'society pre-exists the social practices and social relations it constitutes'. However, in order to understand the relation between older people – both as a social category and empirical referents – and society, a different approach to the concept of political community is needed; an approach that does not see society or the nation as names of a neutral context but as active parts in the constitution of how old age and older people are conceived.

In this chapter I take the position that identities (both collective and individual) and institutions are discursively constituted (Laclau & Mouffe 2001, Torfing 1999). This means that their existence is dependent on iterative practices that rearticulate and stabilize them as entities. This reliance on such rearticulation makes them fragile and ever vulnerable to contestation. A few words on the concept of society from this perspective are in order before tackling the concept of political community. Society is not taken as an objective entity with a positive identity in this analysis. Instead it is 'traversed with antagonism and ... lacks an essence since it is an overdetermined and precarious unity resulting from discursive, articulatory practices' (Norval 2000: 327f). This means that there are competing forces articulating the identity of a society or nation from different perspectives, constructing multiple 'societies' that are partially different and do not always include all State citizens or the entire territory of the nation-state. These various perspectives share some aspects with competing perspectives, and exclude others. Competing perspectives on society also articulate which groups each considers included and part of society: citizens, resident non-citizens, non-resident citizens, only people born in the country, working people, the elite, and so on. Some obvious examples of actors engaged in the struggle to define society include political parties, unions and social movements spanning the nationalist, environmentalist, anti-racist and pensioners movements. Because of this, as Laclau puts it, 'Society does not succeed in constituting itself as an entirely objective order as a result of the presence, within itself, of antagonistic relations' (2014: 111). These antagonisms are not objective relations. Instead they highlight the failures inherent to attempts to constitute society as an objective order. This also means that neither societies nor political communities should be seen 'as empirical referents but as discursive surfaces' instead (Mouffe 1992: 80). The content and meaning of societies and political communities are not empirically given, and instead are always contested and reliant on the active rearticulation of their contents and boundaries. Chantal Mouffe summarizes and further explains the position taken on political community here in this lengthy quote on politics and political community:

> [I]t is necessary to recognize that the *respublica* is the product of a given hegemony, the expression of power relations, and that it can be challenged. Politics is to a great extent about the rules of the *respublica* and their many possible interpretations; it is about the constitution of the political community, not something that takes place inside the political community, as some communitarians would have it. Political life concerns collective, public action; it aims at the construction of a 'we' in a context of diversity and conflict. But to construct a 'we', it must be distinguished from the 'they' and that means establishing a frontier, defining an 'enemy'. Therefore, while politics aims at constructing a political community and creating a unity, a fully inclusive political community and a final unity can never be realized since there will permanently be a 'constitutive outside', an exterior to the community that makes its existence possible. Antagonistic forces will never disappear, and politics is characterized by conflict and division. Forms of agreement can be reached, but they are always partial and provisional since consensus is by necessity based upon acts of exclusion.
>
> (Mouffe 1992: 78)

For the discussion that follows I want to stress Mouffe's position that 'Politics is to a great extent about the rules of the *respublica* and their many possible interpretations; it is about the constitution of the political community', as this is crucial to the discussion to come about how 'older people' appear in public discourse and how the notion of the 'nation-state' or 'society', the taken-for-granted setting, plays an active role in the construction of the moral economy of old age.

Old age and the extreme right

The far right's actions and claims might seem to be entirely unrelated to old age and ageing in Europe – but the activities of the extreme right and radical right political parties, the recent growth of anti-Muslim sentiments across Europe (Boswell & Geddes 2011) and the 'pathological normalcy' of nativism of European societies (Mudde 2010) are highly relevant to the understanding of the moral economy of ageing. The discourses of these groups do not articulate 'society' and 'the nation' according to State borders, but rather along the lines of a political community that is in an antagonistic relationship with what it perceives as an 'external' threat – and older people are often given a prominent role in the rhetoric.

In the 2010 Swedish parliamentary election, the radical right Sweden Democrats party got 5.7 per cent of the vote. This meant that for the first time in the history of the Swedish parliament, it came to include a party whose sole purpose was anti-immigrant rhetoric. The party was formed in the 1980s by activists in the neo-Nazi movement (Ekman & Poohl 2010). Over the last two decades, the party has officially disavowed its links to Nazism and racism (Ekman & Poohl 2010, Baas 2015). Members and elected representatives of the party are regularly caught making racist claims, however, and party rhetoric has to a great extent been focused on Islam as a threat to the nation; the party leader declared Islam to be the biggest threat to Sweden since the Second World War in an opinion piece in one of the biggest newspapers in Sweden (Åkesson 2009). At both the national and local political levels the Sweden Democrats focus mainly on immigration. But when members hold representative positions at the municipal level, which has no jurisdiction over migration issues, they have been very involved in elder care issues (Quensel & Poohl 2011). The welfare of older people also rose to greater prominence during the 2014 national parliamentary election, which ended with the Sweden Democrats becoming the third largest party in parliament with 12.86 per cent of the vote.

In the run-up to the 2010 election, the party produced a television advertisement to promote its message. Significantly, this was the party's only campaign advertisement for television. It starts with two government officials sitting at desks counting the State budget, sorting out money for pensions and immigration. A voiceover says: 'Politics is about making priorities.' The screen flashes and the voice says, 'Now you have a choice.' Simultaneously two emergency brake handles drop down and hang in the near-darkness, one labelled 'pensions' and the other 'immigration' (they allude to the 'brake' in the Swedish pension system that reduces payments when contributions fall). The screen cuts to the squeaking wheel of a walker moving slowly towards the officials' desks. Out of the darkness an older white woman appears, trying to hurry but slow with her walker. She looks over her shoulder and the viewer sees what she sees behind her: a group of burka-clad Muslim women with prams. One cannot see how many there are, just that they are many, and quick. They rush past the elderly white woman with her walker. The camera again cuts to the dangling emergency brake handles and the voice says: 'On the 19th of September you can choose an immigration brake instead of a brake on pensions.' Several hands reach up to pull the brake labelled 'pensions' but just one hand reaches for the 'immigration' brake. The single hand reaching for the brake on immigration represents the Sweden Democrats and the hands reaching for the brake on pensions represents the other parties in parliament. The voiceover says, 'Vote for the Sweden Democrats', and the advertisement ends with a screen showing the name of the party behind the film (the Sweden Democrats) and the party slogan, 'security and tradition'. This is just one example of how older people are used in the far right's political claims, but it is an illustrative one, since the conflict staged in the advertisement is the one the Sweden Democrats chose to represent themselves and their message.

Nationalism is usually seen as being organized around three interrelated logics (Calhoun 1999, Özkirimli 2010). First of all, nationalism has the world consisting of homogeneous and fixed identities such as Swedes, Italians and so on. Second, it articulates a possessive relationship with a certain territory, real or imaginary. The third connects directly to the presence of the white older woman in the Sweden Democrats' campaign ad and the radical right's claims in general. Nationalist rhetoric articulates a national unity over time, a temporal lineage from the past, through the present and, by way of extrapolation, into the future, to conjure the diachronic existence of the nation. The older white woman in the advert serves two functions in its narrative that complement and enhance each other. Her presence is metaphorical, folding one narrative into another and making them indistinguishable. For one thing, the older white woman simply represents older people, an image that comes with conceptions of frailty and an inability to fend for oneself. As such she needs representation and someone to speak for her. But she also represents the history of the nation, the history of the Swedish welfare state as well as the future of its citizens. She is a metaphorical signifier for Sweden, or rather a political community based on ethnicity and nationality. She is a signifier for 'the people', a representative of the 'true' community. Through her whiteness, which contrasts with the faceless Muslim women in black burkas, she represents the Swedish people; those who have been outrun and fooled, whose welfare is threatened. This intertwining of older people and the nation is also shown in the comments to the video on www. youtube.com, as in this comment.

> I agree completely that Sweden is not the same country it once was. There are too many who don't understand Swedish traditions and think that the national anthem and the flag are about racism. Completely wrong. If immigrants are going to move to Sweden, they shall at least understand and appreciate our country, speak our language and understand that Sweden is the country that the old have built, for themselves and their children and so on. I thank the Swedish people for everything.

Continuing on the theme of depicting the welfare of older people as threatened by immigration and immigrants, there are other examples of such rhetoric. The following examples are taken from the Swedish Internet forum 'www.flashback.org', with the stated aim of providing a platform for 'real' freedom of speech. It is a forum where no topic or standpoint is moderated. Topics range from child pornography to philosophy, and racism is frequent. A search on the topic of elder care does not yield many hits, not being a main concern for forum regulars, but there are a few threads dealing with the topic. The comments below come from two different threads, and the vast majority of the comments contain racist or anti-immigrant remarks. The first example is taken from a thread started in 2009 with seven contributions (www.flashback.org/t1007421) and the second from a thread started in 2014 that contains 97 contributions (www.flashback.org/t2430340). The examples show how the antagonism between the rights and welfare of older people and immigration is expressed in the forum.

> I see a conflict of goals in the future between the enormous brown enculturation armies that live off of benefits and the increasing number of Swedish pensioners' pensions and expenses. In the choice between which group to favour, the ethnically Swedish pensioners loose in 100 cases out of 100. This because the realpolitik calculation between people who are dead within a few years and people with a propensity for race riots will always favour the violent elements. (20 September 2009)

> Welcome to the new Sweden, where we cannot afford our old and sick anymore, but spend all our money on well-off refugees from MENA [The Middle East and Northern Africa]. Anyone who wants an easy career should train as an Arabic legal interpreter as soon as possible, because there will be a shortage of them in the future when criminality soars. (20 August 2014)

> Is there anyone who thinks that a record mass immigration will lead to a better life for our elderly, or an even worse situation? Oh my God and fucking shit, what a disgusting country we've become. Our pensioners' grandchildren have now been indoctrinated to starve their grandparents so that more Mahmouds and Alis will be able to rape, kill and drain our tax money. Has there ever been a more easily manipulated, self-hating and spineless people in world history? (20 August 2014)

If one were to look only at what is written in the forum, one might easily conclude that these quotes express extreme views far from public discourse. But read alongside the way that the Sweden Democrats handle these issues (exemplified by the election film), it becomes clear that there are more similarities than differences, not the least in the expression of a political community built on nativism. To this equation we should additionally emphasize that forum contributors are not primarily interested in the welfare of older people; instead 'older people' is used as a signifier for Sweden and ethnic Swedes, and the presumed plight of older people is used to articulate an antagonistic relationship with immigrants (especially Muslims), as we saw in the previously discussed campaign advertisement. In this discourse, the antagonism and its disruptive effects on the moral economy become especially clear when looking at what is written about older immigrants. The signifier 'older people' is reserved for ethnically Swedish people, because in this imaginary, immigrants have not aged, worked, paid taxes or contributed to society, and should accordingly not be allowed to receive welfare.

The Sweden Democrats are not the only party in Europe with an anti-immigrant or racist agenda that have used old age and the welfare of older people in their rhetoric and claims. Right-wing extremist and populist parties across Europe have tried, and with some success, to establish an associative link between migration policies and policies for the elderly. This is exemplified by the British National Front slogan used some years ago: 'Pensioners before asylum seekers'. In Germany the national socialist Nationaldemokratische Partei Deutschlands (National Democratic Party) used the slogan 'Money for grandma instead of Sinti and Roma' in the 2013 elections. Images of older people were also prominent on campaign posters of the Italian Lega Nord party and the French Front National, to name but a few examples. Such use of older people in radical political rhetoric is hardly a new phenomenon, but it has transformed over time.

The way that extreme right parties across Europe use older people in their appeals in itself problematizes the narrow focus on intergenerational relations and serial reciprocity across generations as the basis for the moral economy of ageing, because their framing articulates a nativist logic as the basis for welfare, belonging and deservingness.

Because these anti-immigrant movements highlight and exploit a conception of older people as being 'ours' and thus a national responsibility, there is a need for further exploration and theorization of the ways that older people are signified in relation to conceptions of society. One reason for the far right's interest in the welfare of older people is, of course, related to the general interest for the welfare of older people. As noted earlier, most people think that the welfare of older people is an important issue (van Oorschot 2006). This simple observation is, however, inadequate for understanding specifically how these groups construct older people as a category, not to mention that category's role in their own discursive universe and, perhaps more importantly, how it is communicated and part of broader ways of articulating the moral economy of ageing. This raises the following questions: How did the possibility of using 'older people' emerge as a rhetorical tool for claims from the extreme right? What, if any, is the relationship between the general discussion of the welfare of older people and its presence in nationalist and racist discourses? And in relation to this chapter's focus, how are the moral economy of ageing and its nationalist articulations related? To understand the uses made of older people in radical right discourse, we need to understand whether and in what ways nationalism is present in more general discussions about older people, particularly in mainstream public discourse.

The banal nationalism of the moral economy

A 2012 opinion piece signed by the Swedish prime minister and three other leading politicians stated: 'Strengthening the position and conditions of our elderly, financially and in society at large, is and remains a central priority of the government' Reinfeldt *et al.* 2012). How should this sentence be understood, and what does 'our elderly' mean here? Is the government stating that they have 'their own' older people whose position they aim to strengthen? What society are they writing about? That we already know the answers to these questions without even thinking about them is highly relevant to the moral economy of ageing. The referenced society is, of course, Sweden, and it is the Swedish government that writes about older people in Sweden. We are so accustomed to the nation-state as *the* context that the answers to these questions appear to be both self-evident and devoid of meaning.

Nationalism has largely come to be associated with the more blatant and extreme expressions of national belonging and conceptions of what constitutes the nation as a political community, as shown by the examples in the previous section (Billig 1995). The Sweden Democrats, the Front National and the British National Party are typical examples of this. Likewise the objective existence of nations and nation-states has been taken for granted. As Michael Skey notes, nations and nation-states are often seen as concrete entities 'linked to a particular territory, language, diet, dress and fixed set of values or dispositions shared by all nationals' (2011: 5). On the other hand, some contend that globalization has led the nation-state to lose its integrity and weaken its grip. In fact, nationalism as a force shaping societies and social relations has never been evenly distributed within or among societies (Calhoun 1999, Sörlin *et al.* 2006). And Neugarten and Hagestad's statement (1976) about changing age relations in society is also true at a more general level – the direction of the future is never solely dictated by a single tendency in the present. Nationalism and the way it contributes to constituting 'the people' as a political community and forging mind-sets have never disappeared, as they permeate everyday life (Anderson 1991, Billig 1995, Skey 2011). However, as a substantial amount of research over recent decades has shown, the notion of the nation and nationalism has a profound role in structuring relations and a sense of community among people and is not at all limited to the more overt and extreme forms of nationalism. These studies challenge the taken-for-granted aspect of the nation 'by emphasizing the multiple, often conflicting, ways of talking about the same nation, the arbitrariness of national symbols, the shifting allegiances within and between so-called national groups, and the varying success of nationalist projects' (Billig 1995: 6). Although this view of the nation as overdetermined (and in some ways indeterminate) has gained hold in research, even critics of the traditional view of the nation claim that nationalism, as a sedimented and highly institutionalized discourse, organizes reality in both symbolic and material ways (Özkirimli 2010) and permeates everyday life (Billig 1995). Michael Billig uses the concept of 'banal nationalism' to describe nationalism that functions as a naturalized 'common sense' and 'the ideological habits which enable the established nations of the West to be reproduced' (ibid.: 6), as in the quote above.

The discourse of banal nationalism and the presupposition of the nation-state are present in both gerontology and general public discourse about older people's welfare rights. It is found, in the narrative of the deservingness of older people, for instance, in connection to the stance that they have paid for pensions and other benefits in advance by having worked and paid taxes (cf. Collins 1965, Mau 2003, van Oorschot 2006, Nilsson 2008, Svallfors 2008) or having defended the country in time of war (cf. Skey 2011), as this example from a British study highlights:

> Shunning the identity of the 'deserving poor' – suitable cases for charity – older people prefer to be seen as common members of a national community who expect a pension on retirement and care in old age by virtue of having shouldered the duties of citizenship.
>
> (Vincent *et al.* 2001: 128)

This articulation of citizenship holds that merit is contingent on obligations going back for generations and associated with a contract between citizens, the nation and the state. Among the seniors that Vincent, Patterson and Wale interviewed, poverty among older people was found to be particularly upsetting: 'The idea that people who fought in the war and paid contributions all their lives are now forced to live in poverty was abhorrent to most of the older people we interviewed' (2001: 108). The authors furthermore argue that every political party in Britain has used images of older people as deserving poor in political claims-making, and this also holds in a historical perspective (cf Collins 1965). In Sweden, Jönson (2001) has shown that ever since the 1940s, the logic of deservingness-through-contribution has been central to welfare claims and the actions of pensioners' organizations through the articulation of older people as equal citizens. This idea of merit-based deservingness has explicitly and implicitly been an essential part of the moral economy of old age policy. It has been used to defend care and welfare arrangements, it has framed welfare as redistribution between generations over time and provided a collective identity for older people, and it has also associated older people with the notion of a national community responsible for its older citizens (Jönson & Nilsson 2007, Nilsson 2008).

One way that older people are articulated as both members of the political community and its responsibility in Sweden is through the expression 'our elderly'. In a previous study of the representation of older people in public discourse, I found this expression to be representative of how the relationship between society and older people is articulated (Nilsson 2008). The expression 'our elderly' is mainly used in politically charged texts in the mass media, especially those that criticize how older people are treated as a way of emphasizing the responsibility of the political community. The expression also occurs in texts by representatives of the political establishment as well as non-political texts, although much less frequently. The following example from an opinion piece published in a leading Swedish newspaper provides a good introduction to the national imaginary that the expression 'our elderly' is part of. It very clearly shows how the expression connects older people to notions of national community and national responsibility. The opinion piece deals with the over-prescription of medications to older people, something that does not initially seem related to the nation and nationalism. The main message is that too many medications are given with too little control and knowledge about the effects on 'our elderly' and 'our old [*people*]'. The expressions 'our elderly' and 'our old [*people*]' are used seven times in the article. Here are three examples.

> Despite our desire that our old [people] should have a good life in the autumn of life, be free from the aches and pains that often come with advanced age, something has gone wrong.

> Both research and education are needed on this, but above all greater care in the prescription of drugs to our elderly.

> Stuffing our elderly with loads of pills cannot be the solution to all problems.
>
> (Hedberg & Silvber 2004)

The text very clearly states 'our' responsibility for 'our elderly'. Use of the expression 'our elderly' addresses a 'we', a political community, and that 'we' is ascribed agency. The topic it addresses, the over-prescription of medications, is quite relevant to older people, but instead of being spoken to they are talked about. In the text, 'older people' is a category articulated as the object of the addressed community's care. The opinion piece is written in everyday language instead of the medical terminology that could have been used to present a study of prescription practices. With expressions like 'autumn of life', 'gone wrong', and 'loads of pills', medical experts are not the only ones whose responsibility is evoked and who are addressed as being responsible. Use of this type of language is also an invocation of the nation as a community and its moral responsibility for 'its elderly'. This responsibility is about more than just how medications are to be prescribed and controlled, as this is something allowed only to medical doctors. The text instead addresses the public, an imagined community of non-old Swedes. It emphasizes the responsibility of the community by collapsing the distinction between the medical responsibility of experts and the moral responsibility of the public: this is the function of the expression 'our elderly'.

The above examples of how 'our elderly' is used in articulating the political community and its responsibilities are mundane and in no way remarkable. Instead, the common-sensical function of the nation as *the* context reveals its structuring capacity. The next example of 'our elderly' use is more straightforward in how it relies on a notion of the nation as a political community with a moral responsibility. This quote is also from an opinion piece written by a member of the Green Party who is employed in elder care. The piece voices criticism of the working conditions in elder care and argues that older people as well as the staff and their families suffer from them. It should also be added that the Green Party is not associated with any overt forms of nationalism.

> Sweden is a country where we have promised to take care of each other when we need each other. It is a kind of generational contract. The people that are being cared for in elder care are the people that have built

Sweden and given us the opportunities that we have in life. They have the right to be greeted by a staff that is happy with its job. And those that take care of yesterday's heroes when frailty sets in should be seen as the heroes of today.

We owe this to our elderly. We owe this to everyone that is employed in care services.

(Hell 2013)

This example is exceptional in its very explicit invocation of the nation and national responsibility for its population of older people, something that is rarely seen in general public discourse in Sweden. This quote makes explicit what is implied in the previous examples, which only alluded to it: Sweden is a political community with a moral responsibility for the welfare of its citizens. In all these examples 'our elderly', the category 'older people' comes to signify a conception of the national and societal community, a nation-state where 'our elderly' are made into an object of national responsibility, at the same time as the category 'older people' becomes associated with being Swedish. The category's objectification also deprives it of agency, which in turn creates a need for a community of the non-old to represent older people, a relation I call *including-othering* (Nilsson 2008). The community is implicitly and explicitly evoked by the floating signifiers 'society' and 'nation', and the state is articulated as the supposed instrument of this community. The expression 'our elderly' thus derives its potency from its ability to endow the welfare of older people with great legitimacy and to articulate this as a public responsibility in two ways, as both a moral responsibility of the community of citizens and a financial and organizational responsibility of national authorities. This echoes findings on the normalized and mundane nationalism of other welfare states, where the State (in this case Sweden) is attributed a particular set of moral responsibilities for its citizens (cf. Hall 1998).

The preceding examples should not be seen as special cases. Several studies have noted that the meanings attributed to old age and older people are closely connected to notions of Swedishness (Lundgren 2000, Hyltén-Cavallius 2005, Nilsson 2008). Another, inverted, aspect of this has been demonstrated by Ronström (1996) and Torres (2006), who found that the category 'older immigrants' was articulated as defined by difference from a taken for granted Swedishness, which also functioned as the basis for State welfare interventions.

Discussion: Nationalism as an unexpected guest in the moral economy of ageing

The conception of intergenerational relations as being characterized by both solidarity and the potential for conflict is a key component of the moral economy of ageing. At the core of the moral economy of ageing is the notion that older people deserve welfare because they 'have delivered their contribution to society, and they are seen as belonging to "us", since they are our parents and grandparents and we ourselves will eventually become pensioners' (van Oorschot 2006: 39 fn4) – or, as Vincent, Patterson and Wale (2001: 128) write, 'by virtue of having shouldered the duties of citizenship'. What becomes clear when looking at these tropes positioning older people as esteemed veterans of society and citizens who have done their duty and are now in a position to be repaid for their society-building efforts is that inter-generational relations, despite being central, are just one of many aspects of the moral economy of ageing.

Signifiers of political community such as 'the nation' and 'society' should not be seen as given entities or empirical referents, but instead as overde-termined discursive signifiers that are used in order to stabilize the social (Mouffe 1992). As Ernesto Laclau writes, the imagined community of the nation is 'an always receding horizon' (Laclau 2003: 24) rife with antagonistic relations that pose as a ground, obscuring its active role in what it articu-lates. For that reason 'society', as the site where age relations play out, is not neutral ground, but is instead always complicit in the articulation of what older people are and how they are understood in relation to 'society'. This means that there is often a surplus of meaning in the form of a simultane-ous articulation of the community, its constitution, and its responsibilities when old age and older people are being discussed. Established discourses relating to the concept of the moral economy of ageing are attempts to artic-ulate specific depictions of 'the people' and a delineated political commu-nity, some more benign than others. Because the category 'older people' has been established as a national responsibility in common speech through the banal nationalism of public discourse, and older people's right to welfare is justified by their having built society, being 'ours' and 'yesterday's heroes', the category is also a potential rhetorical tool in the radical right's political claims. This was shown in the examples of the far right's uses of older people in claims-making, how the category is used to articulate antagonism between those said to belong to the community and those who do not but are thought to be unfairly favoured, as well as in the failure of the political community to become a harmonious whole. This was notably shown by the Sweden Democrats' campaign advertisement staging a conflict between the welfare of older people and continued immigration, by Muslims in particular. The articulation of older people's rights in society is thus also a way of constituting the community as such.

For this reason, I argue that we should not merely understand the category 'older people' as a signifier representing a specific age group in society, as an empirical category. Instead, the way that older people surface in both far-right discourse and the banal nationalism of established and 'non-nationalist' actors shows the constitutively metaphorical and metonymical character of the signifier 'older people'. This ability to signify something other than itself, and in so doing also represent the fullness (or rather the absent fullness) of the community, is characteristic of an ideological signifier (Laclau 1996). The category 'older people' must therefore be understood as having the ability to simultaneously refer to a certain group in society as well as signifying the community as such. This is the terrain of the moral economy of ageing.

References

Åkesson Jimmie (2009), 'Muslimerna är vårt största utländska hot', *Aftonbladet* (10 September).

Anderson Benedict (1991), *Imagined communities*. Revised edition, London and New York, Verso books.

Anderson Bo (1993), 'Distributing social goods between generations', *Social Justice Research*, 6.4, pp. 343–355.

Baas David (2015), *Bevara Sverige svenskt: ett reportage om Sverigedemokraterna.* Stockholm: Månpocket.

Billig Michael (1995), *Banal nationalism*. Los Angeles, Sage Publications.

Boswell Christina & Andrew Geddes (2010), *Migration and mobility in the European Union*, Basingstoke, Palgrave Macmillan.

Calhoun Craig (1999), 'Nationalism, political community and the representation of society or, why feeling at home is not a substitute for public space', *European journal of social theory*, 2.2, pp. 217–231.

Collins Doreen V. (1965), 'The introduction of old age pensions in Great Britain', *The Historical Journal*, 8.2, pp. 246–259.

Crepaz Markus M.L. (2008), *Trust beyond borders: Immigration, the welfare state, and identity in modern societies.* Ann Arbor, University of Michigan Press.

Ekman Mikael & Daniel Poohl (2010), *Ut ur skuggan: en kritisk granskning av Sverigedemokraterna.* Stockholm, Natur & kultur.

Elliott Anthony & Bryan S. Turner (2012), *On society.* Cambridge, Polity Press.

Goerres Achim & Markus Tepe (2010), 'Age-based self-interest, intergenerational solidarity and the welfare state: A comparative analysis of older people's attitudes towards public childcare in 12 OECD countries', *European Journal of Political Research*, 49.6, pp. 818–851.

Hall Patrik (1998), *The social construction of nationalism: Sweden as an example.* Lund, Lund University.

Hedberg Lars & Joa Silvber (2004) 'Äldre blir fullproppade med läkemedel'. Ny larmrapport: 25 olika mediciner per dag vanlig dos inom äldrevården. Fyra av tio får antidepressiva medel, *Dagens Nyheter* (6 September).

Hell Kristoffer (2013), Delade turer gör omsorgen sämre, *Aftonbladet* (6 July).

Higgs Paul & Chris Gilleard (2010), 'Generational conflict, consumption and the ageing welfare state in the United Kingdom', *Ageing and Society*, 30.8, pp. 1439–1451.

Jönson, Håkan (2001), *Det moderna åldrandet. Pensionärsorganisationernas bilder av åldrandet 1941–1995.* Lund, School of Social Work, Lund University.

Jönson Håkan & Magnus Nilsson (2007), 'Are old people merited veterans of society? Some notes on a problematic claim', *Outlines. Critical Practice Studies*, 9.2, pp. 28–43.

Kohli Martin (1991), 'Retirement and the moral economy: An historical interpretation of the German case'. In Minkler Meredith & Caroll L. Estes (eds.), *Critical perspectives on aging: The political and moral economy of growing old.* New York, Baywood Publishing.

Komp Kathrin & Theo Van Tilburg (2010), 'Ageing societies and the welfare state: where the inter-generational contract is not breached', *International Journal of Ageing and Later Life*, 5.1, pp. 7–11.

Laclau Ernesto (1996), 'The death and resurrection of the theory of ideology', *Journal of Political Ideologies*, 1.3, pp. 201–220.

Laclau Ernesto (2003), 'On imagined communities'. In Cheah Pheng and Jonathan Culler (eds.), *Grounds of comparison: Around the work of Benedict Anderson*. London and New York, Routledge.

Laclau Ernesto (2014), *The rhetorical foundations of society*. London, Verso Books.

Laclau Ernesto & Chantal Mouffe (2001), *Hegemony and socialist strategy: Towards a radical democratic politics*. London, Verso Books.

Lundgren Eva (2000), 'Homelike housing for elderly people? Materialized ideology', *Housing, Theory and Society*, 17.3, pp. 109–120.

Mau Stephen (2003), *The moral economy of welfare states. Britain and Germany compared*. London and New York, Routledge.

Minkler Meredith & Thomas R. Cole (1992), 'The political and moral economy of aging: not such strange bedfellows', *International Journal of Health Services*, 22.1, pp. 113–124.

Moody Harry (2009), 'The moral economy of retirement', *Generations*, 33.3, pp. 27–33.

Mouffe Chantal (1992), 'Democratic citizenship and the political community'. In Mouffe Chantal (ed.), *Dimensions of radical democracy: Pluralism, citizenship, community*, London & New York, Verso, pp. 225–239.

Mudde Cas (2010), 'The populist radical right: A pathological normalcy', *West European Politics*, 33.6, pp. 1167–1186.

Neugarten Bernice & Gunhild O. Hagestad (1976), 'Age and the life course'. In Binstock Robert H. & Etheland Shanas (eds.), *Handbook of aging and the social sciences*. New York, Van Nostrand Reinhold, pp. 35–61.

Nilsson Magnus (2008), *Våra äldre. Om konstruktioner av äldre i offentligheten*. [Our elderly. On the social construction of older people in public discourse.] Diss. Linköping Studies in Arts and Science nr. 450, Linköping, Linköping University.

Norval Aletta J. (2000), 'Review article: The things we do with words – Contemporary approaches to the analysis of ideology', *British Journal of Political Science*, 30.02, pp. 313–346.

Özkirimli Umut (2010), *Theories of nationalism: A critical introduction*. Basingstoke, Palgrave Macmillan.

Petersen Michael Bang, Slothuus Rune, Stubager Rune & Lise Togeby (2011), 'Deservingness versus values in public opinion on welfare: The automaticity of the deservingness heuristic', *European Journal of Political Research*, 50.1, pp. 24–52.

Quensel A.-S. & Daniel Poohl (2011), *Sverigedemokraterna i kommunerna. En sammanställning av partiets motioner 1991–2011*. Fokusrapport 2011:2, Stockholm, Exporesearch.

Reinfeldt Fredrik, Jan Björklund, Annie Lööf & Göran Hägglund (2012), 'Pensionärernas skatt sänks med en femtilapp per månad', *Dagens Nyheter* (17 September).

Ronström, Ove (1996), Äldre invandrare - från teori till praktik. In Ove Ronström (ed.), *Vem ska ta hand om de gamla invandrarna? Äldre invandrare i Stockholm*. FoU-rapport 1996:3, Stockholm, Stockholm stads socialtjänst.

Skey Michael (2011), *National belonging and everyday life*. Basingstoke, Palgrave Macmillan.

Slothuus Rune (2007), 'Framing deservingness to win support for welfare state retrenchment', *Scandinavian Political Studies*, 30.3, pp. 323–344.

Sörlin Sverker, Hettne Björn & Uffe Östergård (2006), '*Den globala nationalismen: Nationalstatens historia och framtid*'. Stockholm, SNS förlag.

Svallfors, Stefan (2008), 'The generational contract in Sweden: Age-specific attitudes to age-related policies', *Policy & Politics*, 36.3, pp. 381–396.

Svallfors Stefan (2012), 'Welfare states and welfare attitudes'. In Svallfors Stefan (ed.), *Studies in social inequality: Contested welfare states. Welfare attitudes in Europe and Beyond*. Stanford, Stanford University Press.

Torfing, Jacob (1999), *New Theories of Discourse: Laclau, Mouffe and Žižek*. Oxford, Blackwell Publishers.

Torres, Sandra (2006), 'Elderly immigrants in Sweden: "Otherness" under construction', *Journal of Ethnic and Migration Studies*, 32.8, pp. 1341–1358.

Van Oorschot Wim (2006), 'Making the difference in social Europe: Deservingness perceptions among citizens of European welfare states', *Journal of European Social Policy* 16.1, pp. 23–42.

Vincent John A., Guy Patterson & Karen Wale (2001), *Politics and old age: Older citizens and political processes in Britain*. Aldershot, Ashgate.

Will Jeffry A. (1993), 'The dimensions of poverty: Public perceptions of the deserving poor', *Social Science Research*, 22.3, pp. 312–332.

5   Sexual assistance, suicide assistance and the condition of dependent older adults

Alexandre Lambelet

> *Daniel, 74 years old, has been visiting a prostitute in the neighbourhood of Pâquis [in Geneva] at least once a month for twenty-five years. His admission to the nursing home in December changed nothing ... . He says that he feels freer with age. His relations with prostitutes often follow the same scenario. 'First, I take care of her. Then, she takes care of me.' A recent prostate operation has made erections and penetration more difficult but does not affect the desire he experiences when he sees 'generous breasts' and 'beautiful butts'. Preferably young: 'I couldn't with a woman of my age'.*[1]

Thus begins an article entitled 'L'amour jusqu'à la mort' (Love until Death), in the leading Swiss newspaper *Le Temps*.[2] It observes that despite being 'long buried in silence, the sexuality of older adults has an increasing place in nursing homes wanting to allow their residents "personal fulfilment"', and questions the responses institutions give to the sexual demands of dependent older adults in institutional settings. Following this hook of an older adult visiting prostitutes in Geneva's Pâquis neighbourhood, the article goes on to explore the development of the occupation of 'sexual assistant'[3] and recourse to them in various institutions to conclude on a third issue, that of the fulfilment and freedom of dependent older adults' lives. The article does not explore sexual assistance as a practice, but rather as a symptom of an older adult need to which society does not yet know how to respond. Rather than being concerned with sexual assistance's proximity to the practice of prostitution, it addresses the sexual drive (and/or suffering) of these dependent older adults who have lost none of their desire despite their advancing age.

Likewise, the media does not re-examine suicide when discussing assisted suicide.[4] While researchers specialized in suicide (such as Spoerri *et al.*, 2010) and the Swiss federal authorities (Conseil Fédéral, 2011) classify assisted suicide for dependent older adults as a form of suicide and raise questions about it in such terms, media discussion of the subject is very different. The media may not discuss suicide when debating assisted suicide, but it does constantly question the freedom of older adults (or the generally vulnerable, such as those with a dependency) to make their own life choices. In both cases, it is not about suicide or sexuality, assistance or its providers. The issue is old age and growing old perceived in terms of vulnerability and dependency.

This chapter is not concerned with debating the (in)validity of sexual assistance or suicide or passing moral judgement on them. Instead, we examine the construction of these two social issues through the 'frames' (Snow *et al.*, 1986) used in the media. Studying media discourse on these issues reveals how the media portrays and frames later life in the wider context of an ageist society (Davidson, 2012; Ylänne, 2015). Discussing frames requires reconsideration of how participants understand or describe the situations or activities in which they participate. More particularly, the media focus is on how the variety of people involved attempt to impose a cognitive frame in order to come to terms with a social issue, with the knowledge that this frame can affect participants' and observers' understanding of the issue according to how it has been formulated.

We will see that the issues of assisted suicide and sexual assistance both seem to share a paradox that Grignon and Passeron identified almost 30 years ago with respect to the working classes (1989). Namely, when working with groups considered 'dominated' or 'vulnerable', it is difficult to get past the simplistic dichotomy of miserabilism (only seeing the group in reference to the 'dominant' group, thus in terms of their privations) and populism (glorifying this 'dominated' and 'vulnerable' group's ways of being and doing things, while ignoring the domination). In other words, the difficulty in studying certain groups is to avoid conceiving of them as dominated, members of a 'subculture', or even 'heroic victims' (Higgins, 2003). Rowntree and Zufferey (2015) have shown that the recognition of the sexuality of older adults can lead to two types of response, one in terms of 'needs' and the other in terms of 'rights'. This chapter proposes going further; it is less interested in how the elder-care sector acknowledges older adults' hopes for sexual expression or their wish to die than in seeing how assisted suicide and sexual assistance, as specific practices, shed a different light on media-disseminated frames of the rights and needs of dependent older adults.

This chapter, based on analysis of ten TV programmes and articles on sexual assistance and suicide in French-speaking Switzerland published between 2008 and 2015 (see next section for details), reveals that the discussions around these two types of assistance lead to the development of specific rights for concerned populations, rights of a more moral than social order. And while these rights do not explicitly contravene the rights accorded to the population at large (neither prostitution nor suicide are crimes in Switzerland), the fact that sexual and suicide assistance are regarded as rewarding for dependent older adults still shows that they are considered differently than the general population. In other words, discourse about the free choice to die, like that about sexual assistance, is quickly coloured by both populist and miserabilist visions of dependency, placing dependent older adults in a different order than the general population and making old age into a specific subject, clearly demarcated, differentiating old age from other ages of life.

Materials and methods

This chapter is based on a collection of newspaper articles and television reports from French-speaking Switzerland. They were published or broadcast in recent years in the main francophone Swiss newspaper, *Le Temps*, and on its national television network, Radio Télévision Suisse (RTS), and were retrieved through the search engines of their respective websites. It should be noted that this body of programmes and articles also incorporates reports on sexual assistance and assisted suicide for disabled people. Indeed, the development of some disabilities (physical and mental) is what turns some 'young old' into 'old old' and 'dependent', and so the reports' framing is predominantly in terms of a 'vulnerable or dependent condition' that applies to both older adults and people with disabilities.[5]

This chapter is not about whether seniors have sexual desire their entire lives, whether the wish for death increases with age, or whether the tension between Eros and Thanatos is exacerbated in nursing homes, nor does it intend to deny the difficulties nurses have dealing with such desires.[6] We are interested instead in the following three questions, which we address through analysis of newspaper articles and TV programs: 1) Which participants can legitimately speak about these issues? 2) How are these issues framed, and which values are presented as appropriate in the proposed

Table 5.1 Programs and articles on which the analysis is based

---

RTS, 'Métier: assistant sexuel pour handicapés [Profession: Sexual Assistant for
   Disabled People]', *Mise au point* program, RTS 1, 3 August 2008.
RTS, 'Exit aux portes de l'EMS [EXIT at the Door of the Nursing Homes]',
   Temps présent program, RTS 1, 9 October 2008.
RTS, 'Aide au suicide dans les EMS: vers la fin d'un tabou ? [Assisted Suicide
   in Nursing Homes: Towards the End of a Taboo]', *Infrarouge* program, RTS 1,
   14 October 2008.
'L'assistant sexuel donne de l'émotion [Sexual Assistant Gives Emotion]', *Le
   Temps*, Friday, 19 June 2009.
RTS, 'Sexe, amour et handicap [Sex, Love and Disability]', *Temps présent*
   programme, RTS 1, 3 June 2010.
'Je suis convaincue du droit de mon enfant à la sexualité [I Believe in My Child's
   Right to Sexuality]', *Le Temps*, 16 March 2013.
RTS, 'Des prostituées au service des personnes handicapées [Prostitutes at
   the Service of People with Disabilities]', *Faut pas croire* programme, RTS 1,
   22 February 2014.
'L'amour jusqu'à la mort [Love until Death]', *Le Temps*, Saturday, 14 June 2014.
RTS, 'Exit les vieux? [Exit/Out the Elderly]', *Faut pas croire* programme, RTS 1,
   19 October 2014.
'Un professeur du CHUV s'alarme des risques du suicide assisté [A Professor
   Alarmed Risks of Assisted Suicide]', *Le Temps*, Thursday, 27 November 2014.

---

responses? 3) What image of old age emerges from these debates? The presentation and the discussion of the results follow the same structure.

The actors in the debate

An inventory of the individuals that appear in the media reports and which qualifications (position, training and so on) journalists attribute to them reveals which actors the media considers legitimate to address the subject. Media coverage usually interviews or includes the same individuals.

Some, such as the president of EXIT (the francophone Swiss association offering suicide assistance), a sexual assistant, and the president of the association Sexualité et Handicaps Pluriels (Sexuality and Multiple Handicaps Association; SEHP) have public roles and can be characterized as moral entrepreneurs (Becker, 1973), which is to say people who assume the responsibility of persuading society to develop or enforce rules that are consistent with their own ardently held moral beliefs. Others provide sexual assistants' perspective, or represent legitimate professional organizations in the field of ageing, or have spoken out against assisted suicide (professors in palliative care and ethics). Consequently, the limited number of position types to intervene is open to challenge (on this point, see Davidson, 2012). Indeed, with the exception of ethicists, who are only invited to speak on assisted suicide, it is predominantly advocates of these practices (members of EXIT

Table 5.2 The actors in the debate

The president (a man) of French-speaking EXIT, three times;
Six sexual assistants (two men and four women), one of these three times;
The president (a woman) of SHEP, two times;
A co-founder (a woman) of SHEP, one time;
The person (a woman) who started the first training programme for sexual
    assistants in German-speaking Switzerland, one time;
The founder (a man) of the "Coordination Handicap et Autonomie", France,
    one time;
Eight residents (men and women) of nursing homes, each one time;
Four directors (all men) of nursing homes, each one time;
Three disabled people (all men) who don't live in nursing homes, each one time;
Three nurses in nursing homes (all women), one specialized in palliative care,
    each one time;
Two doctors (one man and one woman), one of which two times;
Two professors (both men), heads of palliative care services at two different
    University Hospitals, each one time;
Two mothers of two young disabled people, each one time;
One undertaker (a man), one time;
One sexologist (a woman), trainer of sexual assistance in France, one time;
One geriatrician (a woman) at the University of Lausanne, one time;
One lecturer (a woman) in the field of aging from a school of social work, one time;
One professor (a man) of ethics at the University of Geneva;
One state councillor (a man) responsible for social issues, one time;
One president (a man) of a regional association of nursing homes, one time.

or SEHP), beneficiaries of these 'services',[7] and gerontologists who appear in these articles and programmes. Researchers working on suicide or prostitution are neither interviewed nor represented.

This list demonstrates the significant presence of suicide assistance and sexual assistance advocates in the media. It also reveals the absence of researchers working on suicide or prostitution, which contrasts with the visibility of old-age specialists.

The participation of a geriatrician in an episode of the programme *Faut Pas Croire* entitled 'Exit, les vieux?' (Out with the Old?)[8] is extremely interesting in this regard. She was invited to the roundtable discussion because she conducted a study entitled 'Désir de mort chez les personnes âgées: que savons-nous de cette réalité?' (Desire for Death in the Elderly: What Do We Know of This Reality?) (Monod *et al.*, 2012). She explained that her research found that 14 per cent of older adults have a 'desire to die' and that this percentage rises to 20 per cent for those living in a nursing home. Her contribution shows no continuity between the older population and the rest of the population, nor between assisted suicide and suicide in general, but focuses specifically on dependent older adults, especially those who are institutionalized and would supposedly have a greater desire to die.

Inviting a geriatrician who works on morbidity to such a programme does not lead to the same debate that would result if an expert on teenage suicide were invited. Likewise, none of these programmes and articles ever give equal treatment to sexual assistance or prostitution among the 'healthy' or people in a vulnerable situation due to their age or their dependency, or to assisted suicide and suicide among the 'healthy' or people in vulnerable situations.

The frames and values invoked

Reviewing coverage of sexual assistance for dependent older adults provides a glimpse of their existential needs, which professionals have thus far ignored or denied and whose existence has left institutions feeling largely helpless. The gap between residents' growing needs and the institutions' lack of possible solutions has widened, especially concerning sexual assistance:

> 25 years ago, we reviewed all the needs of seniors. Sexuality did not figure amongst them.
>
> (A nurse in a nursing home)[9]

> It began last summer. He [a resident who thereafter enjoyed the services of a sexual assistant] masturbated frenetically, sometimes violently, and expressed himself in an increasingly uninhibited manner. For those looking after him, it became embarrassing. Faced with the sexual needs of 85 year-olds, there are no prophets to tell us how to act. We are facing challenges that humanity has never experienced before.... . Today, a

> sexual assistant is accepted in our establishment in the same way as an osteopath or a hairdresser.
>
> (A director of a nursing home)[10]

> Why did we do it? It is because people asked us for it, because people expressed this desire to experience their sexuality, as they put it, and my work, my principal task is to respond to the needs of each person and this is a need like any other. ... Requests are always different, regardless of the situation, or the disability, or, in the so-called normal population, the expectations or the vision of sensuality. The challenge is how to respond, but without promoting one approach or another; it's mainly listening.
>
> (The assistant director of a nursing home)[11]

These few quotes illustrate how ill equipped nursing homes are for handling such sexual expression and professionals' regret that there is a lack of written information, guidelines, and policy on the topic (Bauer *et al.*, 2009). They also show that the discourse of sexual expression is framed as a 'need', and this notion of need underpins and permeates staff thinking and practices (Rowntree & Zufferey, 2015). This approach is in line with the conception of the role of nursing home staff members as dispensing care and protection. At the same time, the desire to offer such a possibility is also thought to be part of a broader issue, the necessity of 'deinstitutionalizing' this kind of institution (Loffeier, 2015) and meeting residents' demand for autonomy and privacy. If nursing homes are both hospitals and houses for their residents, professionals should meet all their demands, not just medical ones. If nursing homes are hotels as well as hospitals, care professionals should make rooms more 'ordinary' and consider them as 'hotel rooms' that residents have the right to control. The above-quoted professionals' positions on allowing sexual or suicide assistance places residents at the centre of institutions' concerns. This indicates a break with a conception of an organization focused first and foremost on its mission to provide medical care.

   At the same time, this 'needs' discourse is in competition with another frame – that of 'rights' or even 'human rights'. This 'human rights frame' is not only used by the beneficiaries (as shown by Rowntree & Zufferey, 2015), but also by the moral entrepreneurs of both sexual assistance and suicide assistance:

> I realized that people are unable to experience their sexuality. Sexuality is truly a human right, something that each and every one of us has the right to experience.
>
> (A sexual assistant)[12]

> We should stop turning away from a subject that is serious, that is essential, that is vital. It is not a matter of sexual intercourse, it is a matter

of humanity ... . This is a problem of the incarnation of the person, humanization of the person, the reappropriation of bodies.

(The founder of Coordination Handicap et Autonomie)[13]

We cannot claim to guarantee that people can live the way they wish and, at the same time, deny their sexuality. When you are elderly, you are alone. You are only touched for utilitarian purposes. The human being needs more than that to still feel part of humanity.

(A nurse)[14]

This idea of a need that becomes a right is also omnipresent in the case of suicide assistance. Assisted suicide (called 'self-liberation' by its advocates) also appears to be a basic right, the expression of an individual liberty that, like sexual assistance, no other principle and no person (particularly no institutional employee) should be allowed to oppose.

People assert their self-determination, their autonomy, their free will, and this is a space which we must respect ... . These people wish to avoid a purgatory on earth and we must help them. Allow everyone their freedom and their choice.[15] From the moment when someone is against assisted suicide, this is his dogmatic position, he has the right, but he doesn't have the right to prevent someone when that person still possesses the ability to judge for himself.

(The president of EXIT)[16]

They should let us choose the time of our death; I want to protect myself from all horror, suffering, and degeneration. I often say it's pride, but I don't want to inflict this on my children or my grandchildren.

(A resident of a nursing home)[17]

These quotations demonstrate two things. The first is a miserabilist conception of old age ('purgatory on earth', a time of 'horror, suffering, and degeneration') shared by professionals and dependent older adults alike. The second is a battle not only for the *freedom* to have a sexual life or suicide assistance, but the *actual possibility* of it happening.[18] And institutions seem compelled to respond. Unlike the findings of Rowntree and Zufferey (2015), this is not only a discourse against the general erosion of autonomy and privacy experienced by nursing home residents and their demand to maintain a sexuality[19] or one focused on degeneration and suffering and the need for palliative care. It is also a claim for the right to benefit from sexual assistance or prostitution or the right to commit suicide.

It is interesting to note that our analyses of television and newspaper reports on sexual assistance revealed no references to the commodification of bodies and the vulnerability of practitioners,[20] the most frequently raised challenges to prostitution in the political, scientific, and media arenas. Moral entrepreneurs for both types of assistance therefore hold that the expression of reservations about sexual or suicide assistance is not due to disapproval of suicide or prostitution, but rather results from society's fear when faced with dependent older adults, a fear that should be fought.

> There have been centuries of Judeo-Christian education ... Behind the hostility, there is the fact that the disabled body is frightening. First, there is a human being behind the disabled person and, therefore, a sexual being.
>
> (A sexual assistant)[21]

It is thus not because these practices concern paid sex that they are problematized. Similarly, the problematization of assisted suicide has little to do with suicide. Moreover, although some risks relating to the sexual assistance relationship and the vulnerability of partners might be mentioned, risks to the service providers are never discussed (despite this being a customary concern subject to documentation in discourse on prostitution). In line with a miserabilist conception of ageing, all vulnerability is attributed to the dependent older adults, in situations of sexual assistance or assisted suicide alike.

> The main accusation [against sexual assistance]? The spectre of an abuse of power on the part of the able-bodied individual, especially when it concerns someone with a mental disability. The other source of reservations relates to frustration in case of the beneficiary's attachment or excessive need.
>
> (A sexual assistant)[22]

> Assisted suicide is a right guaranteed by law and no doctor is opposed to this; for me, the trivialization of death, particularly assisted death, is a danger, from the point where it threatens vulnerable human beings, and our role is to be particularly attentive in order to protect the most vulnerable. This is the heart of the question; a particular vulnerability which demands a particular attention on the part of caregivers.
>
> (A doctor in a nursing home)[23]

The question of how sexual assistance relates to prostitution (or the status of suicide assistants, for that matter) is never explicitly addressed, and there is no exploration of why it is legitimate for dependent older adults when it seems to be considered morally reprehensible for other categories of the population. On the contrary, we observe that all forms of sexuality and sensuality can be considered as equivalent where dependent older adults are concerned, thus making little distinction between prostitution and sexual assistance. In the eyes of its beneficiaries and advocates, there is a strong (but never problematic) continuity between recourse to sexual assistance and to prostitution, the former often being requested when the latter seems insufficient to respond to the needs of the dependent older adults.

> Some people can have recourse to sex workers, but they tell me that they go too fast, they take the money, and they do nothing.
>
> (The president of SEHP)[24]

> In the world of prostitution, there are people who absolutely do not want to work with those with disabilities, and we have to respect that. Everyone has their limits. We think that these people don't, but in reality there are also situations that are unthinkable for them; they are just not possible. So we asked ourselves, how to make it happen, why not provide a service? So this led to the training of sexual assistants in French-speaking Switzerland.
>
> (A cofounder of SEHP)[25]

> What we want is to be able to go to the prostitutes, like anyone else, and without necessarily being forced to go with a friend because, when we arrive at the hotel with the prostitute, we find ourselves facing a flight of six steps that have to be climbed with the wheelchair.
>
> (A resident of a nursing home)[26]

These interested parties do not debate the symbolic or policy dimensions of such recourse to prostitution, but speak more about 'freedom' and the right to have access to all kinds of services, including prostitution. Rowntree and Zufferey (2015, p. 24–25) have already linked this idea of a 'right' with the idea of consumption,

> a right that residents choose to exercise … through a model of service provision and consumption that favours privacy and autonomy … A way of thinking which attempts to shift the balance of power towards residents or consumers by reconceptualising residential age-care … towards the concept of a hotel.

In other words: the right to enjoy the opportunities that shopping, leisure and lifestyle consumption offer. Moving from the idea of 'need' to the idea of 'right', residents go from being 'patients' to being seen as – and considering themselves to be – consumers. And in this case, consumption not only has a role in reproducing and refashioning identities and lifestyles but also in offering opportunities for sharing, socializing, and having fun (Gilleard & Higgs, 2011). Prostitution *per se* is not evoked, and the only issue raised is whether the service is provided to dependent older adults in an appropriate manner.

The necessity of responding to this need or right seems to minimize the differences between all forms of contact (commercial, therapeutic and intimate) that could lead to sensual or sexual experiences. This seems to suggest that any moral or values-related discourse must cede when confronted by this absolute need or right of dependent older adults. Sexual assistance above all finds its place as a response to dependent older adults' dissatisfactions stemming from the absence of married life or the quality of services provided by certain prostitutes. The question of commodification of the body, even if it comes up in the remarks, does not appear problematic.

> Personally, I am rather in favour of professional prostitutes intervening. A resident told me that these sexual assistants were great but perhaps not sexy enough for him, and happily they could extend the possibilities of meeting someone to respond to each person's needs.
>
> (A director of a nursing home)[27]

In this situation, the issue of the 'choice' of service provider is not raised to question the status (or the commodification) of the person providing the service but instead, once again, to address the beneficiary's freedom of choice as a consumer. The fact that the similarity between these assistive practices and morally condemned practices (prostitution or suicide) was not made into an issue reflects their advocates' desire to suppress the differences (in symbolic or policy terms, for instance) between these practices and their more common or more socially accepted forms. For example, in the case of assisted suicide, a death becomes a death, regardless of what triggered it.

> If a person died suddenly, everyone would consider this normal, but if this person had chosen the way to die, certain people find this choice highly abnormal. For me, this person merely asserted her philosophy, her personal freedom of choice, her personal ethics.
>
> (The president of EXIT)[28]

A final element should be noted. Because the interested parties cited in newspaper articles and television programmes emphasize the specific nature of old age dependency, they seem to deny and/or ignore the differences between people sharing this condition. There is no discussion of the existence or absence of differences, in social class or gender for instance, in dependent older adults' use of these practices. Concerning the gender dimension more particularly, analysis of newspaper articles and television programs on assisted suicide and sexual assistance reveals that both men and women are engaged in these debates (each practice has moral entrepreneurs of both sexes, and there are sexual and suicide assistants of both sexes). Does this mean that men and women use such practices equally? The dependent older adults who speak in favour of assisted suicide in the media are all women, and the beneficiaries of sexual assistance who speak publicly are all men (although in the case of disability, some mothers tell of their efforts to allow their sons to have sexual assistance, and one article told the story of a woman who received sexual assistance).[29] But participants in the debate never discuss the existence or absence of a gender dimension in the use of these practices. Nobody asks sexual assistants, male or female, if they work with male or female clients. Similarly, the potential gender or class dimension of assisted suicide is never addressed (even though these dimensions are explored in the literature – on this point, see Steck *et al.*, 2014; Pott *et al.*, 2015). It is as if moral entrepreneurs did not want to explore the possibility that social logics other than ageing and vulnerability may be at work in some dependent older adults' use of these forms of assistance, as though highlighting such differences might challenge the framing of dependent older adults as utterly different from the rest of the population.

Conclusion: Between miserabilism and populism, dependent old age as a subculture

Analysis of newspaper articles and television programmes on assisted suicide and sexual assistance led to four striking observations. One is the validation (with a touch of admiration) of the 'sexual drive' of Daniel, who visits prostitutes at over 70 years old, quoted in the newspaper *Le Temps* at the beginning of this chapter.[30] Would Daniel have enjoyed the same sympathy from the journalist if he were 20 or 30 rather than 74? The second is that the parties involved make no connection between sexual assistance and prostitution, or between assisted suicide and suicide; only one person, an ethicist, made the link between the suicide of dependent older adults and suicide more generally.[31] The absence of moral judgement is somewhat astonishing in such debates, especially since such judgements are ubiquitous in coverage of prostitution or suicide among the young. Why, for example, did we not find any coverage of the situation of sexual assistants or people assisting with suicide to inform the audience about their socioeconomic position (for example, Mathieu 2007)? The third point of interest is participants' discourse on the standardization of any form of sexuality or death for dependent older adults. As we have seen, this discourse does not seem to clearly distinguish between death by assisted suicide and a natural death in older adults, since death seems closer; the same is true of sexuality, where the issue of a 'need' or 'right' seems to dominate any question of the forms this sexuality might take. The last observation is that all participants' discourse is above all about dependent older adults. They do not question prostitution *per se*, and the only issue raised is whether prostitutes behave appropriately with dependent older clients. These clients' particular characteristics make it necessary for sexual assistants to specialize so they can act in accordance with this 'specificity'. Adopting a miserabilist point of view, all interested parties seem to think that the dilemma between human rights, needs and dependency can be solved by assuming a consumerist posture.

These four observations – and the lack of any discussion of the existence or absence of social class or gender dimensions in pursuit of such practices – lead us to the conclusion that dependent older adults, as they are represented in the media, no longer seem to be governed by the same social standards as the rest of the population. Review of these articles and programmes showed no equation between the lives of dependent older adults and those of the rest of the population (including the 'young old'). The proposed solutions seem specific to these publics and are never portrayed as generalizable to the population at large.

Dependency in old age is depicted as a very specific condition, incomparable to other phases (or conditions) of life: a time of suffering with its own values and moral judgements due to its specific challenges. While there are specific objective characteristics and types of suffering related to such situations of dependency, making this population into a special 'subgroup' and insisting on its otherness rather than its continuities or similarities with other populations with other social practices amounts to a choice to construct it as a subject – one that is justifiable, but always needing justification and always debatable. Regardless, these constructions of the subject and choices of frames are self-perpetuating and have consequences. The discourse circulating in the current media arena makes ageing and situations of dependency, each in its own way, into specific subjects, defined and with clear boundaries demarcating these periods (or conditions) of life from other periods (or conditions) of life. This makes old age and dependency specific fields of knowledge, differentiating them from other fields of knowledge concerning the entire population.

It seems appropriate to treat 'assisted suicide' and 'sexual assistance' together, as we did here (an original approach, as far as we know), because it is revealing of the world of older and dependent adults, at least in certain sociocultural contexts.[32] It offers particular conceptions (or another illustration of the implication of a 'successful ageing' discourse; Katz, 1996; Katz & Calasanti, 2015) of what it is 'to die well' or 'love well' and the solutions offered to those who are believed (or claim) to be unable to continue enduring their situation. Old age without sexuality and running the chance of dying in suffering seem incompatible with successful ageing. Based on the discourse of the people interviewed in all these television programmes and newspaper articles, we observe a continuum of forms of dying and of sexuality, ranging from 'dying badly' and 'loving badly' to 'dying well' and 'loving well', the latter options seemingly reserved only for those 'who are capable of it': that is, those who are fit, strong and healthy. The 'assisted' forms appear to be the most suitable approaches to 'dying well' or 'loving well' for those who are no longer considered completely able to do so on their own. Furthermore, although the differences between suicide and assisted suicide, and to an even greater extent between resorting to prostitution and sexual assistance, may sometimes appear tenuous (at least in the eyes of those who advocate or resort to them), turning to a 'paramedical solution', with the intervention of specially trained social workers or sex workers for the latter or through the intervention of doctors in the former, seems to ensure some dignity to these assistive practices.

Ultimately, some dependent older adults have access to these special rights that place them in the ranks of those with the possibility of a sexual life or a death 'with dignity'. At the same time, such rights also segregate people by separating dependent older adults from ordinary mortals, thereby attesting to their vulnerability – or reminding us of it.

Notes

1 'L'amour jusqu'à la mort', *Le Temps*, Saturday 14 June 2014, p. 3.
2 I thank the editors for their constructive comments, which helped me to improve this chapter.
3 Sexual assistance is well established in countries such as Switzerland, Germany, the Netherlands, Denmark and Sweden. Sexual assistants provide sexual release to clients who have physical disabilities due to age or other challenges that make attaining sexual pleasure and release difficult. The applicants for the relevant licence have to complete special courses or studies.
4 Swiss law tolerates assisted suicide where the patient commits the act and the helper has no direct interest in the death. There are several organizations in Switzerland, such as EXIT and Dignitas, that help 'terminally ill' and 'polymorbid' patients choose how to die.
5 According to the United Nations Declaration on the Rights of Disabled Persons, 'The term "disabled person" means any person unable to ensure by himself or herself, wholly or partly, the necessities of a normal individual and/or social life, as a result of deficiency (...) in his or her physical or mental capabilities'. It includes dependent older adults.
6 As one of the articles put it, 'harassment of medical personnel constitutes the main impetus within nursing homes to take their residents' urges into account' ('L'amour jusqu'à la mort' [Love until Death], *Le Temps*, Saturday 14 June 2014, p. 3).
7 Is this the sign of the media's ageism? It is interesting to note that these beneficiaries, if they agree to speak with their face visible, are identified only by their first names, which symbolically distinguishes them from the experts, who are identified by their full name.
8 RTS, 'Exit, les vieux?' (Out with the Old?), *Faut pas Croire* television programme, RTS1, 19 October 2014.
9 'L'amour jusqu'à la mort' (Love until Death), *Le Temps*, Saturday 14 June 2014.
10 'L'amour jusqu'à la mort' (Love until Death), *Le Temps*, Saturday 14 June 2014.
11 RTS, 'Des prostituées au service des personnes handicapées' (Prostitutes at the Service of People with Disabilities), *Faut pas croire* television programme, RTS 1, 22 February 2014.
12 RTS, 'Métier: assistant sexuel pour handicapés' (Profession: Sexual Assistant for Disabled), *Mise au Point* television programme, 3 August 2008.
13 RTS, 'Sexe, amour et handicap' (Sex, Love and Disability), *Temps présent* television programme, 3 June 2010.
14 'L'amour jusqu'à la mort' (Love until Death), *Le Temps*, Saturday 14 June 2014.
15 RTS, 'Exit, les vieux?' (Out with the Old?), *Faut pas Croire* television programme, RTS 1, 19 October 2014.
16 RTS, 'Exit aux portes de l'EMS' (EXIT at the Nursing Home Door), *Temps présent* television programme, 9 October 2008.

17 RTS, 'Exit aux portes de l'EMS' (EXIT at the Nursing Home Door), *Temps présent* television programme, 9 October 2008.
18 In other words, it is not only the demand for a 'freedom' but also a 'social right'. By analogy, we can compare this with the right to basic education in Switzerland, which involves not only the right to be educated or to educate one's children but also the right to demand that the State organize the education system so that all children have access to such an education.
19 A large number of practices and emotions can be subsumed under the term of sexuality (Cornelison & Doll, 2012). In the literature, 'sexuality' is broadly defined as the quality or state of being sexual. For Drench and Losee (1996) and Hubbard, Tester and Downs (2003) or the AARP (2005), sexuality is a combination of sex drive, sexual acts, and the psychological aspects of relationships, emotions and attitudes. Expressions of sexuality in nursing homes encompass a broad range of actions, including sexual intercourse, kissing, hugging, sexual touching/caressing, self-stimulation, and oral sex, but also flirtation, affection, making compliments, physical proximity and contact, sentimental intimacy (as a sense of closeness and familiarity with another) and maintenance of physical appearances. The psychological aspects of sex in later life are associated with pleasure, tension reduction, communication, mutual tenderness, passion, a sense of identity, and security when facing risk and loss.
20 The purpose of this chapter is not to discuss the actual or perceived vulnerability of people who work as sexual assistants, or to discuss people's motivations for becoming sexual assistants. According to the studied news reports, sexual assistants may be people who used to be or still are sex workers or practitioners of other occupations (osteopathy, massage and so on). Legally speaking, sexual assistants have a status similar to that of prostitutes, rather than caregivers, since they are paid for their services and the cost is paid by the client.
21 'L'assistant sexuel donne de l'émotion' (The Sexual Assistant Gives Emotion), *Le Temps*, Friday 19 June 2009.
22 'Je suis convaincue du droit de mon enfant à la sexualité' (I Believe That My Child has a Right to Sexuality), *Le Temps*, 16 March 2013.
23 RTS, 'Aide au suicide dans les EMS: Vers la fin d'un tabou?' (Assisted Suicide in Nursing Homes: Toward the End of a Taboo?), *Infrarouge* television program, RTS 1, 14 October 2008.
24 RTS, 'Sexe, amour et handicap' (Sex, Love, and Disability), *Temps présent* television programme, 3 June 2010.
25 RTS, 'Sexe, amour et handicap' (Sex, Love, and Disability), *Temps présent* television programme, 3 June 2010.
26 RTS, 'Métier: assistant sexuel pour handicapés' (Profession: Sexual Assistant for Disabled People), *Mise au point* television programme, 3 August 2008.
27 RTS, 'Des prostituées au service des personnes handicapées' (Prostitutes at the Service of People with Disabilities), *Faut pas croire* television programme, RTS 1, 22 February 2014.
28 RTS, 'Exit aux portes de l'EMS' (EXIT at the Nursing Home Door), *Temps présent* television programme, RTS 1, 9 October 2008.
29 'L'amour jusqu'à la mort' (Love until Death), *Le Temps*, Saturday 14 June 2014, p. 3.
30 'L'amour jusqu'à la mort' (Love until Death), *Le Temps*, Saturday 14 June 2014, p. 3.
31 RTS, 'Exit, les vieux?' (Out with the Old?), *Faut pas Croire* television programme, RTS 1, 19 October 2014.
32 Legislative developments with respect to suicide assistance, like sexual assistance, are recent and may experience some fits and starts. International comparison is thus complicated. Tendentially, it seems that States authorizing assisted

suicide are generally tolerant of sexual assistance; the main ones are Switzerland, Belgium, Luxemburg, the Netherlands and certain states in the United States. Germany and Austria authorize sexual assistance but prohibit suicide assistance, perhaps due to the trauma of the Second World War. More broadly, this comes down to a major division in conceptions of 'dignity', between countries that consider it universal and unequivocal and with precedence over the notion of individual freedom, and others that defend a pluralist conception of dignity that cannot impinge on individual freedom and distinguish between 'dignity' and the 'sanctity' of life or the body. On this point, see Charlesworth (1993) and Hottois (2009).

References

AARP – Amercian Association of Retired Persons (2005), *Sexuality at midlife and beyond: 2004 update of attitudes and behaviors.* Washington DC, AARP.

Bauer Michael, Nay Rhonda & Linda McAuliffe (2009), 'Catering to love, sex and intimacy in residential aged care: What information is provided to consumers?', *Sexuality and Disability*, 27, 1, pp. 3–9.

Becker Howard S. (1973), *Outsiders. Studies in the Sociology of Deviance.* New York, Free Press.

Charlesworth Max (1993), *Bioethics in Liberal Society.* Cambridge, Cambridge University Press.

Conseil Fédéral (2011), *Soins palliatifs, prévention du suicide et assistance organisée au suicide.* Berne, Rapport du Conseil federal.

Cornelison Laci J. and Gayle M. Doll (2012), 'Management of sexual expression in long-term care: Ombudsmen's perspectives', *The Gerontologist*, 53, 5, pp. 780–789.

Davidson Scott (2012), *Going Grey. The Mediation of Politics in an Ageing Society.* Farnham and Burlington, Ashgate.

Drench Meredith E. & Rita H. Losee (1996), 'Sexuality and sexual capacities of elderly people', *Rehabilitation Nursing*, 21, 3, pp. 118–123.

Gilleard Chris & Paul Higgs (2011), 'Consumption and Ageing'. In Settersten Richard and Jacqueline Angel (eds.), *Handbook of Sociology of Ageing.* New York, Springer, pp. 361–375.

Higgins Robert W. (2003). 'L'invention du mourant. Violence de mort pacifiée', *Esprit*, January, pp. 139–169.

Hottois Gilbert (2009), *Dignité et diversité des hommes.* Paris, Vrin.

Hubbard Gill, Tester Susan & Murna G. Downs (2003), 'Meaningful social interactions between older people in institutional care settings', *Ageing and Society*, 23, pp. 99–114.

Katz Stephen (1996), *Disciplining Old Age: The Formation of Gerontological Knowledge.* Charlottesville, University Press of Virginia.

Katz Stephen & Toni Calasanti (2015), 'Critical perspectives on successful ageing: Does it "appeal more than it illuminates"?', *Gerontologist*, 1, 55, pp. 26–33.

Loffeier Iris (2015), *Panser des jambes de bois? La vieillesse, catégorie d'existence et de travail en maison de retraite.* Paris, Presses Universitaires de France.

Mathieu Lilian (2007), *La Condition prostituée*, Paris. Textuel.

Monod Stéfanie, Rochat Etienne, Büla Christophe, Dürst Anne-Véronique & Brenda Spencer (2012), 'Assessing the wish to die in elderly people', *Journal of the American Geriatrics Society*, 60 (Suppl. 4), p. 203.

Grignon Claude & Jean-Claude Passeron (1989), *Le Savant et le Populaire. Misérabilisme et populisme en sociologie and en littérature*. Paris, Seuil.

Pott Murielle, Cavalli Stefano, Stauffer Laeticia & Sarah Beltrami, (2015), *Adhérer à une Association pour le Droit de Mourir dans la Dignité (ADMD): analyse d'une transition et d'une anticipation de la fin de vie pour les membres âgés de 65 ans et plus*. Swiss National Science Foundation, Project 10001A_159378/1, (2015-2018), HES-SO & SUPSI, Ongoing research.

Rowntree Margaret & Carole Zuffferey Carole (2015), 'Need or right: Sexual expression and intimacy in aged care', *Journal of Ageing Studies*, 35, pp. 20–25.

Snow David, Rochford Burke, Worden Steven & Robert D. Benford (1986), 'Frame alignment processes, micromobilization, and movement participation', *American Sociological Review*, 51, 4, pp. 464–481.

Spoerri Adrian, Zwahlen Marcel, Bopp Matthias, Gutzwiler Felix & Matthias Egger, Matthias (2010), 'Religion and assisted and non-assisted suicide in Switzerland: National cohort study', *International Journal of Epidemiology*, 39, 6, pp. 1486–1494.

Steck Nicole, Junker Christoph, Maessen Maud, Reisch Thomas, Zwahlen Marcel & Matthias Egger (2014), 'Suicide assisted by right-to-die associations: A population based cohort study', *International Journal of Epidemiology*, 43, 2, pp. 614–622.

Ylänne Virpi (2015), 'Representations of ageing in the media'. In Twigg Julia & Wendy Martin (eds.), *Routledge Handbook of Cultural Gerontology*. London and New York, Routledge, pp. 369–376.

6   Toward a biopolitics of old age

Vulnerability and aging in postwar France[1]

Richard C. Keller

The devastating heat wave of August 2003 was by every measure an extreme event. Combining unprecedented temperatures with high levels of humidity and ozone pollution, the weather system settled on western and central Europe for over 2 weeks, leaving nearly tens of thousands dead across the continent, and nearly 15,000 dead in France alone, making it the worst meteorological disaster in modern French history. The death toll was also uneven: the heat wave focused its wrath on urban environments and on vulnerable populations. In particular, the elderly bore the brunt of mortality, as more than 80 percent of excess deaths occurred among those over 75 years old. The spectacle of these 12,000 deaths elderly prompted a national conversation about aging in France, raising questions about how such an agglomeration of preventable deaths could possibly have taken place in a nation that the World Health Organization considered to have the best public health system in the world just 3 years earlier. The heat wave revealed the terrible condition of those who often lived in utter isolation and desperate poverty, having aged out of their social networks, and, to an extent, of social citizenship.

The heat wave's devastating effects for an aging population provoked an extensive debate about the place of the elderly in French society. Politicians, social scientists, and the general public demanded explanations of how a particular segment of the population could be so vulnerable as to suffer such extensive and preventable deaths in a contemporary industrialized nation. Panels and news documentaries engaged in extensive examinations of the social condition of the elderly and the apparent fractures in social solidarity that the heat wave deaths revealed. Yet concerns about aging and society were far from an emergent problem of the early twenty-first century. Instead, aging was a demographic phenomenon that had troubled French politicians and social scientists for decades. Such figures saw old age as a fundamental problem of modernity for which society was ill equipped to cope. Since the early twentieth century, an increasingly strident discourse framed the elderly as a population at the limits of citizenship and a burden for an emerging postindustrial nation. The aging of France threatened the republic's integrity: it menaced its economic vitality, it sapped its physical strength, and it generated an unproductive—and increasingly feminine—demographic that promised to break the welfare state.

The "problem" of aging between economics and population science

There has long been an implicit tension in French attitudes toward aging. As the sociologist Isabelle Mallon has argued, perspectives on aging have "oscillated between admiration and pity" (Mallon, 2004). There is the image promoted by advertisers and the leisure industry, catering to a new demographic: one of a fit, tanned class of successful early retirees, enjoying the first phases of grandparenthood and deserved leisure. Yet this image is counterbalanced with the figure of the vulnerable, yet also parasitic senior, a victim of poor economic circumstances and a failing body. The former notion is an artifact of postwar prosperity, which witnessed the development of the new figure of the youthful retiree (Levet & Pelletier, 1988; Rochefort, 2000). The latter, by contrast, has been more prevalent in twentieth-century political discourse. As Hervé Le Bras (1993; see also Keller, 2016) has argued, the pervasiveness of this notion is in part a product of language: in contrast to the English term "aging," which connotes a natural chronological process in a subject of any age, the French term *"viellissement,"* or "getting old," signifies a process of decay specific to the end of life. *"Viellesse,"* or old age, is always a "degradation." It is a step toward death, rather than a process of maturation.

Much of this attitude originated in a perceived demographic crisis over a century ago. While fears of depopulation in France date to the late nineteenth century and the shocking loss in the Franco-Prussian War (Nye, 1984; Pick, 1993), the realization of a birth gap between France and Germany and the staggering death toll of the First World War gave these concerns a fresh impetus. Pronatalist policies informed much of French political discourse through the interwar period on both sides of the political spectrum (Bourdelais, 1993; Roberts, 1994; Koos, 1996). But after the German Occupation of 1940–45, some of the critics who had led the pronatalist charge between the wars took up the cause of aging, which they also saw as a critical factor in the development of a national vulnerability.

For nationalist demographers and politicians in the postwar era, aging threatened the vitality of the population. As Alfred Sauvy, another pronatalist who became the founding director of the Institut National d'Etudes Demographiques (INED, National Institute for Demographic Research) in 1945, argued, the population could "grow" or it could "grow old," but not both (Parant, 1992). For nationalist demographers, and politicians consequently, by growing older and withdrawing from productive activity, the elderly became a drain on a society desperate for economic recovery from the War; as parents of too few children, they bore responsibility for the nation's depopulation. In the aftermath of the Occupation, the elderly had become an icon of national weakness. "The conditions of modern warfare," one demographer argued in 1948, demanded armies comprised of "the young, in full possession of their physical means" (Daric, 1948). As two of his colleagues concurred, an "invasion" by the elderly had preceded the invasion of the Germans; thus "the terrible failure of 1940, as much moral as it was material, should be linked in part to this sclerosis" (Feller, 1998, 2005).

For Fernand Boverat, the sheer magnitude of aging constituted France's major population problem. A political crusader of the far right, Boverat became the secretary general of the *Alliance nationale pour l'accroissement de la population française* in the interwar period. For Boverat depopulation was a problem at both ends of the life cycle: low birth rates and the aging of the population were the source of national weakness (Boverat, 1939). In 1951, Boverat prepared a substantial report on "The Aging of the Population and its Repercussions for Social Security" for France's *Haut-Comité Consultatif de la Famille et de la Population* (HCPF), which sounded the alarm about a national demographic emergency. He noted that since 1775, the proportion of those under 20 had declined by 50 percent, while the proportion of those over 60 had increased by 228 percent. More troubling was the increase in the "very old." The past century had witnessed a 65 percent increase in the number of those in their sixties, but a 122 percent increase of those in their seventies and a whopping 200 percent increase in those in their eighties. As a consequence, "the French population is currently the oldest in the world." Particularly alarming for Boverat was that "the number of elderly women" was "much more considerable and has grown more than that of elderly men." Since women traditionally spent fewer years as wage earners than men, they were therefore "a heavier burden for the collective" (Boverat, 1951a).

Boverat attributed the rise in the number of elderly citizens to advances in medicine. Although such progress was commendable, caring for the very old came at the expense of the working-age population and constituted an increasing burden for the nation that should dampen enthusiasm for longevity. As a consequence, the elderly became a parasitic population, "consum[ing] a share of national production without contributing to it." For Boverat, "by slowing economic activity, aging halts production and impoverishes the country" (Boverat, 1951a). Moreover, aging was a problem with cascading effects: aging slowed national rates of marriage and reproduction, while increasing rates of mortality.

Much of Boverat's concern was economic—which makes sense in light of France's development of a comprehensive social security system in the mid-twentieth century. Likewise, much of the historiography of aging in modern France has focused on relationship between labor, economic security, and old age (see, e.g. Lenoir, 1979; Guillemard, 1993; Caradec, 2005; Feller, 2005; Guillemard, 2010). But although the economic framing of aging is critical, it leaves important cultural and political dimensions of aging unquestioned, including the fundamental devaluation of the lives of the elderly as marked by their economic transition into retirement. For even if a new category of "retiree" had begun to replace that of the dependent elderly, it still marked a way station between working adulthood and what critics came to call true old age. As an inevitable biological phenomenon, the aging of the population threatened to sap national economic and political strength, calling for the deployment of an arsenal of legislation designed to manipulate the state of the population and restore national vigor. For Boverat and others, only the state was equipped to remedy this problem through prophylactic action in order to immunize the nation against the dangers of shifting demographics.

The philosopher Michel Foucault's introduction to the concept of biopower as a technique of modern sovereignty provides a useful frame for interpreting Boverat's language and the strategies he advocated. This notion marks a new direction in Foucault's thought, away from the concept of discipline, which operates at the level of the individual body, and toward the concept of a biopolitics of population, which operates on a broader scale with the goal of shaping large demographic trends. The security of the state depended on its ability to manage the endemic conditions of humanity within its borders. The capacity of the state to direct life, as Foucault argued in his lectures at the Collège de France in the late 1970s, employed a biopolitics of populations that operated at the aggregate level: it aimed at massaging or manipulating the edges of enormous problems, gradually influencing means rather than enforcing norms (Foucault, 2007). Moreover, it operated explicitly within a context of liberal democracy through a subtlety of action. Population did not respond to decree: it was instead a "thick natural phenomenon," something that could be adjusted rather than coerced by the agency of the state and capital. As Foucault argued, population "varies according to the laws to which it is subjected, like tax or marriage laws for example." Population is "accessible to agents and techniques of transformation, on condition that these agents and techniques are at once enlightened, reflected, analytical, calculated, and calculating" (Foucault, 2007). Biopolitics acts at the level of statistics: rates of mortality and morbidity, yields of internment and rehabilitation, a management of risk, and a maximization of reward are its principal registers. It also operates in an often extra-legal fashion, reliant on policies and practices designed to influence or incentivize population measures rather than coercion or legislation.

One lecture in 1976 explicitly engaged the question of a biopolitics of aging. Here, for Foucault, the rise of the industrial sector initiated a deep concern for the ineluctability of the process of aging and its inevitable extraction of subjects from "the field of capacity, of activity." But this transition was not merely economic. Illness, death, and aging were "phenomena affecting a population." Like illness and death, aging was "something permanent, something that slips into life, perpetually gnaws at it, diminishes it and weakens it," a problem that "can never be eradicated," that acts to "incapacitate individuals," and that demands the development of new techniques of management: "subtle, more rational mechanisms" of "insurance, individual and collective savings, safety measures, and so on" (Foucault, 2003).

Aging was thus a natural biological phenomenon that could not be eradicated, but which was subject to state intervention and manipulation. The state's institutions had the capacity to direct life and so influence the course of national demographic trends. As Boverat argued in his report, "it is not possible to modify chronological age and prevent a man who has lived 64 years from being in his 65th." Instead, the most important mechanism the state and its institutional allies could adopt was its capacity to shape life constructively in order to combat the pathogenic forces that aged the population prematurely. Boverat argued that "certain significant factors in premature aging can be eliminated, the influence of many others can be reduced." Effective self-discipline was important for the individual, but required complementary action by the state. Alcohol prevention policies, infectious disease control, labor protections, and housing policies could all combine to inhibit the dangers that aging presented to the population (Boverat, 1951b). Boverat offered draft legislation that promised "to halt the statistical aging of the French population" by developing family and housing legislation that would encourage young families to reproduce. The legislation also recommended "that the struggle against infant and child mortality be intensified" and advocated for the "select immigration of young foreign workers, easily assimilable and by preference the heads of households" (Boverat, 1951a).

The direction of life represented one side of biopower; the other involved allowing death. As Foucault argued in *The History of Sexuality*, the manipulation of population involved both of these possibilities: the fostering of youth, adulthood, and vigor, and the disallowance of life that had reached the limits of its vitality (Foucault, 1981). In directing resources toward the lives of some, the state develops and fosters a "negative biopolitics" that effectively cuts off the lives—and social citizenship—of others (Esposito, 2008).

Reflecting on the disproportionate increase of the elderly in France's population, Boverat insisted in a 1951 report that "only a significant increase of young foreigners or a massacre of the old could perceptibly reduce this growth" (Boverat, 1951b). At the beginning of the report, he acknowledges the human decency that would prevent a wholesale consignment of the elderly poor to death. But he presents such humanism as a costly indulgence:

> At least if we do not want to leave a very considerable number of the old in the street in 10 or 15 years, or if we don't want to condemn them to finish their lives lamentably in the slums, we will have to build or refit retirement homes for hundreds of thousands of them.

In addition to the staggering cost of such a proposition, he asks, how could the country staff these facilities, given the decline of the working-age population? By the end of the discussion, he reframes the question of insuring the health—and lives—of the aged: "Could we," he asks, "refuse to give the old treatments that are capable of prolonging their life for several years?" (Boverat, 1951b). What he considered unimaginable at the report's beginning has now become a rhetorical possibility.

Pierre Laroque and "the problem of aging"

In 1960 the HCPF established the *"Commission d'étude des problèmes de la vieillesse,"* directed by Pierre Laroque. Laroque was a specialist in social welfare, having served on a social insurance board in the French cabinet in the early 1930s and as the director general of the French social security division since 1944. The Commission's report, submitted to the HCPF in 1962 and published widely, is ambivalent about aging. It vacillates between a sympathetic analysis of the real difficulties faced by the elderly and the possibilities of the state to manage those difficulties, and a language of objectifying difference portraying the elderly as a drain on social resources and a stultifying force. From its outset, it betrayed a significant bias: the very name of the Commission conceived of aging as a "problem" for the nation, rather than a "question" or an "issue." The report concerns itself with the demographic reality of an aging population and its meanings for the welfare state: its principal focuses are issues such as the retirement age and pensions, housing for the elderly, and social assistance. Its opening lines signal that "the aging of the population entails consequences in all domains of national life; progressively, but in an unavoidable way, it is burdening the conditions of existence for the French collectivity." Although aging had been on the rise incrementally, it had now achieved such a scale as to transform French culture and society. As the report frames the problem, "it is striking to note that if, in a century, the total population has accumulated nearly 3 million old people, it has only gained 53,000 children" (HCPF, 1962). It was thus the magnitude of aging that demanded a state response.

The project represented a massive expansion of social citizenship that targeted the elderly for state intervention. While a 1905 law mandating state assistance to the elderly represented the first welfare provision for seniors, that law had a low economic threshold for eligibility, and offered minimal assistance. This new project promised to go far beyond the provisions of the 1905 law. Yet in so doing, it also designated the elderly as a group apart. The report—and the state programs that ensued in the following decades—fell into a double bind: its efforts at inclusion created a fundamental segregation. The Commission had sought from the outset to avoid this trap, indicating that it aimed "at an adaptation without segregation": a policy that would provide for the elderly without rendering them a population apart (HCPF, 1962). Combined with the documentation produced in the Commission's work on the report, such language indicates a painful awareness of this dividing practice in action: that society was remaking itself through the marginalization of the elderly, pushing a growing population to the limits of citizenship. The demographer Alfred Sauvy's wry comment during the

Commission's deliberations captured the biopolitical dimensions of a segregative mentality that would push the elderly out of consciousness. This, he said, "has long been the norm for social programs for the elderly: get rid of the old—humanely of course—but cut them out of the loop because they get in the way" (CEPV, 1960).

The data were sobering. Far from imagining old age as a future stage of humanity—that all citizens were potentially elderly—the results of polls and reports showed that the bulk of the nation framed old age as a state of alterity, and many elderly experienced aging as a process of increasing isolation and marginalization. Many elderly expressed a desire to live with their adult children and their families upon retirement. But the younger groups surveyed thought this would work only in "strictly utilitarian" conditions; that is, if their aging parents could provide domestic service and baby-sitting for the family. Perhaps the starkest indication of a segregative mentality among the young was a dissonance on the question of nursing homes: 72 percent of French adults saw the expansion of nursing homes and senior communities as "desirable," but only 22 percent imagined themselves living in one: they were too "brutal," too "sad," "demoralizing," and in them "the old are treated too much like animals" (IFOP, n.d.).

The magnitude of aging, a baby boom that rendered natalism moot, and the development of a national social security system indicate why aging became a preoccupation of the state. The more complex question is why not only a state concern with the development of a new aging policy emerged in the 1960s (despite state inaction following the report), but why a sort of negative biopolitics emerged alongside it. That is, how did the aged begin to lose their humanity, to creep firmly toward the margins of citizenship and no longer count as part of the population in the social imagination? As a number of historians and sociologists of aging have noted, the denigration of the elderly was nothing new in this period. Yet there is a kind of renewed vigor to these representations that emerged alongside a comprehensive welfare state in the mid-twentieth century. At the moment that the "old" had become "retirees" (on their way to becoming "seniors"), a broad social contempt created a significant obstacle to the state's efforts at inclusion of the elderly (see, e.g. Stearns, 1976).

The Laroque Report signaled that this was in process in its concerns about the segregation of the elderly. One critical element of the notion of the elderly as a population at the edge of humanity was the idea of their unproductivity, their "non-utility" in the late industrial economy (*France-Soir*, 1962). While many viewed retirement as a well deserved benefit that capped a lifetime of labor, others saw the elderly as an unproductive drain on society. As the sociologist Robert Castel has argued, the modern period has witnessed the rise of the *société salariale*, in which social citizenship has become affixed to status in the marketplace of labor. Castel describes a mechanism of *disaffiliation* from labor characterized by "passing from integration to vulnerability, or sliding from vulnerability to social nonexistence" (Castel, 1995). As such privileges of citizenship as health coverage, family assistance, and pensions became closely linked with one's place in the workforce, distance from wage labor through disability, immigration status, or age marked a degree of segregation from full social investment. Retirement—a life stage defined by the absence of work (albeit with a pension in many cases)—framed the elderly as fully outside the labor market, and therefore pushed to the margins of a new society organized around economic productivity. In addition, in the transformation to a consumer economy that marked the *Trentes Glorieuses*, the elderly were non-consumers in the market—a population on fixed incomes who "saw their savings disappear bit by bit" (*Association nationale des assistantes sociales et des assistants sociaux* 1961)—who disproportionately consumed public resources. Although there was a modicum of understanding that the elderly had aged beyond the capacity for self-sufficiency, Castel notes, a lingering market-based logic also saw the dependent elderly as responsible for their own lot, a result of insufficient saving during the period of work (Castel, 1995).

Given the emphasis that the Laroque commission and the social debate that ensued placed on the economic dimensions of aging, it is tempting to cast the issue in a frame that privileges the market and the alienation of the traditional family. Yet the Laroque commission's work and the debates within which it operated also engaged questions that went beyond economics: questions of vitality, humanity, and citizenship. In its depictions of the elderly as a suffering demographic segregated through both policies and social isolation from the rest of the population, the report questioned and reified the notion of old age as a limit of social citizenship, and bore witness to a prominent representation of aging as decay, dependency, and devaluation of life. The question—the problem—of aging in this period therefore also merits a biopolitical framing that examines the conditioning of life at its limits and its links to processes of dehumanization, as well as the ways in which the state and other institutions both deploy and instrumentalize discourses of health and hygiene toward the end of encouraging, nurturing, and developing the lives of some and allowing others to exist outside of its frame: how they make live and let die.

"A corpse under a suspended sentence": Growing old in the 1970s and 1980s

The Laroque Commission concluded with extensive policy recommendations, many of which the state implemented in the decades to follow. The state added significantly to social spending on the elderly. Through the 1960s and 1970s, the national assembly had created new spaces in hospices for the elderly poor, had passed legislation on hospital reform that guaranteed the elderly a right to their choice of physicians and caregiving institutions, and had begun issuing housing allowances for the elderly as a right of retirement, such as the laws of 31 December 1970 on hospital reform and the law of 16 July 1971 on lodging allocations. The state also developed new activity policies that created institutions such as "lifelong universities" to allow for the productive use of retirees' expanded leisure time, and *"Clubs de troisième âge"* to provide a social space for fighting isolation.

Yet for many little had changed. Simone de Beauvoir, for example, saw the provisions of the Laroque Commission as an insufficient security mechanism that preserved the elderly at the status of bare life. As she argued in her 1970 volume *La Vieillesse*, the elderly in France were a population at the edge of humanity. Like the child, the old person was a dependent being who relied on social intervention for survival. Yet given a choice between investing in the future and rewarding the past, society chose youth over old age. Beauvoir foreshadows Foucault in eerie ways when she points to the operation of a capitalist society that relegated a population to death: that allowed some to die as it compelled others to live. While it did not quite eliminate its "useless mouths," the state's provisions only sustained a bare survival. And while big labor always kept one eye on retirement, its major concern was future employment rather than aging. Therefore, Beauvoir argued,

> society imposes a hideous choice: either sacrifice millions of the young, or allow millions of the old to waste away miserably.... . It is not only the hospitals and the institutions: it is all of society that is, for the old, "death's antechamber."
>
> (Beauvoir, 1970)

As Beauvoir wrote, things were changing somewhat. The population was aging ever more rapidly: between 1962 and 1974, the number of retirees doubled in France, and the number over 65 grew by 25 percent (Lenoir, 1979), but the amount of state aid to the elderly grew six-fold. At the national and local levels, the French further promoted social opportunities for the elderly. Publishers developed magazines, books, and advice manuals for the elderly, and broadcasters produced radio and television programs geared toward an expanding audience of those in the early stages of their retirement. Yet Beauvoir's meditations on the cultural condition of aging in France foreshadowed more empirical work by social scientists on the economic and social precarity of the elderly. Although state spending improved the economic fortunes of many French seniors and the private sector offered new social possibilities, at the levels of both experience and representation things were getting worse if anything. One 1976 study conducted by researchers at a center funded by the Centre National de Recherche Scientifique indicated that the state's protections amounted to little more than "asylumization" in a network of hospices. Poor elderly women with no surviving family in particular were likely to end up in state institutions with medical diagnoses that marked them for social "exclusion" and "segregation" from society; worse, the authors described Paris's hospices as draconian institutions whose disciplinary atmosphere sought submission more than they delivered care, and in which suicides amounted to "a final act of liberty and the only conduct that could check the power of the institution" (Benoît-Lapierre et al., 1980).

Outside of formal institutionalization, many elderly also experienced a widespread sentiment of worthlessness and dehumanization. The sociologist Anne-Marie Guillemard, for example, noted in her 1972 study *La retraite, une mort sociale*, that although many French retirees flourished in their post-work life, others, principally those with lower incomes and insufficient accumulation of social capital, found themselves socially "paralyzed" after retirement (Guillemard, 1972). Between the mid-1970s and the early 2000s, a CNRS-funded team of sociologists led by the demographer Françoise Cribier in Paris conducted an extensive longitudinal study of over 2000 retirees, nearly all in the Paris region, to document the experiences of aging in contemporary France. The interviews reveal a population in deep reflection over its condition on the margins of citizenship. Participants talk about aging in place in a dramatically changing world, one that menaces them with physical and social insecurity. They discuss their increasing isolation from that world, and that world's increasing contempt for them. Perhaps most disturbing, they show an internalization of that contempt: a self-hatred and devaluation of old age as a condition at the limits of humanity.

One woman desperately wanted to avoid moving into a nursing home.

> Old folk's homes, I see them on TV, but that's not really true, TV, because it's not reality. They show us what we want to see.... I went to see a lady in one of these homes.... It was disgraceful.
>
> (LASMAS BI06).

Hearing problems were another disability that affected social life. One man stopped going to church because he couldn't hear the services, and said he no longer liked the company of others, because "it's tiresome to make people repeat themselves two or three times" (LASMAS PL04).

Many complained of isolation as a consequence of a dying social network. Speaking of his friends, one man said, "We see them die one after the other" (LASMAS PL04). Another Parisian man echoed the sentiment: "I don't have a lot of friends because you know at 76 years! There are those who are gone" (LASMAS CO24). The participants also indicated their awareness of rampant ageism, sometimes from youths, sometimes from the middle-aged. One woman who lived in the rue Mouffetard complained about one shopkeeper as indicative of a larger rejection of the old in contemporary Paris: "he's awful with old people. There was a woman who asked him for a paper bag, an old woman, and he said to her, 'How did you carry things in 1914?!'" (LASMAS KE04). Others spoke of being insulted by teens on the street, and about the "demoralizing" depictions of the elderly on television (LASMAS MA51). This was also a product of a changing time; in one participant's view, "The young don't have the respect for the elderly like they used to" (LASMAS "Poussot"). More disturbing is the internalization of ageism. Many participants displayed a near self-hatred in the interviews. One man refused to "watch shows for seniors: I have enough of my own age to deal with without having to deal with that of others" (LASMAS "Giron"). Another man refused to socialize with those his own age because of their constant griping about pain and suffering: "one will complain about this, another about that" (LASMAS "Delattraz"). One woman said that she had to "accept" aging: "It doesn't do anything to cry, to moan, or to complain. Because those around us don't like the old much. They don't like the old very much at all.... . I can't cry about it, that wouldn't help anything" (LASMAS "Guitard"). The participants also described their experiences in *"clubs de troisième âge"* with a contempt that belied the intent behind their development. Most found them "demoralizing." For one woman, "to see these little old people trying to do gymnastic movements, it's enough to make you cry" (LASMAS "Castaing"). In the eyes of one married couple, the senior centers were a symptom of elderly isolation rather than its solution: "The center, oh no, that's for those who are alone, we're two, we don't bother with that" (LASMAS LE12). Another couple agreed, saying, "That doesn't interest us" (LASMAS AU06).

The sentiments of the elderly who participated in this project reveal simultaneously a profound, if veiled, suffering and its disavowal. Few of the participants admitted their isolation directly, providing instead important suggestions of its depth: they mentioned the increasing frequency of their friends' deaths; the difficulty of seeing their children, now busy with their own families; steadily mounting problems navigating staircases and public transportation, leading to longer periods of confinement to the home; increasing fears of changing neighborhoods and environments that exacerbated their reclusion. But many indicated a deeply ingrained self-abnegation that a discourse of aging originating in the postwar era had initiated. As Cribier herself argued in 2004, since the 1970s the French had greeted their dramatic increase in life expectancy not with celebration, but with a sense of "crisis" (Cribier, 2004). If society embraced retirement as a part of adulthood, it did so while rejecting old age as a costly social burden. Yet while Cribier argues that a moral economy of age should trump a fiscal one, it is also clear that the language of aging cast the elderly not merely as a threat to national solvency, but also to humanity: "corpses under a suspended sentence." At the turn of the millennium, national and social rhetoric closely linked to a political economy of marginalization had pushed the elderly to the boundaries of the human.

Marked for death: The elderly and the heat wave

"Depression overtakes me, but I'm used to it. I have no visitors, before I knew the old neighbors, we saw each other a bit, but the new ones I don't know."

Madame Jeanne R., 1995 (d. 14 August 2003, Clichy)

By the summer of 2003, most of Cribier's initial cohort had died: only 145 remained. Only one of them, Madame Jeanne R., died during the heat wave. Jeanne was emblematic of those who had died in many ways. She had been born in 1912, and was 91 when she died on 14 August in a nursing home in Clichy. The study had lost touch with her after interviewing her in 1995. But at that stage she had begun to experience profound disability and isolation. Then in her early eighties, she lived in a tiny apartment in Saint Denis that she had purchased with her husband in the 1930s; she had lived there alone since his death in 1972. By 1995 she was losing her eyesight due to cataracts that surgery had failed to correct, and was diabetic. Despite her two knee replacements, she lived on the third floor with no elevator and had no toilet or running water. She had no children, and her only social contacts were a distant niece and a social worker, without whose help she could not leave the apartment. She was also desperately poor, living below the threshold of taxation (LASMAS RO14). She was a typical victim in a number of ways. Her poverty, disability, age, and sex imprinted her with risk. Like many in her cohort, she was also nearly completely isolated, and had internalized this condition—as well as her poverty—as her natural state.

The one condition that rendered her somewhat less typical was her residence in a nursing home at the time of her death. Only about one in five of those who died during the heat wave died in nursing homes. This is largely due to the fact that closer monitoring of subjects in those environments prevented many unnecessary deaths (Holstein et al., 2005). Far more common were deaths at home, symptomatic of lives lived in desperate isolation as a consequence of a broader social abandonment. This is both an economic and a biopolitical consequence of aging that has linked a devaluation of the elderly with their dehumanization. Claims about the economic threats of aging have accompanied a negative biopolitics—a thanatopolitics—that has at least implicitly suggested death as a technique for influencing population: Boverat's "could we let them die?" of 1951. The heat wave cast this problem in high relief. The expenses of managing the health of an aging population have steadily increased in France (Smith, 2004). By the end of the 1980s, one journalist went so far as to declare the elderly "gluttons" of the health care sector, more interested in preserving life at the limits of existence than in the solvency of the state (Badou, 1989) In an example of particularly bad timing, the French finance minister Francis Mer announced at the end of July 2003 his "solution" to this "problem of health insurance" costs in France: "Quite simply, get rid of the last year of life, because that's what costs the most for social welfare" (*Le Canard enchaîné*, 2003a). Within 2 weeks, this vision had come true. Given the high death toll among the elderly from the heat, the satirical newspaper *Le Canard enchaîné* declared that the ministry of health should be renamed the "ministry of economy" (2003b).

Health minister Jean-François Mattei erred arguably even more greatly. On 11 August, aware of the crisis, he appeared on the news from his vacation home, urging calm and dismissing the numbers as a few hundred excess deaths of those who likely would have died soon anyway. On 14 August, upon his return to Paris, he indicated how little value the elderly held as a constituency. When a reporter asked him why early warning systems for heat risk were not in place, he replied, "You know, the elderly, as they don't have very good memories, often from one moment to another, so the preventive messages that we could air … well, they'd forget them the same day!" (Canal + 2003).

These sorts of sentiments write the elderly poor out of existence as fully human. Isolation of the elderly is an important social reality, one often compounded by poverty. According to recent census data, this is particularly a problem for aging women. Whereas among Parisian men 65 and older, some 30 percent live alone, 90 percent of Parisian women 65 and older are married (Insee, 2011). And the economic circumstances of the elderly, although improved since Beauvoir's day, remain difficult. According recent data, some 10 percent of those above 65 live below the poverty line, and the percentage increases with age (Arnold and Lelièvre, 2015). Above age 75, women are half again as likely to live in poverty (10 percent) as men (7 percent) (Insee, 2016) Living in isolation explains much of this disparity: elderly women, far likelier to live alone than elderly men, cannot benefit from the economies of scale that life as a couple or in a family provides, thus stretching their already smaller disposable income further than among men in the same age group (Arnold and Lelièvre, 2013).

Eugénie offers a useful case for thinking through the realities of isolation and poverty. Eugénie was one of nearly 100 victims of the 2003 heat wave in Paris whose bodies remained unclaimed by family or friends, and who were buried at public expense in the aftermath of the disaster. In the course of my research on the heat wave, I interviewed neighbors and building caretakers about these victims in an attempt to curate their social histories. At 87, Eugénie had lived for as long as anyone can remember in her apartment in the Boulevard Poniatowski in the twelfth arrondissement. Eugénie had a daughter, the building caretaker and neighbors told me, but she had never visited in their recollections. "She was really all alone," the caretaker insisted. She had once had some financial means, but gradually her resources began to dwindle precisely when she began to suffer from increasing disability. Her failing sight had left her "practically blind," her next-door neighbor told me. Her neighbors, quite elderly themselves when I interviewed them in 2007, said that they had tried to do what they could for her. They did shopping for her and ran small errands when they could. But she had stopped leaving her apartment at all, relying exclusively on the charity of her neighbors and of the grocer on the ground floor of the building, who delivered much of what she needed. One of her neighbors told me, "we were nice to her, because she deserved to be liked." But "she lived on very little." She had no social assistant to help her with day-to-day tasks. But with no one to discover her she remained dead in her apartment for more than a week after she died. It was only the stench in the hallway that alerted neighbors to her death. When I visited in 2007, there was still a mark on the door from where health authorities had sealed the apartment until a disinfection team could sanitize it.

Such cases attest to a broad social problem of isolation: an epidemic of elderly vulnerability in a period of extreme crisis. But following the dehumanizing rhetoric of Mattei and others, isolation is less a social problem than it is a function of a growing disablement that excludes the elderly from full membership in the community. Such isolation is therefore inevitable, rendering their deaths also inevitable and merely hastened by extreme temperatures: the biology of aging in modern culture has opted the elderly out of the social contract. By this logic their aging, poverty, and isolation constitute transgressions against citizenship. They exist in a state of exception—as Beauvoir said, in death's waiting room—outside the domain and protections of the human polity. Their lives are those of social abandonment, effectively "invisible," as one journalist put it after the heat wave (France 3, 2003).

Conclusion

Neither high heat mortality nor an aging population were unique to France in 2003. The factors that influenced high mortality were also similar throughout Europe. Elderly populations—the highest risk group for death by heat stroke and dehydration—are on the rise throughout Europe as a result of low fertility rates and increased life expectancy. French women, for example, can now expect to live to over 84, while women in Spain and Italy can expect to live to 83, compared with 80 in the United States (Adveev et al., 2011). Although for much of the twentieth century, France had the oldest population in the world, now Spain, Italy, and Germany have surpassed the nation. These countries also have some of the highest old-age dependency ratios in the world (defined as the ratio of those of retirement age to those in the working-age population), which exceed 35 percent in some regions (European Union, 2013). To this extent, France's experience of aging, isolation, and heat mortality constitutes a case study of western demographic vulnerability in a period of climate instability.

Yet only in France did the heat wave engender a social and political crisis, as well as an impassioned debate over the plight of the elderly in postindustrial urban society. This is one reason that the biopolitics of population offers a useful frame for imagining old age in contemporary France. From a Foucauldian perspective, aging and its social knowledge constituted a dividing practice that measured inclusion and exclusion by reifying social phenomena as biological expressions. Population management signaled aging as a problem to be solved, a phenomenon that generated a broader social knowledge about the elderly as a marginal demographic. Yet whereas other dividing practices have spawned enormous scholarship, historians have been relatively slow to engage with aging, leaving critical questions about the culture of aging in France underexamined.

Yet social knowledge about aging is clearly historically contingent. Between the 1960s and 1980s a new discourse of old age emerged in France, of which the Laroque Report, Beauvoir's *Vieillesse*, Foucault's outline of biopolitics, and Cribier's longitudinal surveys are both artifacts and sources of evidence. Capital, state, and society took a significant interest in the problem of aging for population, linking economic implications to a devaluation of life. Recent interventions on existence at the margins of life, at the margins of citizenship, at the margins of representability in all its senses, suggest ways in which we can consider aging outside of its strictly economic and physiological domains, and in a more broadly cultural one. The humanist crisis that the heat wave engendered prompted a desire to imagine a possibility of an old age at peace after a lifetime of labor. But the grotesque realities of Mattei's and Mer's language, and of a broader language of abnegation of the elderly in contemporary France, belie such a framing by figuring old age primarily as an existence unworthy of life.

Note

1 This is an edited version of a previously published chapter that originally appeared as "Vulnerability and the Political Imagination: Constructing Old Age in Interwar France," in Richard C. Keller (2015), *Fatal Isolation: The Devastating Paris Heat Wave of 2003*, Chicago, United States, University of Chicago Press, pp. 115–49.

References

Adveev Alexandre, Eremenko Tatiana, Festy Patrick, Gaymu Joëlle, Le Bouteillec Nathalie & Sabine Springer (2011), "Populations et tendances démographiques des pays européens (1980–2010)," *Population-F*, Vol. 66, no.1, pp. 9–133.

Arnold Céline & Michèle Lelièvre (2013), "Le niveau de vie des personnes âgées de 1996 à 2009: Une progression moyenne en ligne avec celle des personnes d'âge actif, mais des situations individuelles et générationnelles plus contrastées", *Les revenus et le patrimoine des ménages*, Paris, France, Insee, pp. 33–53.

Arnold Céline & Michèle Lelièvre (2015), "Niveau de vie et pauvreté des personnes âgées de 1996 à 2012", *Retraite et société*, no. 70, pp. 17–40.

Association nationale des assistantes sociales et des assistants sociaux (1961), "Etude sur les réactions et attitudes individuelles des personnes âgées en face des problèmes de la vieillesse et sur les difficultés que rencontrent les assistantes sociales dans leur action auprès des personnes âgées", *Centre des Archives Contemporaines*, 19860269–004.

Badou Gérard (1989), *Les nouveaux vieux*. Paris, France, Le Pré aux clercs.

Beauvoir (de) Simone (1970), *La Vieillesse*, Paris, France, Gallimard.

Benoît-Lapierre Nicole, Cevasco Rithée & Markos Zafiropoulos (1980), *Vieillesse des pauvres: Les chemins de l'hospice*. Paris, France, Editions Economie et Humanisme.

Bourdelais Patrice (1993), *L'âge de la vieillesse*. Paris, France, Odile Jacob.

Boverat Fernand (1939), *Comment nous vaincrons la dénatalité*. Paris, France, L'Alliance nationale contre la dépopulation.

Boverat Fernand (1951a), "Le Vieillissement de la population et ses répercussions sur la sécurité sociale", Haut-Comité Consultatif de la Population et de la Famille, 30 October, 1–3 ter, *Centre des Archives Contemporaines*, 19860269–001.

Boverat Fernand (1951b), "Projet de motion concernant le vieillissement de la population," unpublished manuscript, *Centre des Archives Contemporaines*, 19860269–001.

Canal + (2003), "Canicule 2003," 26 December.

Caradec Vincent (2005), "'Seniors' et 'personnes âgées': Réflexions sur les modes de catégorisation de la vieillesse". In Cribier Françoise & Élise Feller, *Regards croisés sur la protection sociale de la vieillesse*, Paris, France, Comité d'histoire de la sécurité sociale, pp. 313–26.

Castel Robert (1995), *Les métamorphoses de la question sociale: Une chronique du salariat*. Paris, France, Fayard.

CEPV: Commission d'Études du problème de la vieillesse (1960), Procès-Verbaux de la réunion du 8 Octobre 1960, *Centre des Archives Contemporaines*, 19860269–006.

Cribier Françoise (2004), "Vieillesse et citoyenneté". In Cribier Françoise (ed.), *Villes et vieillir*. La Documentation française, pp. 312–19.

Daric Jean (1948), *Vieillissement de la population et prolongation de la vie active*. Paris, France, Presses Universitaires de France.

Esposito Roberto (2008), *Bíos: Biopolitics and Philosophy*. Trans. by Timothy Campbell, Minneapolis, United States, University of Minnesota Press.

European Union (2013), *Eurostat Regional Yearbook 2013*, Luxembourg, Publications Office of the European Union.

Feller Elise (1998), "Les femmes et le vieillissement dans la France du premier XXe siècle," *Clio*, Vol. 7, pp. 199–222.

Feller Elise (2005), *Histoire de la vieillesse en France, 1900–1960: Du vieillard au retraité*. Paris, France, Seli Arslan.

Foucault Michel (1981), *The History of Sexuality, Volume 1: An Introduction*. Trans. by Alan Sheridan, New York, United States, Vintage.

Foucault Michel (2003), *"Society Must be Defended": Lectures at the Collège de France, 1975–1976*. Trans. by David Macey, New York, United States, Picador.

Foucault Michel (2007), *Security, Territory, Population: Lectures at the Collège de France, 1977–1978*. Trans. by Graham Burchell, New York, United States, Picador.

France 3 (2003), *Vieillir ensemble ?*, France 3, 23 September.

France-Soir (1962), "Les personnes âgées ont-elles oui ou non le droit de vivre ?", *France-Soir*, 20 June.

Guillemard Anne-Marie (1972), *La retraite, une mort sociale*. Paris, France, Mouton.

Guillemard Anne-Marie (1993), "Emploi, protection sociale et cycle de vie: Résultats d'une comparaison internationale des dispositifs de sortie anticipée d'activité," *Sociologie du travail*, Vol. 2, no. 63, pp. 4–22.

Guillemard Anne-Marie (2010), *Les défis du vieillissement*. Paris, France, Armand Colin.

HCPF: Haut-Comité Consultatif de la Population et de la Famille (1962), *Politique de la vieillesse: Rapport de la commission d'étude des problèmes de la vieillesse*, Paris, France, La Documentation française.

Holstein Josiane, Canouï-Poitrine Florence, Neumann Anke & Alfred Spira (2005), "Were Less Disabled Patients the Most Affected by 2003 Heat Wave in Nursing Homes in Paris, France?" *Journal of Public Health*, Vol. 27, no. 4, pp. 359–65.

IFOP: Institut Français d'Opinion Publique (n.d.), untitled poll, *Centre des Archives Contemporaines*, 19860269–006.

Insee (2011), Couples - Familles - Ménages en 2008, Département de Paris (75), 30 June 2011, www.insee.fr/fr/statistiques/2017003?sommaire=2133755&geo=DEP-75), accessed 6 February 2017.

Insee (2016), Taux de pauvreté selon l'âge et le sexe en 2014, 6 September 2016, www.insee.fr/fr/statistiques/2408170, accessed 6 February 2017.

Keller Richard C. (2015), *Fatal Isolation: The Devastating Paris Heat Wave of 2003*. Chicago, United States, University of Chicago Press.

Keller Richard C. (2016), "Social geographies of sickness and health in contemporary Paris: Toward a human ecology of mortality in the 2003 heat wave disaster". In Jackson Mark (ed.), *The Routledge History of Disease*. New York, United States, Routledge.

Koos Cheryl (1996), "Gender, Anti-Individualism, and Nationalism: The Alliance Nationale and the Pronatalist Backlash against the Femme modern, 1933–1940", *French Historical Studies*, Vol. 19, no. 3, pp. 699–723.

LASMAS: Laboratoire d'Analyse Secondaire et de Méthodes Appliquées à la Sociologie, Centre Maurice Halbwachs, Paris.

Le Bras Hervé (1993), *Marianne et les lapins: L'obsession démographique*. Paris, France, Hachette.

Le Canard enchaîné (2003a), "Le comique de Bercy", 6 August.

Le Canard enchaîné (2003b), "Francis Mer, devin d'honneur", 20 August.

Lenoir Rémi (1979), "L'invention du 'troisième âge," *Actes de la recherche en sciences sociales,* Vol. 26. no. 1, pp. 57–82.

Levet Maximilienne & Chantal Pelletier (1988), *Papy boom*. Paris, France, Grasset.

Mallon Isabelle (2004), *Vivre en maison de retraite: Le dernier chez-soi*. Rennes, France, Presse Universitaire de Rennes.

Nye Robert (1984), *Crime, Madness, and Politics in Modern France: The Medical Concept of National Decline*. Princeton, United States, Princeton University Press.

Parant Alain (1992), "Croissance démographique et vieillissement", *Population*, Vol. 47, no. 6, pp. 1657–76.

Pick Daniel (1993), *Faces of Degeneration: A European Disorder*. New York, United States, Cambridge University Press.

Roberts Mary Louise (1994), *Civilization without Sexes: Reconstructing Gender in Postwar France, 1914–1939*. Chicago, United States, University of Chicago Press.

Rochefort Robert (2000), *Vive le papy-boom*. Paris, Odile Jacob.

Smith Timothy B. (2004), *France in Crisis: Welfare, Inequality and Globalization since 1980*. New York, United States, Cambridge University Press.

Stearns Peter (1976), *Old Age in European Society: The Case of France*. New York, United States, Holmes and Meier.

Part III

Bridges between science and policy

7 Connecting categories

Age, gender and archaeologies of knowledge

Nicole Kramer

Age and gender are key markers of social difference, but scholars of ageing and of gender studies were slow to seriously engage with each other. Their differing approaches – the former preferring an empirical quantitative approach, the latter more theory-driven – led them to ignore one other for some time. Since the 1990s, however, a growing number of scholars have been calling for the inclusion of gender in ageing studies, and vice versa (Arber & Ginn, 1995; Kampf *et al.*, 2013). This old lacuna is about to be filled – at least in the disciplines of sociology and psychology, as historians are still rather reluctant to integrate perspectives from gender and ageing studies. So far only a few historical studies focus on gender in old age. Most prominent are Pat Thane's extensive writings on the stereotypes and experiences of elderly women in the past using sources ranging from censuses to qualitative survey data, diaries, and memoirs (Botelho & Thane, 2001). Other scholars have focused on elderly men and the debate over the existence of a male climacteric, also known as andropause, that had already become popular among medical experts and the lay press in the 1930s and experienced a resurgence in the 1990s (Siegel Watkins, 2007). Their studies emphasised that the model of female menopause inspired reconsideration of male ageing, changing conceptions of masculinity in the process. Finally, Stephen Katz' work is somewhat relevant here, showing how the category of gender can be useful in analysing the emergence of geriatrics and gerontology. He convincingly highlights how Jean Charcot's *Clinical Lectures of the Diseases of Old Age*, a very influential study of geriatrics published in 1867 (Achenbaum, 1978) that painted a negative image of old age, was shaped by negative stereotypes of elderly women, as indeed most of the patients whose bodies and minds he studied in the Salpêtrière hospital of Paris were female (Katz, 1997).

In line with these pioneering studies, this chapter explores how the production of expert knowledge shaped ageing and older people's lives as new kinds of problems, through ideas and notions of gender. It reflects the current research agenda to study the history of expert knowledge and social reform beyond the boundaries of the nation-state (Herren, 2006). When have gerontologists taken interest in gender issues and ideas of femininity/ masculinity, and to what effect? How have feminist approaches impacted the knowledge of ageing? Answers to these questions should emerge by focusing on two concepts and the debates surrounding them. The chapter first addresses the debate about the 'feminisation of old age' that was active in the second half of the twentieth century. Data produced by demographers stressed the life expectancy differences between men and women and old-age gender differences in general. In doing so, they drew particular attention to elderly women, many of whom are at risk for poverty late in life, resulting in a problematisation of old age. The chapter then turns to how feminist theorists have influenced knowledge of ageing and the elderly with the emergence of the concept of care in the 1980s. Drawing attention to the overlooked unpaid personal services that are mainly carried out by women within the family, an exploration of the carer's movement in Britain will show how their fight also contributed to framing ageing as a problem.

Following the example of other scholars, the use of case studies serves to shed light on a vast issue from different perspectives (Black, 2010). By using in-depth examples of the production of knowledge on age and gender, the chapter is intended to elucidate the history of the 'appropriation of the social by science' (Raphael, 1996; Ash, 2002). Based on examples from Great Britain, the Federal Republic of Germany and international organisations, it aims to map the relationship between expert knowledge and policies concerning ageing and gender. It therefore covers the roles of academic networks and political institutions (namely the Council of Europe), and voluntary organisations like the British Carers National Association and its predecessors are examined in greater depth. In the process, the chapter also draws upon the literature, which adapts Foucauldian concepts such as the archaeology of knowledge (Foucault, 1971) to the exploration of understandings of ageing (Powell & Biggs, 2003). Primary sources from German and British Archives, including correspondence, minutes and surveys, provide insights into how knowledge of age and gender was created in a variety of places, exploring the highways and byways of the processes of making systems of thought and practice. The article will discuss the extent to which expert knowledge informs policy-making, while at the same time exploring how the discourse on ageing and gender was influenced by social and political changes.

The following analysis is focused on the latter half of the twentieth century, especially the decades of the 1960s through the 1980s when the social sciences and psychology entered the field of ageing studies and broke the hegemony of biological and medical approaches to the field (Katz, 1996; Thane, 2000). Moreover, during this period, Western industrial countries were marked by a massive expansion of social security programmes directed at older people (among other population groups), and pensioners and those suffering from frailty chief among them (Nullmeier & Kaufmann, 2012). Finally, the decades of the 1960s throughout the 1980s were the heyday of activism by social movements for the rights of women, the elderly, and disabled persons. All in all, this period was characterised by a growing number of actors producing statements about old age and gender.

The feminisation of old age

Over the course of the twentieth century, the national population statistics of most industrialised countries showed a gender gap in life expectancy, and women outnumbering men at advanced ages. Study of long-term data demonstrates that gender differences started to widen early in the century in countries such as France and England. This trend came to a halt during the 1970s, since improvements in the life expectancy of men at the time led to a decrease in the gender gap (Thorslund, 2013). After the Second World War, politicians and academic experts alike became very aware of this 'feminisation of old age', although the term was not coined until later.

Demographic knowledge and the gender gap in life expectancy

Demographers interested in the European region were among the first to discuss the significance of the gender gap in life expectancy and its consequences for population developments in depth. The phenomenon was one of the main topics at the first European Population Conference, which was organised in cooperation with the Council of Europe in 1966. Demographers' reasons for paying so much attention to the population ageing process and gender differences in old age become clear upon study of the conference papers. They reflect a major shift in demographic discourse that started after the First World War. The leading demographic paradigm had long been informed by the thinking of Thomas Robert Malthus, feeding fear of overpopulation. After the First World War, decreasing fertility and the high number of deaths from the conflict fostered a change in thinking. Theories about shrinking populations gained some popularity, and not only in right-wing circles (Szreter, 1993; Lengwiler, 2007), while discourse on population ageing became part of the new demographic paradigm. Increasing life expectancy and the growing number of elderly continued to concern demographers in the second half of the century. Even more so as this topic helped to shift the focus of academic discourse back to Europe: international conferences were mainly concerned with developing countries, where overpopulation was still a significant phenomenon. Therefore, when Jean Bourgeois-Pichat, president of the European Population Conference and a leading French demographer, gave his keynote speech he justified narrowing the scope to Europe by citing its specific features, including the population-ageing trend. He moreover saw Europe as a laboratory for the whole world:

> It is in Europe that solutions will first have to be found to the economic and cultural problems which the end of the demographic revolution will bring. Perhaps it is no exaggeration to say that it is in Europe that the future of the human race will be decided.[1]

Papers given at the 1966 conference stressed that alongside phenomenon like declining fertility rates and a growing number of elderly, increasing gender differences also characterise the populations of European countries. The demographers' discussions eventually contributed to the Council of Europe's decision to add population ageing to its topics of concern. The council established a commission headed by Pierre Laroque, a French social security expert, to develop a resolution on social and medico-social policy in old age.[2] The Council of Europe, founded in 1949, was important in the circulation of ideas and models for social reform, as its 1965 adoption of the European Social Charter defining social rights attests. While in the 1960s and 1970s social policy was secondary to the main aim of economic harmonisation and collaboration in the integration process of the European Union and its predecessor organisations (Kingreen, 2014), the Council of Europe already provided a platform for discussing social reforms. It worked alongside organisations like the International Labour Organization (ILO), whose role as forum for thought on transnational social policy is widely recognised (Kott & Droux, 2012). Experts working for both organisations contributed to their close ties. Pierre Laroque, for example, was a leading figure in the ILO's efforts to restructure European countries' social security systems in the 1950s (Guinand, 2014), so he had already earned credentials as transnational social policy expert when he was appointed chairman of the Council of Europe's commission on the elderly in 1966.

The commission started by gathering data on population ageing and the situation of the elderly from every member state. The commission's research revealed, among other things, that old women were an especially vulnerable group. Many of them lived in poverty and depended on benefits from state welfare programmes. These findings echoed those of national surveys; for instance, in 1965 Peter Townsend and Dorothy Wedderburn stated that single and widowed women in Britain 'are the poorest among the old today' (Townsend & Wedderburn, 1965). Many studies had discovered that gender not only affected life expectancy, but also social status and living situation in old age (Cole & Utting, 1962; Shanas *et al.*, 1968). Women might have the chance of living longer, but they did so under poor conditions.

Gender inequalities in pension systems

The explanation for female poverty in old age pointed to the fact that women were burdened with disadvantages accruing from their position on the labour market. In general, they earned less and thus could not build up savings. Moreover, older women's poverty reflected gender-specific inequalities produced by state welfare programmes. First and foremost, pension systems were known for creating and reinforcing gendered differences, especially when benefits were related to wage labour. Absence of employment experience led to reduced benefits for women or their not being entitled to benefits at all. For example, until the 1970s women in Britain were worse off than men under state schemes, although William Beveridge had already recommended tackling gender inequalities by extending pension system coverage to housewives. His endeavours were unsuccessful, and many women continued to have difficulty earning entitlements in their own right and were consequently dependent on their husbands (Thane, 2006). In the (West) German Welfare state, which is often seen as counter-model to the British, the majority of the female population was confronted with the same disadvantages, and were in some respects even worse off.

West Germany exemplifies a pension system tailored to fit a standardised labour profile, thus reinforcing the male-breadwinner model and excluding housewives from the pension insurance coverage. They had, in fact, gained access to the pension system for a short time, when the Nazi government opened the pension programme to voluntary enrolment for all Germans in 1937. This development fitted the Nazi conception of a people's community, but it also brought in more revenue. The inclusion of housewives was clearly not lawmakers' intent, but rather an unforeseen consequence. In 1957, housewives' voluntary ability to enrol was withdrawn by one of the most important pensions acts in the history of the German welfare state (Haerendel, 2007). This is even more remarkable because the reform is widely known for improving pensioners' situations by changing how benefits were calculated (pensions were tied to gross wages), so although it generally fought old-age poverty it proved to aggravate the gender gap. Low women's pensions also resulted from the fact that until 1967 women could opt out of pension insurance when they got married and left employment (Noll, 2010). This had severe long-term implications that feminist politicians had been pointing out since the 1920s.

All in all, most countries – except Sweden, known for its generous and gender-neutral old age social security system – established welfare state schemes that favoured male workers and were not designed to meet the needs of most women, especially those who performed informal care work. The expansion of the welfare state in the post-war period did little to change this fact, but the improvement of social security for women did become a major topic in many industrial countries over the 1960s and 1970s.

The Council of Europe's resolution on social and medico-social policy in old age is a case in point. The first draft of the Laroque commission report contained far-reaching recommendations for welfare benefits for housewives; indeed Laroque himself was a strong advocate for improving the pension rights of women (Laroque, 1972; Brocas, 2004). The first draft's innovative recommendations were nonetheless stripped from the document over the course of negotiations. Representatives of member-state governments set out to remove the parts that clashed with the main principals of their respective social security systems. Additionally, the German delegate was among those fearing that the resolution might someday justify binding supranational decisions and intervention by international organisations.

Eventually, most member states did introduce provisions directed at the female population. Great Britain (like France) had already implemented such reforms in the 1970s. The Social Security Act (1975) and the introduction of state earnings-based pensions significantly improved women's entitlements in their own right. However, the second pillar of the pension system, occupational schemes, still supported the male-breadwinner model (Thane, 2006). In West Germany it was not until the mid-1980s that the Christian Democratic/Liberal government began to remedy the pension system's gender bias by allowing women to accumulate pension credit based on their unpaid caregiving work (Kuller, 2007).

Demographisation of the gendered social

It can thus be concluded that the concept of the feminisation of old age at that time was a collection of diverse observations, from the gender gap in life expectancy and the poverty of female pensioners to the fact that women were more likely to enter residential care facilities than men. Demographic knowledge on gender differences in life expectancy was connected to findings about the characteristics of women's lives in old age. Such a 'demographisation of the social', a term coined by Eva Barlösius, was quite common in the twentieth century. Demographers entered the field of sociology, which led social risks and needs to be identified as consequences of demographic developments, making them seem inevitable. Moreover, demographic changes leading to sex ratio and age cohort imbalances were perceived as problematic (Barlösius, 2007; Messerschmidt, 2014). The 'surplus' of elderly women is a case in point.

Similar to what Stephen Katz described in his exploration of the writings of Jean Charcot, the discourse on the feminisation of old age also shows how gender and age discrimination influenced each other. This time, however, it was the other way around: the negative realities facing the elderly, such as poverty, frailty and institutionalisation, were conceived as only concerning women. Those talking about a feminisation of old age led elderly women to emerge as a problematic group.

This discourse furthermore led to actions to counter the described phenomena. While the overrepresentation of women in residential care was a rather recent observation that experts only came to realise in the 1950s and 1960s, the discrimination against women in social security programmes had been decried by first-wave feminist activists in several countries since the First World War. Feminists continued stressing elderly women's hardships after 1945 as well, although some gerontologists accused second-wave feminism of having neglected such issues, and some notable exceptions are worth mentioning. In 1970 Simone de Beauvoir published her famous account *La Vieillesse* (translated as *The Coming of Age*), which today is considered to be one of the first writings uniting gender studies and gerontological approaches (de Beauvoir, 1970; Katz, 1997). The French philosopher uncovered the many ways in which older women are materially and culturally stigmatised and penalised. Moreover, in the mid-1970s some women's groups launched the 'wages for housework' campaign, which was inspired by the writings of Selma James and Mariarosa Della Costa (Zellmer, 2011; Bracke, 2014). They criticised the gendered division of paid wage labour and informal care work, which they saw as a consequence of the capitalist order in society. By demanding salaries from the state for women performing family care and household duties, they also touched on issues like pensions schemes' discrimination against female caregivers.

This time, unlike earlier in the century, the voices decrying elderly women's disadvantages no longer went unheard. It seems that the hardships of the female population in later years only began to draw interest outside feminist circles when demographers contributed to the discourse by pointing to the feminisation of old age.

Caring in an ageing society

Although scholars from women's and gender studies long neglected study of the elderly, they certainly showed considerable interest in the people caring for them. Their research on care and carers did not study them as a field where the interests of gerontology and gender studies overlap, however, as will be seen in the following case study of the carer's movement in Great Britain. After the Second World War the country adopted far-reaching social policy reforms originating in the 1942 Beveridge Report. The welfare state's choice to take a universal approach in expanding its reach was partly intended to help the elderly population. Despite increasing state intervention, however, the voluntary sector remained important in the provision of social welfare, especially for groups that were at the margins of the welfare state, and a strong carer's movement based in voluntary organisations began to emerge in the 1960s. Finally, British university scholars played a key role conceptualising ageing and care work. Altogether, these circumstances make Great Britain a good site for the following exploration.

Gerontology and the social ties of the elderly

How did the experts' interest in care and carers shape views on old age and the elderly? Female carers became the focus of surveys and studies as gerontologists started exploring the social status and social relations of older people. In Great Britain, Peter Townsend, mainly known for his poverty research and child poverty activism, was one of the first to focus on the elderly and their caregivers (Phillipson, 2010). Before going on to become one of the most influential sociologists and gerontologists in Britain, he began research on the family relations of the elderly in 1954. Three years later he published his seminal book *The Family Life of Old People* (Townsend, 1957). The study was part of a larger research programme and should be understood in relation to the newly founded Institute of Community Studies in East London.[3] The Institute soon gained influence as one of the main empirical social research centres, which examined the working-class town of Bethnal Green as 'site for social change' (Savage, 2011).

Alongside its role of knowledge production as a research centre, the Institute of Community Studies should also be seen as a major public policy think tank. The initial scope of the research organisation was to examine the effects of the expanding post-war welfare state on community and family structures. While Michael Young and Peter Willmott explored family relations by looking at couples with children, Townsend turned towards old people.

The study stressed the active family life most elderly in Bethnal Green experienced. Townsend demonstrated that the proximity of relatives meant that old people received care. But perhaps his most striking findings concerned the help that the elderly, primarily older women, gave to younger generations; a grandmother who did some cooking, cleaning and child-minding came in very handy for some couples. Like Michael Young, Townsend stressed the female-centric character of the close-knit extended family, as most care was provided by female family members and the findings pointed towards a 'special bond between grandmother, daughter, and daughter's child' (Townsend, 1957, p. 228). Relying on the anthropological concept of matriliny, Institute of Community Studies researchers laid the groundwork for discussing the value of female family care work.

Asserting the intensity of family ties, the researchers challenged the arguments of politicians lamenting the 'loosening of family ties and insistence on individual rights and privileges' (King, 1955, p. 45). Willmott, Young and Townsend also took a stand against sociological theorists, especially Talcott Parsons and his claim that the process of industrialisation had put an end to kinship-based society. Parsons believed modern industrial societies were based on isolated nuclear families with no obligations to wider kin.

Around that time many researchers rediscovered family and kinship as an issue worth examining in more detail, and there were many surveys concerning family and kinship structures in Britain and other Western industrialised countries. Townsend's work influenced other researchers testing his conclusions in other areas and social configurations, especially among the middle classes. Their studies found Townsend's conclusions held up to the challenge – family reciprocity applied well beyond the working classes. Townsend himself expanded the scope of his research beyond Bethnal Green. Along with Ethel Shanas, who studied the elderly and their families in the United States (Shanas, 1962), he joined a group of pioneer gerontologists working on a multi-national survey assembling data about old people and their housing conditions, health status, income, and personal relationships in the US, Great Britain and Denmark. *Old People in Three Industrial Societies* became a landmark in gerontology stressing universal developments in ageing in Western industrial countries (Shanas *et al.*, 1968).

Social scientists may have shifted the focus from the aged body to older peoples' lifestyles and social networks, but they stuck to the question of defining good/bad ageing. Being integrated into close-knit family networks became a criteria distinguishing normal from pathologic forms of ageing. As Townsend stated in his conclusion:

> The poorest people, not only financially, were those without an active family life. They had the fewest resources in time of need. Yet many of them denied they were lonely.... . Elderly isolates seemed likely to make disproportionately heavy claims on health and welfare services.
>
> (Townsend, 1957, p. 229)

By using the term 'poor', Townsend made it very clear that missing kinship ties were as problematic as bad economic conditions. He moreover highlighted that loneliness in old age was not merely a private matter but became a collective concern as soon as elderly had to rely on provisions of the welfare state. The study drew attention to the fact that the older people who entered geriatric hospitals or old people's homes generally had no relatives. And yet living in an institution was seen as a stopgap, as Townsend eventually demonstrated in his follow-up study on residential care, *The Last Refuge* (Townsend, 1962).

In general, sociologists and other commentators (most of them male) at that time were taking female carers for granted (Struthers, 2013). Townsend was no exception, not giving much thought to the gendered nature of care. In contrast, his colleagues Young and Willmott were among the few to admit that working-class women face risks linked to their role as wife and mother, and pointed to the problem of their economic dependence on male family members (Willmott & Young, 1960).

The interest gerontologists developed in family and kinship ties has to be seen in a broader context. In England as in other Western industrial countries, the post-Second World War period is known for a discourse on marriage and family as the backbone of a stable society. Against the background of wartime experiences such as evacuation, psychologists and social scientists (John Bowlby notable among them) argued strongly for the importance of close mother–child relations and the danger of separation. Their ideas and concepts spread beyond scientific circles into discussions among politicians and ministers as well as in the media (Thane & Evans, 2013). Townsend and others looked at the family from the opposite end of the life course, but they elevated family relations in the same way, calling them decisive to the wellbeing of old people. This appreciation of strong kinship ties is all the more interesting because it indicates that the post-war family discourse was not exclusively limited to conservative circles. Townsend and Young are known as left-wing social scientists and campaigners, yet both were critical of the left (and more pointedly of the Labour Party) for its neglect of family care (Townsend, 1958; Butler, 2015). They asked for a reconsideration of socialist conceptions of society, which were centred on the workplace.

Hence, research like Peter Townsend's has contributed to the popularity of the idea of community care. In Great Britain, as in other countries, it became very influential in welfare state policies for the elderly. It not only seemed less expensive than residential care, but it was also seen as better choice regarding old people's wellbeing (Struthers, 2013).However common it became in gerontological research to praise family networks' valuable role in old age and community care, the number of critical voices would begin to grow in the 1970s. Feminist and gender-studies approaches played a crucial role in this shift.

The British carers' movement and the down-sides of community care

Organisations advocating the interests of carers played a highly significant role in shifting the focus from the family lives of old people to family caregivers for the elderly. The National Council for the Single Woman and her Dependants (NCSWD) had been founded in 1965 by Mary Webster, who worked as a minister and teacher. She had cared for her frail parents for many years, which motivated her to found the organisation. It was initially exclusively for unmarried women,[4] but in the late 1970s the organisation had to rethink its focus.

Another organisation was founded around the same time: established in 1981, the Association of Carers was much more inclusive and addressed all carers' rights from the outset. It was founded by Judith Oliver, who cared for her disabled husband. These two organisations had a great deal in common, and they merged in 1987 to become the Carers National Association. In 2001 it was renamed Carers UK (Barnes, 2001).

These organisations were part of the voluntary sector, offering services and giving voice to carers who supported disabled – mainly elderly – relatives or friends. Most members were carers themselves, and so the organisation's local branches qualified as support or mutual aid groups. Matthew Hilton and others have shown that the voluntary sector is very important to the history of twentieth-century Britain, thus challenging the older theory of a decline in voluntary action due to the expansion of the welfare state. According to Hilton, it is quite the contrary: the number of registered charities rose, as did the number of volunteers (Hilton, 2011). Those exploring the history of voluntary action in the latter half of the twentieth century stress the flexibility of this so-called third sector to address new needs and the emergence of new social problems. Charities offered help for groups that were neglected by public policy, like single mothers or drug users (Crowson, 2011).

Many of these more general developments apply to the carers' organisation, too. They succeeded in organising people whose needs and rights had been largely overlooked in the post-war period. At first the main aim was to provide services like sitting-in schemes and respite care that offer short-term relief for carer hardship, but trying to influence policy grew to be very important alongside this practical work. The voluntary sector was increasingly characterised by a considerable professionalism that was reflected in the pursuit of scientific research to lend legitimacy to their claims as well as the employment of trained staff and the adoption of professional fundraising and lobbying methods (Hilton *et al.*, 2013).

The campaigning was mainly aimed at improving financial provisions, and single women who cared for an adult relative were initially the focus of their efforts. The NCSWD fought against the discriminatory regulations confronting single women as opposed to men and married women. They also attacked welfare state schemes that were mainly based on paid labour, as well as entitlements earned through marriage. The invalid care allowance, which was introduced by the Labour Government in 1976, thus became one of its main objectives. The new benefit was explicitly designed to meet the needs of single persons who had given up work in order to care for severely disabled persons for at least 35 hours a week, meaning that married women were ineligible for it. Only in 1986 did the British Government review its position and decide to include them, anticipating the ruling of the European Court of Justice on the matter.[5] The Association of Carers chose Jackie Drake, carer for her mother suffering from dementia, as a test case. The trial was based on European Economic Community directive concerning social security systems.

Internal carers' movement discussions about the campaign for an invalid care allowance tell us much about shifting gender roles and the reconception of assumptions about family relations. To be clear, the Carers National Association and its predecessors did not participate in the women's liberation movement, and in fact some representatives even distanced themselves from any feminist agenda. These organisations nevertheless tackled feminist issues like discrimination against unmarried women, the exploitation of women's unpaid care work, and the blind eye the welfare state turned towards domestic labour. This reflects the picture recent research has drawn of a vibrant and diverse feminism in the 1970s and 1980s (Segal, 2013), showing that one need not look far beyond the core of the women's liberation movement to see many forms of feminist identities and ideas in Great Britain. Although it is difficult to identify a direct influence from the feminist movement, widening the scope of feminist research exposes situations that may independently manifest feminist thinking. I argue that the carers' organisations are key sites for studying changing conceptions of gender-specific divisions of labour and the rights of women that stay at home. They cultivated a rather pragmatic brand of feminism that corresponded to the day-to-day concerns they had to deal with and the plain and simple solutions they had to deliver. This is in line with Matthew Hilton's research findings on British non-governmental organisations (NGOs), concluding that such a pragmatic approach characterises the voluntary sector in general (Hilton, 2011).

Carers' identities and the feminist conception of 'social care'

The NCSWD started conducting surveys among single women in 1965, when a small group of 47 respondents was interviewed in the Southampton area.[6] This early survey served mainly as a way for the founding members of NCSWD to get in touch with a wider group of single women and learn about concerns that lay beyond their own experience. The surveys were important to the rather small voluntary organisation, allowing them to claim to represent all single women, or at least the majority of them. Mike Savage has emphasised that 'surveys were used to delineate the characteristics of particular social groups' (2011), to which I would add that this was not only a process of external ascription but also a self-description technique in order to create a carer identity.

Scholars studying carers' experiences and care policies have stated that the term 'carer' is a social invention of the later twentieth century, and that carers' organisations can be credited with shaping it (Bytheway & Johnson, 2008). In 1995 the Carers (Recognition and Service) Act defined a carer as 'an individual providing or intending to provide care on a regular basis'. This act gave carers a legal status when only a few decades earlier the term had not yet entered use in the English language, or at least not in such a specific way.

But why did the term carer become so popular, and what did the people using it mean by it? In studying the carers' organisation's memoranda and pamphlets, one finds the term carer is used to describe a group within society and a category to which individuals could claim membership. The organisation's surveys helped to define this group and more importantly produced quantified information that became very important in media and political discourse. In the late 1980s survey results spoke of six million carers, a fact which drew some attention. Statistics also constructed the average carer, who was female and middle aged, and had to quit her job, was hindered from entry into the labour market, or at least had to reduce her working hours in order to devote her time to the person in her charge. There was a strong feminisation of care, which led to the neglect of male carers (who did exist) as well as other categories of social inequality, racial in particular. The speech of carer's organisation members and people seeking their help show that the term carer became part of their language and their self-description. Carers' organisation surveys marked the beginnings of conceptualising care as a 'labour of love'. This strand of research was picked up by feminist theorists who taught us much about the gendering of and by welfare states. It is no coincidence that in the 1980s one of the main feminist thinkers on the welfare state, Jane Lewis, had conducted a study based on interviews with carers whom she found through the NCSWD and the Association of Carers. Her book *Daughters Who Care* launched her into the research field of care under the welfare state (Lewis & Meredith, 1988).

The carers' organisation helped shape the carer identity in a positive way. The carer was not someone in need of assistance, but someone who provided assistance to others. Emphasising the carer's performance was important to claiming welfare entitlements, a strategy that benefitted greatly from feminist researchers' conception of care as labour. This development is even more interesting in the light of the concept of dependency, which, as Nancy Fraser and Linda Gordon demonstrated, had been stigmatised and feminised over the course of the twentieth century (Fraser & Gordon, 1994). But the carers' movement challenged the view of female carers as dependent by pointing to the fact that they cared for someone else who was dependent on them. In doing so, however, they retained the negative conception of dependency and reinforced the dependent/independent dichotomy.

This leads to the question of which concepts of ageing the carers' organisations produced, and more generally, how feminist concerns shaped the idea of dependent elderly.

The surveys paint a very different picture than the studies by gerontologists like Peter Townsend, mentioned earlier. Although they agreed on the importance of family care for the elderly, the carers' organisation challenged their assertions concerning extended family networks. They maintained that caring was not a team effort, but a one-woman show. Many carers felt abandoned rather than supported by other relatives.[7] They felt alone.

Finally, focusing on the needs of carers significantly changed perceptions of the elderly, as indicated by a 1979 report called 'The Loving Trap', which was based on 700 questionnaires from female carers. The authors were anxious to shed light on the hardships of female carers.

Talking about carers 'sacrifices' and 'hardships' they had to face, let alone references to their risk of 'isolation' also reflect back on those who were at the receiving end of the care relationship. While Townsend and others had portrayed old people as active family members, emphasising the reciprocity of support structures, the carer surveys went back to shaping negative images of old age which many gerontologists believed they had proven wrong. Looking at the carers' organisation's reports and surveys, they have a discernable tendency to portray the elderly as destitute persons clinging on the carer in a childlike, sometimes tyrannical manner.

The carers' movement thus created a discourse marginalising old age. It contributed to shape the idea of the fourth age, 'a social imaginary realised and revealed in the discourse and practices of third persons' (Gilleard & Higgs, 2013, p. 376).

Conclusion

The chapter began by stating that scholars of ageing and gender studies had ignored each other for quite some time, but the subsequent historical perspective went on to show that ideas of gender have influenced conceptions of age, and vice versa. The chapter retraced the work of Stephen Katz and others in the study of the discourses of the feminisation of old age and care, offering new insights into how conceptions of gender and age are interrelated. The first observation is that when life expectancy data shows a widening gender gap, 'elderly women' as a group become a target public for research and policy. The so-called feminisation of old age not only reflects a surplus of women among the elderly, but also risks of poverty, health problems and institutionalisation that accentuate with advancing age, ultimately leading the negative aspects of old age to become associated with the older women. In contrast, the term was less used for describing the phenomenon of older people, for the most part women, taking on care duties for their grandchildren.

The focus then shifted to the debate on care and carers in the 1970s and 1980s. If after the Second World War gerontologists claimed that the best way of growing old was to live with family, taking women's care obligations for granted, feminist thinkers later challenged the idealisation of the concept of community care. Pointing to the vulnerability of female carers had some implications for the people in their care, however: while carers were presented as carrying the burdens of ageing, the elderly were portrayed as needy and dependent. This observation is all the more interesting because it shows how the interests of two vulnerable groups, and the movements fighting for their rights, could stand in the way of each other. It raises questions about the ambivalence of social rights activism, especially in the 1970s–1980s, which is considered to be the golden age of new social movements.

As for the relationship between politics and expert knowledge, the chapter provided ample evidence as to how they contributed to each other. It first became clear that expert knowledge drew governmental awareness to social problems. The way in which seemingly incontrovertible evidence such as demographic or survey data was presented proved to be a key to successfully setting the agenda. Second, the actors involved in knowledge production are not only found within governmental bodies of the nation-state, but also in international and voluntary organisations. Study of the latter and how they were involved in knowledge production of old age made it clear that they participated in enacting governance by shaping perceptions of social problems and reforms.

In concluding this chapter, it should be said that the road to exploring interactions between ageing and gender studies is still wide open. One such new research agenda might be to explore men and masculinities in old age, which would widen the scope of both gerontologists interested in gender issues and historians interested in twentieth-century masculinity.

Notes

1 Speech of Jean Bourgeois-Pichat, Conseil de l'Europe, Conférence demographique européenne, 30 August 1966, Official Documents of the Conference, vol. IV, Strasbourg 1966, p. 4.
2 Draft of the Resolution 'on social and medico-social policy for old age', 12 July 1968, BArch Koblenz, B 189/2398, Bd. 2.

3 The Institute of Community Studies was established in 1953 and was mainly financed by the Nuffield Foundation and the Elmgrant Trust. In 2005 it was renamed The Young Foundation, but it is still located in Bethnal Green.
4 Report 'Caring Single Women: 10 Years Later', February 1976, Derby Branch NCSWD, Derbyshire Record Office, D3132/20/1-17.
5 House of Lords, Debate, 23.6.1986, Historical Hansard, vol 477 cc26-31.
6 Report on a Survey in the Southampton Area, 1965, Greater Manchester Record Office G/CA/1/2.
7 'The Dynamics of Informal Caring', Report prepared by MAS surveys Ltd for NCSWD, June 1979, Greater Manchester Record Office G/CA/1/8.

References

Achenbaum Andrew W. (1978), *Old Age in the New Land: The American Experience since 1790*. Baltimore, The Johns Hopkins University Press.

Arber Ann & Jay Ginn (1995), *Connecting Gender and Ageing: A Sociological Approach*. Buckingham and Philadelphia, Open University Press.

Ash Mitchell (2002), 'Wissenschaft und Politik als Ressourcen für einander'. In vom Bruch Rüdiger, *Wissenschaften und Wissenschaftspolitik – Bestandaufnahmen zu Formationen, Brüchen und Kontinuitäten im Deutschland des 20. Jahrhunderts*. Stuttgart, Franz Steiner Verlag, pp. 32–51.

Barlösius Eva (2007), 'Die Demographisierung des Gesellschaftlichen'. In Barlösius Eva & Daniela Schiek, *Demographisierung des Gesellschaftlichen. Analysen und Debatten zur demographischen Zukunft Deutschlands*. Wiesbaden, VS Verlag für Sozialwissenschaften, pp. 9–34.

Barnes Marian (2001), 'From Private Carer to Public Actor. The Carers' Movement in England'. In Daly Mary, *Care Work. The Quest for Security*, Geneva. International Labour Office, pp. 195–209.

Black Lawrence (2010), *Redefining British Politics: Culture, Consumerism and Participation, 1954–70*. Basingstoke, Palgrave Macmillan.

Botelho Lynn & Pat Thane (2001), *Women and Ageing in British Society Since 1500*. New York and London, Longman.

Brocas Anne-Marie (2004), 'Les femmes et les retraités en France: un aperçu historique', *Retraite et société*, vol. 43, no. 3, pp. 11–33.

Bracke Maud Anne (2014), *Women and the Reinvention of the Political. Feminism in Italy, 1968–1983*. New York & London, Routledge.

Butler Lise (2015), 'Michael Young, the Institute of Community Studies, and Politics of Kinship', *Twentieth Century British History*, Vol. 26, no. 2, pp. 210–234.

Bytheway Bill & Julia Johnson (2008), 'The Social Construction of Carers'. In Johnson Julia & Corinne de Souza, *Understanding Health and Social Care. An Introductory Reader*. London, SAGE, pp. 223–232.

Cole Dorothy & John Edward George Utting (1962), *The Economic Circumstances of Old People*, Welwyn, Codicote Press.

Crowson Nicholas (2011), 'Introduction: The Voluntary Sector in 1980s Britain', *Contemporary British History*, Vol. 25, no. 4, pp. 491–498.

Daly Mary & Jane Lewis (2000), 'The Concept of Social Care and the Analysis of Contemporary Welfare States', *British Journal of Sociology*, Vol. 51, no. 2, pp. 261–298.

De Beauvoir Simone (1970), *The Coming of Age*. New York, W.W. Norton.

Fraser Nancy & Linda Gordon (1994), 'A Genealogy of Dependency: Tracing a Keyword of the U.S. Welfare System', *Signs*, Vol. 19, no. 2, pp. 309–336.

Gilleard Chris & Paul Higgs (2013), 'The Fourth Age and the Concept of a Social Imaginary', *Journal of Aging Studies*, Vol. 27, no. 4, pp. 368–376.

Guinand Cédric (2014), 'A Pillar of Economic Integration: The ILO and the development of Social Security in Western Europe'. In Mechi Lorenzo, Migani Guia & Francesco Petrini, *Networks of Global Governance. International Organisations and European Integration in Historical Perspective*. Newcastle upon Tyne, Cambridge Scholars, pp. 111–133.

Haerendel Ulrike (2007), 'Geschlechterpolitik und Alterssicherung. Frauen in der gesetzlichen Rentenversicherung von den Anfängen bis zur Reform 1957', *Deutsche Rentenversicherung*, Vol. 62, no. 2/3, pp. 99–124.

Herren Madeleine (2006), 'Diskussionsforum: Sozialpolitik und die Historisierung des Transnationalen', *Geschichte und Gesellschaft*, Vol. 32, no. 4, pp. 542–559.

Hilton Matthew (2011), 'Politics is Ordinary: Non-governmental Organizations and Political Participation in Contemporary Britain', *Twentieth Century British History*, Vol. 22, no. 2, pp. 230–268.

Hilton Matthew, McKay James, Crowson Nicholas & Jean-François Mouhot (2013), *The Politics of Expertise. How NGOs Shaped Modern Britain*. Oxford, Oxford University Press.

Kampf Antje, Kampj Antje, Marshall Barbara & Alan Petersen (2013), *Aging Men, Masculinities and Modern Medicine*. New York, Routledge.

Katz Stephen (1996), *Disciplining Old Age. The Formation of Gerontological Knowledge*. Charlottesville, University of Virginia Press.

Katz Stephen (1997), 'Charcot's Older Women: Bodies of Knowledge at the Interface of Aging Studies and Women's Studies', *Journal of Women and Aging*, Vol. 9, no. 4, pp. 73–87.

King Geoffrey (1955), 'Policy and Practice'. In *Old Age in the Modern World. Report of the Third Congress of the International Association of Gerontology*. London, Livingstone, pp. 36–45.

Kingreen Torsten (2014), 'Epochen der Europäisierung des Sozialrechts'. In Masuch Peter et al., *Grundlagen und Herausforderung des Sozialstaats. Denkschrift 60 Bundessozialgericht*. Berlin, Erich Schmidt Verlag, pp. 313–332.

Kott Sandrine & Joëlle Droux (2012), 'Introduction: A Global History Written from the ILO', in Kott Sandrine & Joëlle Droux, *Globalizing Social Rights. The International Labour Organization and Beyond*, Basingstoke, Palgrave Macmillan, pp. 1–14.

Kuller Christiane (2007), 'Soziale Sicherung von Frauen – ein ungelöstes Strukturproblem im männlichen Wohlfahrtsstaat. Die Bundesrepublik im europäischen Vergleich', *Archiv für Sozialgeschichte*, Vol. 47, pp. 199–236.

Laroque Pierre (1972), 'Droits de la femme et pensions de veuve', *Revue internationale du travail*,Vol. 106, no. 1, pp. 1–13.

Lengwiler Martin (2007), 'Vom Überbevölkerungs- zum Überalterungsparadigma. Das Verhältnis von zwischen Demographie und Bevölkerungspolitik in historischer Perspektive'. In Barlösius Eva & Daniela Schiek, *Demographisierung des Gesellschaftlichen. Analysen und Debatten zur demographischen Zukunft Deutschlands*. Wiesbaden, VS Verlag für Sozialwissenschaften, pp. 174–191.

Lewis Jane & Barbara Meredith (1998), *Daughters Who Care. Daughters Caring for Mothers at Home*. London, Routledge.

Messerschmidt Reinhard (2014), 'Garbled Demography or Demographization of the Social? – A Foucaultian Discourse Analysis of German Demographic Change at the Beginning of the 21st Century', *Historical Social Research/Historische Sozialforschung*, vol. 39, no. 1, pp. 299–335.

Noll Dorothea (2010), '*...ohne Hoffnung im Alter jemals auch nur einen Pfennig Rente zu erhalten...' Die Geschichte der weiblichen Erwerbsbiographien in der gesetzlichen Rentenversicherung*. Frankfurt a.M., Vittorio Klostermann Verlag.

Nullmeier Frank & Franz-Xaver Kaufmann (2010), 'Post-War Welfare State Development'. In Castles Francis G., Leibfried Stephan, Lewis Jane, Obinger Herbert & Christopher Pierson, *The Oxford Handbook of the Welfare State*, Oxford, Oxford University Press.

Phillipson Chris (2010), 'Older People. Introduction'. In Walker Alan, Gordon David & Ruth Levitas, *The Peter Townsend Reader*, Bristol, The Policy Press, pp. 405–411.

Powell Jason L. & Simon Biggs (2003), 'Foucauldian Gerontology: A Methodology for Understanding Aging', *Electronic Journal of Sociology*, Vol. 7, no. 2, www.sociology.org/content/vol7.2/03_powell_biggs.html, accessed 31 January 2017.

Raphael Lutz (1996), 'Die Verwissenschaftlichung des Sozialen als methodische und konzeptionelle Herausforderung für eine Sozialgeschichte des 20. Jahrhunderts', *Geschichte und Gesellschaft*, Vol. 22, no. 2, pp. 165–193.

Savage Mike (2011), *Identities and Social Change in Britain since 1940: The Politics of Method*. Oxford, Oxford University Press.

Segal Lynne (2013), 'Jam today. Feminist impacts and transformations in the 1970s'. In Black Lawrence, Pemberton Hughes & Pat Thane, *Reassessing Seventies Britain*. Manchester, Manchester University Press, pp. 149–166.

Shanas Ethel (1962), *The Health of Older People: A Social Survey*. Cambridge, Harvard University Press.

Shanas Ethel, Townsend Peter, Wedderburn Dorothy, Friis Henning, Milh.j Poul & Jan Stehouwer (1968), *Old People in Three Industrial Societies*. London, Atherton Press.

Siegel Watkins Elizabeth (2007), 'The Medicalisation of Male Menopause in America', *Social History of Medicine*, Vol. 20, no. 2, pp. 369–388.

Struthers James (2013), 'Historical Perspectives on Care and the Welfare State. The Rise, Retreat, Return, and Reframing of a Key Concept'. In Armstrong Pat & Susan Braedley, *Troubling Care. Critical Perspectives on Research and Practices*. Toronto, Canadian Scholars' Press, pp. 159–170.

Szreter Simon (1993), 'The Idea of Demographic Transition and the Study of Fertility Change: A Critical Intellectual History', *Population and Development Review*, Vol. 19, no. 4,pp. 659–701.

Thane Pat (2000), *Old Age in English History. Past Experiences, Current Issues*. Oxford, Oxford University Press.

Thane Pat (2006), 'The "Scandal" of Women's Pensions'. In Hugh Pemberton, Pat Thane & Noel Whiteside, *Britain's Pension Crisis. History and Policy*, Oxford, Oxford University Press.

Thane Pat & Tanya Evans (2013), *Sinners, Scroungers, Saints? Unmarried Motherhood in Twentieth-Century England*. Oxford, Oxford University Press.

Thorslund Mats, Wastesson W. Jonas, Agahi Neda, Lagergren Mårten & Marti G. Parker (2013), 'The Rise and Fall of Women's Advantage: A Comparison of National Trends in Life Expectancy at Age 65 Years', *European Journal of Ageing*, Vol. 10, No. 4, pp. 271–277.

Townsend Peter (1957), *The Family Life of Old People. An Inquiry in East London*. London, Routledge & Kegan Paul.

Townsend Peter (1958), 'A Society for People'. In Norman Ian MacKenzie, *Conviction*. London, MacGibbon & Kee.

Townsend Peter (1962), *The Last Refuge. A Survey of Residential Institutions and Homes for the Aged in England and Wales*. London, Routledge & Kegan Paul.

Townsend Peter & Dorothy Wedderburn (1965), *The Aged in the Welfare State*. London, G. Bell.

Willmott Peter & Michael Young (1960), *Family and Kinship in East London*. London, Routledge & Kegan Paul.

Zellmer Elisabeth (2011), *Töchter der Revolte? Frauenbewegung und Feminismus in den 1970er Jahren in München*, München, Oldenbourg Verlag.

8 The breakdown of consensus on pro-natalist policies

Media discourse, social research and a new demographic agreement

Antía Pérez-Caramés

The autonomous community of Galicia, situated in the northwest of the Iberian Peninsula and with little more than 2,700,000 inhabitants (6 per cent of the total Spanish population[1]), has been framed as a paradigmatic model of population ageing in the Spanish mass media. According to indicators used to describe the population ageing process, the average age in Galicia is 46 years, and around 25 per cent of its population is aged 65 or over. This situation led the regional authorities to develop the 'Plan for the Demographic Revitalisation of Galicia' (Plan para a Dinamización Demográfica de Galicia, PDRG), passed by the Galician regional parliament in 2013,[2] which analyses the Galician demographic situation and aims to reverse population ageing by raising the total fertility rate to 1.59 children per woman (Xunta de Galicia, 2013). This document is unique in that it is the first explicitly natalist policy to be introduced by a Spanish regional government since Spain's transition to democracy, thus breaking with an implicit consensus among all political orientations to shun intervention in this domain.

This chapter will look into how the foundations for this policy were laid, rooted in media and political discourse but also with academic support, to foster not only the adoption of this plan but also a reorientation of demographic consensus towards an alarmist perspective that problematises the ageing of the population. The empirical materials for this chapter consist of the text of the PDRG, political speeches by members of the Galician parliament, academic texts and news clippings. As we will detail in the methods section, these materials were mainly analysed using content and frame analysis.

The structure of this chapter is as follows. The following section will provide a brief analysis for understanding Galicia's specificity in the wider Spanish and European Union (EU) demographic contexts. It will be followed by a review of the concept of apocalyptic demography and the problematisation of population ageing that appears in certain demographic works and is influential on Galician social researchers. We shall then briefly present the methodology. The fourth section contains analysis of the results and allows us to understand how the previous implicit consensus rejecting explicit pro-natalist policies in Spain came to break down and be replaced by another consensus holding that the population ageing process was negative. The chapter closes with a few brief conclusions.

Population ageing in Galicia in a wider context

According to the most recent Eurostat data available for the total population in the EU of 28 Member States (EU-28), dating to 2013, Spain does not stand out as the most aged country in Europe. In fact, the two most frequently used indicators for population ageing, the proportion of population aged 65 or over and the old-age dependency ratio, place Spain in fourteenth place for its share of population aged 65 or over (17.7 per cent, compared to 21.2 per cent for Italy and 20.7 per cent for Germany, the first two countries) and seventeenth according to the old-age dependency ratio (26.3 per cent, compared to 32.7 per cent for Italy and 31.3 per cent for Germany).

But once this data is broken down by region, several Spanish autonomous communities stand out for being among the most aged regions in the EU-28. In Spain, the regions of Galicia and Castile and León placed among the 20 most aged of the EU's 276 regions.[3] In fact, given that the demographic growth of many European countries depends largely on migratory movements, the unequal distribution of immigrants in Spain (as well as the uneven impact of the recent upsurge in migration flows) leads to a situation where some regions are relatively demographically dynamic while others are more prone to a decrease in the number of inhabitants and accelerated ageing. Table 8.1 compares several standard indicators used to measure population ageing in the 17 Spanish autonomous communities, revealing strong differences between

Table 8.1 Indicators of population ageing in the autonomous communities (2015)

	Share of population aged 65+	Share of population aged 85+	Average age	Old-age dependency ratio
Andalusia	16.2	2.1	40.7	24.5
Aragon	21.0	3.8	44.0	32.7
Asturias	24.0	4.2	47.2	37.4
Balearic Islands	15.1	2.0	40.7	22.2
Canary Islands	14.8	1.6	41.2	21.5
Cantabria	20.3	3.5	44.4	31.1
Castile and León	24.1	4.7	46.4	38.1
Castile-La Mancha	18.3	3.3	42.0	28.1
Catalonia	18.1	2.8	42.2	28.5
Valencian Community	18.4	2.4	42.4	28.4
Extremadura	19.8	3.2	43.2	30.4
Galicia	24.0	4.0	46.2	37.9
Madrid	16.8	2.5	41.5	25.6
Murcia	15.0	2.0	39.7	22.9
Navarra	18.9	3.2	42.6	29.7
Basque Country	21.1	3.3	44.7	33.6
La Rioja	19.9	3.5	43.5	31.2
SPAIN	18.4	2.8	42.5	28.3

Source: Author's own based on data from the Municipal Register of Inhabitants, 2015 (Spanish Statistical Institute, INE).

certain regions and the rest. We can thus identify a rough cluster of what are considered the most 'aged regions', composed of Aragon, Asturias, Cantabria, Castile and León, and Galicia; all are located in the north and sustain the north–south demographic divide within Spain that stems from regional differences at the outset of the first demographic transition (Livi-Bacci, 1991).

In the Galician case, population ageing is accompanied by a very low fertility rate (32.7 per cent in 2014, according to Instituto Nacional de Estadística (INE) calculations) and negative migratory growth, due to its weak attractivity for immigration in addition to a recent rise in emigration flows (in the form of return migration of foreign residents and emigration of young autochthones), thus making it a paradigm for population ageing.

Apocalyptic demography at the service of natalism: academic influences in the framing of population ageing as a political problem

The overwhelming number of academic publications concerning depopulation and demographic ageing in recent years has had significant resonance in the media and has also penetrated political speech, influencing the design of public policy, social policy in particular. And as Gendreau and Véron have already stated,

> In principle, the demographer describes what is or, if he is more daring, indicates possible futures. Then it is society's turn to say what must happen and act accordingly. But this division of tasks is not always respected: the description of population trends usually leads to identifying problems in the population and recommending population policies.
>
> (Gendreau & Véron, 1998, p. 309).

This surge of demographic analysis into planning policy has been accompanied by a feeling of impending demographic doom and gloom that has acquired an alarmist and apocalyptic tone.

The term 'apocalyptic demography' was coined by Robertson (1990) to define an ideology of population ageing. One of its fundamental pillars is treating older people as scapegoats for social spending increases, thus justifying arguments of intergenerational injustice and limiting access to the healthcare system. Since then, the concept has enjoyed popularity among researchers in the sociology of ageing and critical gerontology. Gee and Gutman further elaborated on their definition, indicating that apocalyptic demography 'demonstrates that population can become intertwined with politics to serve a political agenda' (p. 14) and that the 'holy writ' of apocalyptic demography is to accept that:

> population ageing has negative consequences for society and intergenerational relations, i.e., that increasing numbers and proportions

of elderly translate into the need for major cuts in social policies and programmes, and that generational tensions are bound to escalate... . [Apocalyptic demography] is the oversimplified idea that population ageing has catastrophic consequences for a society.

(Gee & Gutman, 2000, p. 3–5).

It is also necessary to understand Foot's related concept of 'voodoo demography' (2002, p. 149, 151), which he defines as 'the equivalent of combining population dynamics (or population ageing) with static (or unexplained) social behaviour' to explain how apocalyptic demography arises when voodoo demography is applied to issues such as welfare, pensions or health. The term voodoo demography is similar to the process of 'demographisation of the social' that Messerschmidt (2014; also this volume) identifies when he analyses German population projections alongside media discourse on population issues. Still other designations have been proposed for academic contributions along these lines, such as Katz's demographic alarmism, which he defines as 'ideological, fuelling a politics of difference that exempts the State from meeting its life course commitments' (1992, p. 207). For his part, Domingo believes that the political discourse around population, as well as a certain part of the scientific production, travel paths already frequented by literary dystopias[4] borrowed from certain fictional works where demographic issues are central to the plot (2015, p. 64), so that one may speak of 'demodystopias' and 'demodystopic speeches' (2008, 2015).

At the heart of these alarmist perspectives on population change is the seed for advocating measures that alter the seemingly inexorable course of population ageing.

Ageing as the epitome of disaster

One of the consequences of demographic pessimism is the academic emphasis that has been given to 'population ageing', a fraught term and powerful organismic metaphor that makes it seem like populations age like human beings (Bourdelais, 1999). In fact, the organismic conception of populations is inherited from social Darwinism, one of most influential currents of thought in the late nineteenth and early twentieth century (Pérez Díaz, 2005). According to the historian of old age Patrice Bourdelais (1993, 1994), this is because the birth of the very concept of demographic ageing is linked to the metaphor of the organism. He warns of the dangers of the simile, as its 'pedagogical temptation results in explanations that oversimplify and mislead because they overlook most dynamics of human societies' (1994: 176). The Belgian demographer Michel Loriaux goes further and mentions the existence of an 'insidious displacement of the biological concept of individual ageing to the collective concept of demographic ageing' (1995a, p. 1612).

Likening individual and population ageing has direct rhetorical consequences. Since human ageing is associated with a certain vital decline, demographic ageing ends up inherently connected to depopulation. In strictly analytical terms, population decline is reflected in gradual population loss through a total growth of a negative sign, but at a more abstract level it can suggest a society's moral decline and loss of identity.

'Wrinkled France', 'demographic winter', 'grey dawn', 'the cancer of Europe', 'stopwatch feast' and 'demographic crash' are some of the poetic epithets for the ageing population used in the titles of some renowned demographers' works (Dumont *et al.*, 1986; Geinoz *et al.*, 1990; Dumont, 1991; Peterson, 1999; Schooyans, 1999). With a few exceptions, ageing has been approached fatalistically as a hopeless situation, often from an apocalyptic perspective. Ageing seems to epitomise a certain demographic conception of evil, defined by falling birth rate, depopulation and decline, and many papers do not take the trouble to detail the causal relationships and dynamics between all these processes (Le Bras, 1991).

Galician demographers have a tradition of drawing upon French demography, either because their academic background links them to France or due to the influence of certain French demographers (such as Louis Henry) in the development of certain demographic sub-fields such as historical demography (Sullivan, 2000). So to a certain extent, the pessimistic view of population ageing found in the texts of certain French demographers has made its way into the prognosis for the Galician population.

It is undeniable that the increase in the number and proportion of people who have left the working age poses certain challenges to the social structure, which contributes to troubling the tone of the debate on ageing outside of the strictly demographic field. And if the onus is on demography in some regards, researchers like Loriaux (1995a, 1995b) deflect the blame back to social institutions, which are accused of not adapting to the changes in demographic dynamics.

In summary, population ageing is no longer regarded as a mere consequence of the first demographic transition. It is perceived as a notoriously negative process that must be corrected to avoid an even more disastrous situation.

Methods

The methodology used in this research takes a qualitative approach. Hermeneutical content analysis was conducted to interpret the discourse emanating from the PDRG text and the political speeches published in the *Journal of Sessions of the Regional Parliament*[5] concerning the development and approval of this plan. In addition, the main academic contributions to the demographic debate in Galicia were analysed to determine how they align with political and media discourse.

A frame analysis of the demographic issue was conducted on Galician print media, using articles published in the autonomous community's widest-circulating and most-read newspaper, the socially liberal, fiscally conservative *La Voz de Galicia*.[6] It was selected for its relevance and the size of its readership relative to other newspapers in Galicia according to the General Media Survey. Relevant news and opinion articles were systematically gathered from the beginning of the debate on the need for a plan (late 2010) until a year after passage of the PDRG by Parliament, a period of 4 years. A total of 1,333 articles were compiled for this period.

According Scheufele's typology of framing research (1999), this study focuses on 'media frames', which we will consider as dependent variables. He takes the definition of media frames from Gamson and Modigliani (1987, cited in Scheufele, 1999, p. 106) who conceive of them as 'a central organising idea or story line that provides meaning to an unfolding strip of events ... The frame suggests what the controversy is about, the essence of the issue'. Considering media frames as dependent variables, we wonder what factors influence journalists' framing of certain issues (along the same lines as Scheufele [1999, p. 109]: social values and regulations, organisational coercion, pressure of interest groups, journalistic routines, and journalists' ideological orientations or policies), and above all, which frames they choose for demographic issues.

Pro-natalism boosted by overlapping media and social research discourse

Policies and programmes of public social intervention in Spain have avoided an explicitly natalist orientation since the beginning of the democratic period. At a time when population growth trends were not seen as problematic, the desire to escape ideological identification with the Franco regime was more important. The Francoist regime had inflated the importance of family and used social intervention to reward people for having numerous children (Meil, 1995). The regime's collapse led to the emergence of an implicit political consensus between all political forces present in Spanish regional parliaments, even conservative ones, to avoid population policies. Some authors (Valiente, 1995; Cousins, 2005) also believe this is the main reason for the underdevelopment of family policies in Spain as compared to other countries of the EU.[7] That an autonomous parliament approved a PDRG with a clear natalist orientation, its main objectives being to invest in countering the downward trend in the number of inhabitants by increasing the number of children per woman, thus represents a distinct break with this post-democratic transition consensus.

How could an autonomous regional government in Spain formulate and implement population policies clearly directed at increasing fertility[8] in such a historical context? The PDRG provides an interesting case study of a complete policy reversal, in how it was developed and approved with barely any criticism. In other words, although the media and academic research were both already depicting population ageing as a social problem before the regional government decided to intervene, the decision to bring it into the political arena further boosted alarmist discourses.

In the first place, various governmental authorities of the autonomous community of Galicia have had some success with demographic arguments in budgetary negotiations with the State on investment in issues such as long-term care, infrastructure, and healthcare policies. Galician politicians put forward factors related to the density, distribution and ageing of the population to obtain more funding from the Spanish State. In fact, Galicia was at the forefront among demographically similar autonomous communities in forming a common front in budget negotiations to demand more funding to address issues such as population ageing or an isolated and scattered population. Despite the fact that service provision is more expensive when the population is more scattered, and more resources are needed for healthcare and dependency if the number of older people is higher (Hortas-Rico & Solé-Ollé, 2010), these policy strategies have created a good climate among all Galician political parties through a shared recognition that demography matters. The first milestone in the demographic consensus was thus achieved when the full ideological spectrum of political parties wielded population factors to obtain more funding from the State.

Second, the media has played an important role problematising the Galician population situation and creating a context conducive to demographic alarmism. *La Voz de Galicia* has devoted considerable attention to the demographic issue, through news pieces as well as opinions (opinion columns and editorials). Its approach to demographic issues approach reveals the repetition of a few frames: some of the organismic metaphors are of their own creation, and others are picked up from political discourse or demodystopic academic publications, as we will see in the following paragraphs.

Throughout the period analysed (late 2010–late 2014), a total of 1,333 articles on demographic issues were published in *La Voz de Galicia*. Of them, 240 were opinion pieces (written either by journalists or by experts, mainly academics). This means that 18 per cent of the published materials on population issues were opinions, a high number that is explained by the very common practice of accompanying a news piece on the issue with an opinion piece. There is a slight difference, however, between opinion pieces written by journalists and academics. The former serve to transmit the newspaper's stance, whereas those by researchers tend to convey alarmist academic explanations to the general public, thus creating a link between academic and media discourses. The newspaper frames these academic contributions as the voice of experts, and so it mainly requests written opinion pieces from university professors and researchers, but it may solicit freelance researchers and intellectuals as well.

The newspaper is organised in several sections classifying news thematically (such as the Economy and Society pages) or geographically (International, Spain, Galicia). Nearly 40 per cent of all articles related to demographic issues were located in the 'Galicia' section. This distinctive feature serves to convey the message that population 'problems' are Galician 'problems', thus making the issue of population ageing in something idiosyncratic.

Demography was the subject of 5 per cent of all articles in this section and of all opinion pieces, while population issues were less present in other sections of the paper (1.5 per cent average presence in the whole paper during the studied period).

Images, stereotypes and metaphors were identified by selecting topical expressions that went beyond describing and providing facts in order to convey a particular message on the studied phenomenon. Those expressions were then searched in the whole newspaper, and noted according to the section where they appeared, the type of article in which they were used, and whether they were used metaphorically or literally. Many opinion articles, drawing upon aforementioned alarmist demographers, advanced some images that were later recovered by journalists in their news articles. This is the case for the expression 'demographic suicide', for example, which appeared first in an academic voice in an opinion piece only to be found later in non-opinion articles.

Five of the identified images and metaphors were especially salient, either because of their repetitive nature (appearing frequently in news pieces on population issues) or for the aforementioned particularity of emerging from expert opinion pieces and entering the vernacular by regular use in news pieces on population issues. These images are the following: demographic bloodletting, demographic suicide, demographic winter, demographic haemorrhage and demographic desert (also in the form of demographic desertification). Additionally, journalists rarely used two of these image-words (bloodletting and desert) metaphors not related to demography.

Two of the frames adapted from academic publications corresponding to the apocalyptic demography paradigm stand out in particular: 'demographic winter' and 'demographic suicide'. The latter may be relatively specific to Spain, as it is derived from an essay entitled 'The demographic suicide of Spain', written by Macarrón Larumbe (2011), who heads the ultra-conservative Demographic Renaissance Foundation (Fundación Renacimiento Demográfico). Another of these commonly recurring images was coined by the newspaper itself: 'demographic bloodletting' was repeated 198 times (in

Table 8.2 Presence of demographic metaphors in La Voz de Galicia (2010–2014)

Concept	No. Mentions in sections 'Galicia' and 'Opinion'	No. of metaphorical uses	No. uses as demographic metaphor
Bloodletting	180	109	71
Suicide	201	72	7
Haemorrhage	72	33	7
Desertification	31	31	20
Winter	484	21	9

Source: Author's own.

both news and opinion pieces) in the studied period. The image has become so common that even the President of the autonomous government, Alberto Núñez Feijoo (Partido Popular (Popular Party)), adopted it into his demographic discourse with the expression 'demographic haemorrhage'.

The use of these expressions, clearly linked to the loss of inhabitants, might appear to be more related to emigration than to demographic ageing, but in political and print media discourse, causal analyses using these expressions 'magically' erase migratory growth's contribution to population change, thus displacing all responsibility for 'bloodletting' onto natural growth by emphasising the size of the aged population and the reduced number of children per woman.

Third, in 2011 the autonomous Parliament created a commission for the study and development of a demographic revitalisation plan, the future PDRG. All political parties in parliament participated.[9] The commission worked for months preparing the plan, hearing from experts in demography, public officials of different levels and domains of public administration, and representatives of social and cultural organisations. With slight nuances, parliamentary speeches demonstrate that all political parties shared an alarmist analysis of the demographic situation in Galicia, and although the PDRG was ultimately only approved thanks to votes of the Partido Popular (the party in power with the majority of seats in Parliament), opposing votes were more due to formal issues than its content.

It is interesting to note that the plan could have benefited from the findings of an EU-funded INTERREG programme called DART (Declining, Ageing and Regional Transformation), since the Galician regional government was one of its 13 participants.[10] This programme defined indicators for measuring demographic change and population decline in European regions to facilitate comparisons and policy recommendations, and it resulted in a study (IFAD, 2012) that curiously was not used in preparing the plan.[11]

The combination of all these factors has led the population question to burst onto the political, media and research agenda. Using Google Scholar to search for the number of papers containing the words 'demographic ageing' and 'Galicia' produces 185 publications in the 2004–2009 period, and 228 for 2010–2015, representing an increase of 23 per cent. Additionally, PDRG initiatives have led to numerous conferences and symposia on the demographic subject in recent years,[12] and some have led to publications re-enforcing the apocalyptic tone. Among them, we should mention the multi-author work edited by Manuel Blanco Desar (2014) entitled *Galicia: un pobo con futuro? O noso devalo demográfico* (*Galicia: A Land with Future? Our Demographic Decline*). The transformation of 'demographic ageing' into a political problem implies an increase in public funds for research initiatives (research programmes, conferences, etc.) that in turn simultaneously keeps the topic on the agenda while allowing the 'alarmist imagination' to develop.

From alarmist discourse to pro-natalist policy:
PDRG content analysis

Thus far we have presented the main elements from the political, media and research realms that led to the emergence of a new demographic consensus, inspired by apocalyptic demographic literature and framed in alarmist terms, that paved the way for public intervention in this arena. We will now explore the main political tool designed to deal with population ageing with a pro-natalist approach.

The PDRG is a document of little over 100 pages, the result of 3-years' work by the Galician parliamentary commission created for this purpose, and was passed in 2013. After an analysis, it presents a series of measures to be carried out in the 2013–2016 period intended to make a discernable impact in Galician population structure and dynamics by 2020. Content is divided into three major sections. The first, entitled 'Necessity of the plan', contains the political arguments and the demographic analysis justifying the proposal. The second, 'The Plan for the Demographic Revitalisation of Galicia 2013–2016, Horizon 2020', is divided into four subsections that present the plan's principles, structure, objectives, thematic areas and measures to be taken. The third section, more brief, sets outs the plan's monitoring and evaluation system.

We begin our analysis with the first section. The conceptual framework justifying the need for a plan starts by characterising the Galician demographic situation with one of the terms most used by Galician politicians as well as the media, experts and academics: 'demographic winter'. The genealogy of this expression is interesting, because it appears for the first time in a multi-author work entitled *Europe. L'hiver démographique* (*Europe. The Demographic Winter*) (Geinoz *et al.*, 1989) which had little academic impact.[13] However, French demographer Gérard-François Dumont quickly adopted the term to describe the process of population decline due to sustained reduced fertility below the generational replacement level (see, among many other publications, Dumont, 2006, 2008). Although the concept has little academic relevance, it has found fertile ground in the political and media arenas; it was even taken as the title of a documentary filmed in the United States in 2008 that was produced by organisations linked to conservative religious activism (Joice, 2008).

Beyond describing such a Galician demographic winter, the plan seeks legitimacy in EU political strategy. Specifically, the plan almost exclusively highlights the relevance of an 'exploratory opinion' from the European Economic and Social Committee entitled 'The role of family policy in relation to demographic change with a view to sharing best practices among Member States' (EESC, 2011), requested by Hungarian ambassador to the EU, Peter Györkös. The report urges the promotion of family policies to increase fertility and curb the demographic decline, since any 'reversal of this trend would hinge predominantly on significantly improving the total fertility rate'. That is to say, the solution to population loss should be sought exclusively in recovering fertility. They indicate that demographic projections include an 'alarmist' hypothesis:

> In the 'catastrophe' scenario, demographic winter would intensify, with births considerably outstripped by deaths! ... 'catastrophe' scenario would result in skilled young people leaving an ageing European Union for more entrepreneurial nations ... and in immigration falling.

The language of this opinion clearly refers to the work of the demographer who promoted the expression 'demographic winter', Gérard-François Dumont, who is also the only academic reference mentioned in the report.

The plan's final argument relies on a demographic analysis of recent trends in the structure and evolution of the Galician population in comparison with Spain and the EU. This section is precisely where it becomes clear that French alarmist demography was imported to frame demographic ageing as a global problem that can be addressed using pro-natalist measures. This assessment is based on the following main elements:

1   The European comparison is made with France, a country with virtually the highest fertility rate of all EU Member States, with the exception of Ireland. We find that this comparison is somewhat misleading because the dilated French demographic transition bears little resemblance to the rapid and intense Spanish demographic transition, which has implications for the resulting age structure (Chesnais, 1990).

2   Comparison with other autonomous communities is based on Asturias, Murcia and Andalusia. While Asturias shares certain demographic characteristics with Galicia, both Murcia and Andalusia are autonomous communities that historically have a higher number of children per woman and a younger age at the birth of the first child. In addition, they (and especially Andalusia) are communities that have received large influxes of immigration in the 1990s and the first decade of the twenty-first century, which contrasts with Galicia's situation. Despite the fact that migratory growth is taken into account in the total population of all compared regions, the comparative statement ignores the relevance of the different roles such immigration flows can have in the considered regions.

3   The dependency ratio was used as the main indicator to describe the population structure by age, although it has been challenged and criticised for its deficiencies in assessing the impact of an ageing population (Sanderson & Scherbov, 2010; Donoghue, 2003).

4   When addressing the issue of population growth, only the natural balance is considered and there is no mention of the migration balance. This implies that one of the two main drivers of demographic change (migratory growth) is completely excluded from the analysis, thus giving

readers the impression that migratory movements are rather irrelevant to the observed population trends. Furthermore, the indicators chosen to analyse the temporary evolution of the natural balance refer almost exclusively to natality, and give considerably less attention to mortality.

To summarise, the demographic analysis that is presented in the plan is intended to give an alarmist problematisation of demographic ageing and present recovery of the fertility rate as the only way to affect population change.

The plan's second section, which develops measures to reverse the described demographic trends, indicates five guiding principles: raising awareness of the 'delicate' demographic situation, equality between men and women, protection of the family, participation and cooperation, and a transversal dimension (involvement of all domains of the autonomous government). Following these principles, the plan's main objective is defined as follows:

> To promote the demographic revitalisation of Galicia by raising its position in the ranking of the 303 European regions according to total fertility rate, moving towards the goal of increasing the average of 1.08 children per woman registered in Galicia closer to the European average, which is 1.59 children per woman.
>
> (Xunta de Galicia, 2013)

In other words, the plan not only explicitly targets a higher fertility rate, but also demonstrates an understanding that the average number of children per woman must approach the European average if Galicia is to be removed from the regions with the lowest fertility rate.

Furthermore, the stated objective's proposal overlooks the fact that the total fertility rate is an indicator of a given moment in time (thus not longitudinal), so it refers less to the number of children per woman than to the number of children that would be borne by each woman in a fictitious cohort not exposed to mortality risks during their fertile period and following the fertility intensity observed in the year of calculation. It is therefore a hypothetical measure whose results are distorted by changes in the maternity calendar – as Bongaarts and Feeney have already indicated (1998) – which causes underestimation of fertility intensity when age of maternity rises (as is the case of Galicia).

There is a dimension of natalist propaganda in the measures the plan develops to reach this single main objective, expressed through the initiatives to raise awareness of demographic revitalisation that frame advertising campaigns on the importance of having offspring.[14] In addition, it includes a set of actions to facilitate maternity/paternity and support families, some of which already existed in regional regulations or State precedent and others that are more recent (including housing and transport assistance, lowering the automobile tax for families with children, and priority in consultations for assisted reproductive care). On the whole, the measures aim to strengthen support for large families and help parents reconcile work and family life – measures that, to paraphrase Stratigaki's critique of this term (2004), constitute a co-optation of gender relations' potential for change to the benefit of a 'demography-oriented' objective.

It is nonetheless striking that barely any measures are designed to promote immigration, and even more so considering that the generation of women currently in the middle of their fertile period is a reduced cohort, because they were born during the period of the greatest decline in fertility, the 1980s.

Conclusions

Over the course of this chapter we have analysed how demographic discourse has substantially changed in the political and media spheres, resulting in the approval of a plan containing measures intended to reverse population ageing and depopulation solely by increasing the average number of children per woman. In order for this change to take place, it was necessary to dismantle an implicit consensus to avoid explicitly pro-natalist policies that had been in place since Spain transitioned to democracy. It was replaced by a new consensus that is based on demonisation of the demographic ageing process, disinterest in the demographic contribution of immigration, and insistence on an increase in the birth rate as salvation.

As the analysis demonstrated, this new consensus is built on and expressed through an apocalyptic view of Galician population change that was created in academia and reproduced (and sometimes recreated) in media and political discourses, ultimately leading to the main measure proposed by the Galician government for tackling the phenomenon of population ageing. Over the course of this process, demographic ageing became a political problem, something that authorities had to address and try to resolve by proposing ways of increasing fertility. For this to happen, alarmist analysis of population processes had to be validated, promoting a new demographic consensus among scholars, mass media and the political realm.

Acknowledgements

The author is very grateful to the editors of this volume for their careful, thorough, and valuable work reviewing this chapter.

Notes

1 The population figures used in this introductory section date to 1 January 2015, and come from the Municipal Register of Inhabitants (Padrón Municipal de Habitantes) of the National Institute of Statistics (Instituto Nacional de Estadística, INE).

2 As we will see later, the plan was elaborated by a parliamentary commission including representatives of all political parties present in the regional Parliament and gave audience to experts, most of whom were academics but also including policymakers and stakeholders.

3 According to Eurostat figures, the proportion of people aged 65 or over in EU regions in 2013 gives the following ranking (in descending order): Liguria (Italy), Chemnitz (Germany), Sachsen (Germany), Ipeiros (Greece), Sachsen-Anhalt (Germany), Friuli-Venezia Giulia (Italy), Dresden (Germany), Tuscany (Italy), Alentejo (Portugal), Umbria (Italy), Piedmont (Italy), Severozapaden (Bulgary), Limousin (France), Thüringen (Germany), Castile and León (Spain), Galicia (Spain).

4 According to *The Oxford Dictionary of Literary Terms*, dystopia is a 'term coined to convey the opposite of Utopia: the dystopian mode, which projects an unpleasant or catastrophic future, is frequently used by Science fiction writers'. (www.oxfordreference.com/search?q=dystopia&searchBtn=Search&isQuick-Search=true, accessed 11 February 2016).

5 The *Journal of Sessions of the Galician Regional Parliament* (*Busca de Boletíns Oficiais e Diarios de Sesións*) publishes the verbatim transcripts of sessions of the Galician Regional Parliament. They can be consulted at www.parlamentodegalicia.com/sitios/web/contenidogal/Procuras/Boletins.aspx, accessed 10 August 2015.

6 According to the latest available General Media Survey (Estudio *General* de Medios, EGM) (October 2014 to May 2015), *La Voz de Galicia* is the most-read newspaper in the autonomous community (sixth in Spain) with about 600,000 readers (www.aimc.es/-Datos-EGM-Resumen-General-.html, accessed 17 September 2015).

7 According to the Organisation for Economic Co-operation and Development's (OECD) Social Expenditure database preliminary data for public spending on family benefits in cash, services and tax measures for 2011, Spain invested 1.51 per cent of its total gross domestic product (GDP) on family policies whereas the average expenditure in other EU countries in the OECD was 2.83 per cent (bearing in mind that only 20 of the current 28 EU Member States are in the OECD (United Kingdom, Denmark, Ireland, Hungary, Luxembourg, Sweden, France, Belgium, Finland, Germany, Estonia, Czech Republic, Slovak Republic, Slovenia, Netherlands, Italy, Poland, Spain, Portugal and Greece).

8 The Spanish State is decentralised to a certain extent. Although it varies according to the development of each community's Autonomy Statute, autonomous communities have responsibilities in education, health and social services.

9 The work of this commission ran from the end of the 8th Term of the Galician Regional Parliament (2009–2012) until the first year of the 9th Legislature (2012–present), a period during which the Partido Popular was in power and held an absolute majority. In addition to the Partido Popular, the commission named by the 8th Legislature also included the PSdG-PSOE (Socialist Party of Galicia (Partido dos Socialistas de Galicia)-Spanish Socialist Workers Party (Partido de los Socialistas de *Galicia]*) and the NBG (Galician Nationalist Bloc [Bloque Nacionalista Galego)). The 9th Legislature additionally incorporated the party AGE (Alternative Galician Left (Alternative Galega de Esquerdas)), an electoral coalition of Anova Irmandade Nacionalista (Anova Nationalist Brotherhood) and Izquierda Unida (United Left).

10 The other participating European regions were: Brandenburg and Saxony (Germany), West Region (Ireland), Central Bohemia (Czech Republic), Kainuu and North Karelia (Finland), Limburg (The Netherlands), Veneto (Italy), Lower Austria (Austria), Gorenjska (Slovenia), Silesia (Poland) and Centru (Romania) (www.dart-project.eu, accessed 13 August 2015).

11 The report contained detailed demographic analysis of the regions participating
   in the project and proposed new indicators for measuring demographic change,
   as well as some general public policy recommendations. Its conclusions had no
   impact in the Galician press. The comparison of several European regions with
   similar demographic characteristics was contrary to one of the purposes of the
   PDRG, which was to make Galicia stand out as the paradigm of demographic
   ageing.
12 Among them are: 'Conference on demography and development: keys to a
   reversal policy of the demographic inertia in Galicia' (Santiago de Compostela,
   26–28 October 2011), 'International Congress of Demography' (Santiago de
   Compostela, 21 March 2014), 'Natality Forums and Old Age in Galicia. A people
   with a past, a people with a future?' (Several Galician cities, between June 2012
   and January 2013), 'International Day of Demographic Awareness' (Santiago de
   Compostela, 29 November 2013).
13 A Google Scholar search of works using the expression in French, English or
   Spanish, reveals that it is uncommon in academic journals (129 results in French,
   290 in English and 112 in Spanish). The search was conducted on 14 August 2015.
14 Some samples of the advertisements can be seen on the autonomous government's YouTube channel: www.youtube.com/watch?v=a2IEnAEcMgU, accessed
   10 August 2015.

References

Blanco Desar Manuel (2014), *Galicia: un pobo con futuro? O noso devalo demográfico*.
   Vigo, Xerais.
Bongaarts John & Griffith Feeney (1998), 'On the Quantum and Tempo of Fertility',
   Population and Development Review, 24(2), pp. 271–291.
Bourdelais Patrice (1993), *L'âge de la vieillesse*. Paris, Odile Jacob.
Bourdelais Patrice (1994), 'Le vieillissement de la population: question d'actualité
   ou notion obsolète?', *Le Debat*, 85, pp. 173–192.
Bourdelais Patrice (1999), 'Demographic Aging: A Notion to Revisit', *The History
   of the Family*, 4(1), pp. 31–50.
Chesnais Jean-Claude (1990), 'Demographic Transition Patterns and Their Impact
   on the Age Structure', *Population and Development Review*, 16(2), pp. 327–336.
Cousins Christine (2005), 'The development of a gendered social policy regime'. In
   Threlfall Monica, Cousins Christine & Celia Valiente (eds.), *Gendering Spanish
   Democracy*. London, Routledge, pp. 55–77.
Domingo Andreu (2008), '"Demodystopias": Prospects of Demographic Hell', *Pop-
   ulation and Development Review*, 34(4), pp. 725–745.
Domingo Andreu (2015), 'Sonen les trompetes: discurs demodistòpic en el tercer
   mil·leni', *Documents d'Anàlisi Geogràfica*, 61(1), pp. 49–66.
Donoghue Chris (2003), *Deconstructing Aged Dependency: An Assessment of the
   Dependency Ratio as an Indicator of Population Ageing*. Paper presented at the
   annual meeting of the American Sociological Association, Atlanta Hilton Hotel,
   Atlanta, GA, 16 August 2003. Available at: www.allacademic.com/meta/p106377_
   index.html (accessed 14 August 2015).
Dumont Gérard-François (1991), *Le festin de Kronos: réalités et enjeux des évolutions
   socio-démographiques en Europe*. Paris, Fleurus.
Dumont Gérard-François (2006), *Les territoires face au vieillissement en France et en
   Europe. Géographie-Politique-Prospective*. Paris, Éllipses.

Dumont Gérard-François (2008), 'Les conséquences géopolitiques de "l'hiver démographique" en Europe', *Géostratégiques*, 20, pp. 29–46.

Dumont Gérard-François, Chaunu Pierre, Legrand Jean & Alfred Sauvy (1986), *La France ridée*. Paris, Hachette.

EESC (2011), 'The Role of Family Policy in Relation to Demographic Change with a View to Sharing Best Practices among Member States'. Opinion of the European Economic and Social Committee. SOC/399 Family Policy and Demographic Change. Available at: http://toad.eesc.europa.eu/viewdoc.aspx?doc=ces/soc/soc399/en/ces804-2011_ac_en.doc (accessed 28 May 2016).

Foot David K. (2002), 'Voodoo and Apocalyptic Demography – Conceptual and Methodological Issues', *Canadian Journal on Aging*, 21(1), pp. 147–151.

Gamson William A. & Andre Modigliani (1987), 'The changing culture of affirmative action'. In Braungart Richard G. & Margaret M. Braungart (eds.), *Research in Political Sociology*. Greenwich, CT, JAI Press, pp. 137–177.

Gee Ellen & Gloria Gutman (2000), *The Overselling of Population Aging. Apocalyptic Demography, Intergenerational Challenges, and Social Policy*. Oxford, Oxford University Press.

Geinoz François, De Siebenthal François, Suarez Antoine & Michel Tricot (1990), *Europe. L'hiver démographique*. Paris, L'âge d'homme.

Gendreau Francis & Jacques Véron (1998), 'La démographie, objet de fantasmes ?'. In Schlemmer Bernard (ed.), *Terrains et engagements de Claude Meillassoux*. Paris, Karthala, pp. 309–323.

Hortas-Rico Miriam & Albert Solé-Ollé (2010), 'Does Urban Sprawl Increase the Costs of Providing Local Public Services? Evidence from Spanish Municipalities', *Urban Studies*, 47(7), pp. 1513–1540.

IFAD (2012), Indicators and Standards of Demographic Cange. Study by the Institute for Applied Demographics (IFAD) under the DART Project. Available at: www.dart-project.eu/fileadmin/OrdnerRedakteure/0103_Achievements/Indicator_Study/IFAD-Study_DART_long_eng_Nov2012_final.pdf (accessed on 13 August 2015).

Joice Kathryn (2008), Review: Demographic Winter. The Decline of the Human Family. Available at: http://kathrynjoyce.com/articles/review-demographic-winter-the-decline-of-the-human-family/ (accessed 14 August).

Katz Stephen (1992), 'Alarmist Demography: Power, Knowledge, and the Elderly Population', *Journal of Aging Studies*, 6(3), pp. 203–225.

Le Bras Hervé (1991), *Marianne et les lapins. L'obsession démographique*. Paris, Hachette.

Livi-Bacci Massimo (1991), *Modelos regionales de la transición demográfica en España y Portugal*. Alicante, Asociación de Demografía Histórica.

Loriaux Michel (1995a), 'Du vieillissement démographique à l'intégration des âges : inconvénients et adaptation', *Population*, 50(6), pp. 1611–1625.

Loriaux Michel (1995b), 'Perspectives démographiques et prospectives sociales. Un autre regard sur le vieillissement', *Revue Française des Affaires Sociales*, 48(1), pp. 191–199.

Macarrón Larumbe Alejandro (2011), *El suicidio demográfico de España*. Madrid, Homo Legens.

Meil Gerardo (1995), 'Presente y futuro de la política familiar en España', *Revista Española de Investigaciones Sociológicas*, 70, pp. 67–90.

Messerschmidt Reinhard (2014), '"Garbled demography" or "Demographization of the Social"? – A Foucaultian Discourse Analysis of German Demographic Change at the Beginning of the 21st Century', *Historical Social Research*, 39(1), pp. 299–335.

Pérez Díaz Julio (2005), 'Consecuencias sociales del envejecimiento demográfico', *Papeles de Economía Española*, 104, p. 210–226.

Peterson Peter G. (1999), *Gray Dawn: How the Coming Age Wave Will Transform America*. New York, Random House.

Robertson Ann (1990), 'The Politics of Alzheimer's Disease: A Case Study in Apocalyptic Demography', *International Journal of Health Services*, 20(3), pp. 429–442.

Sanderson Warren C. & Sergei Scherbov (2010), 'Remeasuring Ageing', *Science*, 10(5997), pp. 1287–1288.

Scheufele Dietram A. (1999), 'Framing as a Theory of Media Effects', *Journal of Communication*, 49(1), pp. 103–122.

Schooyans Michel (1999), *Le crash démographique. De la fatalité à l'espérance*. Paris, Sarment-Fayard.

Stratigaki Maria (2004), 'The Cooptation of Gender Concepts in EU Policies: The Case of "Reconciliation of Work and Family"', *Social Politicsxi*, 11(1), pp. 30–56.

Sullivan David-Sven (2000), 'La investigación en demografía histórica: pasado, presente y futuro', *Boletín de la Asociación de Demografía Histórica*18(2), pp. 15–78.

Valiente Cclia (1995), 'Rejecting the past: Central government and family policy in post-authoritarian Spain (1975–94)'. In Hantrais Linda & Marie-Thérèse Letablier (eds.), *The Family in Social Policy and Family Policy*. Loughborough, Cross-National Research Papers, European Research Centre, pp. 80–96.

Xunta de Galicia (2013), *Plan para a dinamización demográfica de Galicia 2013–2016, horizonte 2020*. Available at: http://benestar.xunta.es/export/sites/default/Benestar/Biblioteca/Documentos/Plans_e_programas/PLAN_DINAMIZACION_DEMOGRAFICA_DE_GALICIA_2013-2016_V2.pdf (accessed 12 August 2015).

9 The social construction of dependency controversies around an assessment instrument in France

Nicolas Belorgey

Interest in the notion of dependency has been growing in France and elsewhere in Europe since the late 1970s. The term is not a reference to the accepted fact that people are (inter)dependent on each other in society (Durkheim 1893, Elias 1991 [1987]), but instead designates the risk that upon ageing some people might lose the ability to perform everyday activities like dressing, bathing or using the toilet. The issue of dependency (or 'lack of autonomy', a more positive term used by left-leaning administrations) gave rise to a number of official reports eventually informing public policies. Central to the discussion is an assessment instrument known as the AGGIR scale (standing for Autonomie Gérontologique – Groupes Iso-Ressources).

The usual approach takes dependency as a given: people are assumed to be more or less dependent, and the AGGIR scale only serves to assess their status. This chapter argues to the contrary, that dependency does not exist prior to and without its assessment instrument.[1] Far from merely measuring dependency, the scale contributes to its invention, doing so in a particular way and to great controversy. But the scale acts as a black box linking people to public subsidies, and consequently many want to leave it untouched. This chapter opens the black box to show how it works; how, why and by whom it was built; and what its strengths and weaknesses are. In a word, it shows the social construction of dependency as a public policy issue (Becker 1985 [1963], Gusfield 1986 [1966]) through the statistical tool that serves as its foundation (Desrosières 1993).

The data informing this chapter primarily comes from the United States, as the origin of much of the framing of dependency in both medicine and public policy. The chapter then focuses on France for a European case study of the implementation of dependency policy. There is some highly enlightening work (Ennuyer 2002, Frinault 2005, 2009) in the existing literature, but it has yet to address assessment issues in depth as I do here, using legal sources, medical journals, media reviews and ethnographic observations of street-level bureaucrats handling applicants for public benefits.[2]

This text describes the emergence of dependency as a social risk in France in the 1990s, first through the action of geriatricians, then of the State, despite the criticism of opponents. It then shows how this new issue has fluctuated since the 2000s, comforted by the action of street-level bureaucrats, and supported but eventually threatened by insurers and geriatricians themselves.

Geriatricians: From the medical perspective to the cost perspective

A retrospective consideration of the story is the best way to understand the current situation, and especially the form the scale has taken.[3] The first stage took place in the United States. Gerontologist Sydney Katz and his team published 'Studies of Illness in the Aged' (1963) in the leading *Journal of the American Medical Association* (JAMA). It proposed an Index of Independence in Activities of Daily Living (ADL) to advance study of the elderly and chronically ill. Six ADLs were assessed – bathing, dressing, going to toilet, transferring (switching between seated, in the bed, straight positions), continence and feeding – and each was coded as dependent, independent or intermediate depending on the individual's abilities. This index, originally derived from observations of elderly people with hip fractures, was then tested on 1,000 persons. It produced a stable, ordered ranking of eight degrees of dependency.

Two other scales should be mentioned alongside Katz's. The first is that of Powell Lawton and Elaine Brody (1969), of the Geriatric Center of Philadelphia, who added *instrumental* ADLs (IADL) like housekeeping, laundry and the ability to handle finances. Another dependency assessment instrument was developed by Exton-Smith, a physician in a major London hospital, little used in France so not worth describing here. The origins of these scales indicate dependency assessment's deep roots in the medical world.

The second stage occurred in France in the 1980s, when reflections on dependency assessment first began there (Ennuyer 2002: 111–115). Among the numerous studies of the time, Robert Leroux *et al.*'s (1981) is of particular interest. Geriatrician in a small hospital far from the capital, he developed a tool to depict his patients' disabilities and named it 'Géronte', meaning 'old man'. The instrument consists of an outline of a person broken into parts, each representing a potential disability (see Figure 9.1).

Parts of the body are grouped according to activity type (top to bottom): 'mental disabilities', 'sensorial functions', 'exterior activities', 'domestic activities', 'bodily activities', 'locomotive activities'.

The potential disabilities were shown in six groups, each represented by a region of the body: physical ambulation inside or outside the home by the legs, bodily activities like continence by the torso, domestic activities like communication by one arm, public activities like shopping by the other arm, sensory activities like seeing or hearing by the head, and mental disabilities by an added hat. Like Katz, assessment is made into three categories, black shading meaning no disability in an area, white indicating disability, and grey indicating partial disability. The resulting picture gives the patient's situation at a glance, useful when a nurse or a physician needs to sum up the case for a colleague (see Figure 9.2).

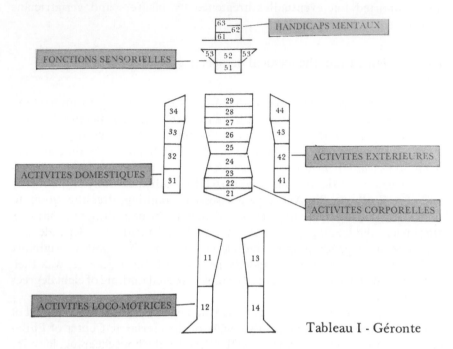

Tableau I - Géronte

Figure 9.1 Géronte. Source: Leroux *et al.* 1981.

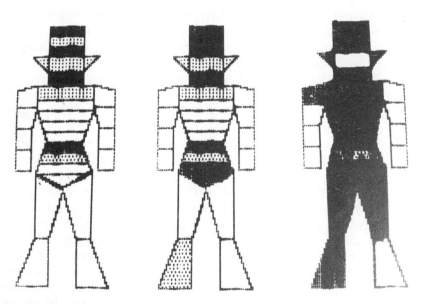

Figure 9.2 Three people dependency assessed using Géronte. Source: Leroux *et al.* 1981.

Géronte is therefore clearly intended for medical use, which I will call 'the medical perspective'. R. Leroux explains it thusly:

We built a simple, easy-to-use instrument for:
- helping the nursing team to know about elderly patients
- following changes in their health condition
- evaluating the effectiveness of treatments
- assessing their potential for returning home, or helping to direct them to another place or kind of treatment.

Other papers in the thematic journal issue containing Leroux's presentation of Géronte address how it could be used by the nursing team, its potential in developing physical therapy programmes, and how it could be computerized to automate image-making. This last point is destined to develop greatly with time.

Indeed, computerization issues are the hallmark of the third stage, which began in 1993. There were two important publications in French geriatrics that year. The first was a special issue of the *Revue de Gériatrie*, published by the national geriatricians' association, the National Clinical Gerontology Union (Syndicat National de Gérontologie Clinique; SNGC), entirely devoted to 'Computing in geriatrics'. One of the papers reminds readers of an important event that had happened in the interim, in 1982: the advent of a governmental programme enhancing the role of computing in hospitals, called the 'PMSI' (see below). Briefly, this programme was intended to boost hospitals' transparency and accountability to the government, which had long been striving for better control. This paper was written by the director of a Medical Information Department (DIM), one of the new government-created medical records offices responsible for implementing this program. Like all DIM directors, he was a physician. Here are some extracts (Lardy 1993):

The PMSI has created the DIMs, given them financial resources, created jobs.... Physicians must remain vigilant with regards to their future role.

It would be dishonest to physicians to claim that they could use computing for following up on their patients or evaluating the effectiveness of a medical treatment. [It] might at best give a very basic overview of the illnesses present in the hospital. However... , the compulsory reporting to the government does not prevent it from being used to develop a broad computing framework, and from there computing solutions for each hospital department, meeting its real needs.

[Conclusion] The PMSI is real and won't be terminated. It is compulsory. Should we be afraid of it? Perhaps. But in order to salvage the situation, we must:
- Be part of the system
- Participate in evaluation committees, should they exist
- If they do not, or if the government does not want to establish them, to denounce the situation.

This text illustrates the strategic posture some geriatricians adopted towards the government. The gist is that the government has imposed a programme, the PMSI, which they oppose as an intrusion on their profession (on this point, see Freidson, 1988 [1970]), but it is inescapable. They should therefore develop their own conception of computing systems and their uses instead of having them imposed from outside. The issue's editor, geriatrician Jean-Marie Vetel, expressed a similarly ambivalent position in the journal's introduction (Vetel 1993):

> Like every physician, the geriatrician must learn computing. Here are the basics... . Controlling our budgets, evaluating health care quality, knowing our patient's pathologies and degree of dependency, etc.: these target specifications must be set before any implementation. It is of the utmost importance that the medical community participate in this kind of project from the outset and acquire some computer literacy. Otherwise, our hospital administrations would be alone and obliged (doubtless reluctantly) to make decisions without us. For what purpose and to whom shall that data be of use... ? Better information will save time, making us more efficient so we can optimize our scant resources.

There are thus two reasons for geriatricians to develop dependency assessment instruments. There are medical reasons, such as improved knowledge of pathologies and better treatments, and there are managerial reasons, like the ability to 'optimize our scant resources'. All papers in this special journal issue reflect this duality, some rather fatalistically (like the DIM director) and others more reluctantly, as seen in R. Leroux's contribution or another article suggesting a positive correlation between patients' dependency levels and the burden they represent for the nursing staff (Manciet *et al.* 1993).

This paper is also interesting because, like Katz's (where it was implicit), it expresses the idea that dependent patients require more work and are therefore more costly than 'merely' sick ones for a given pathology. This reveals a managerial tendency that emerges sporadically in this literature and that could be termed the 'cost perspective'.

In another key text, J.-M. Vetel and J.-M. Ducoudray (who will be presented in greater detail below) expressed their deep discontent with the Anglo-American criteria for assessing dependency. They found the Katz–Lawton approach ignored patient behaviours connected with potential mental disorders (a factor that is taken into account in Géronte's hat), reduced functional indicators to sheer binary variables, induced a highly heterogeneous 'other' patient category and did not allow supplementary resources to be given to dependent elderly.

This criticism did not stop these geriatricians from working towards developing their own dependency assessment scale. The same year, in the more social-science-oriented journal *Gérontologie et Société*, they overtly proposed creating a 'PMSI for geriatrics'. The goal would be to evaluate the economic and human resources necessary for the care of elderly people with given pathologies and levels of dependency. The dependency dimension is clearly propelled by the cost perspective highlighted earlier:

> If we give priority to the [dependency criteria rather than the medical ones], it is because economic studies on several institutions have shown that ... the level of resources used was, in a determinant manner, linked to the lost of autonomy.

The text went on to describe how the French scale was built. It used Géronte and its three-level coding in a way that would remain virtually unchanged right through its adoption into law:

- Black: the elderly person does the activity alone completely, usually, correctly.
- Grey: he or she does it only partially.
- White: he or she does not do it.

The instrument was tested on 2,533 individuals from a wide range of nursing homes and homecare associations. A draft showing an algorithm for performing the classification confirms the binary structure of the process (see Figure 9.3). But their procedure induced a heterogeneous 'other' patient category like the one they had critiqued in Katz *et al.* (1963) so it was abandoned.

The physicians then considered another statistical method, the Principal Component Analysis (PCA). It allows multi-dimensional observations to be summarized into a set of just a few variables (typically two or three), making it seem to be the perfect tool for transforming a multi-dimensional phenomenon, like dependency, into one with fewer dimensions (ideally only one) to yield a 'level of dependency'. And indeed, the geriatricians discovered that a single constructed variable explained '85% of all the information'. Moreover, they used a statistical property of PCA to deem that some of the initial dependency variables were not explanatory of the result but merely 'illustrative'. In the ensuing years, the separation between explanatory and illustrative variables of dependency led to a heated controversy whose origin lies at this precise stage of the story. Eventually the result of the constructed aggregate variable, which had 13 levels, was grouped into only five ranks, 'for the sake of evaluation simplicity'.

This undertaking led the medical and cost perspectives to become mixed. In the conclusion, the geriatricians stated, 'the system will allow the creation of permanent indicators for the departments and hospitals ... and give a better conception of the financial resources to be allocated at both individual and collective levels'. Those indicators were then quickly transformed into the final version of the scale. The following year, in April 1994,

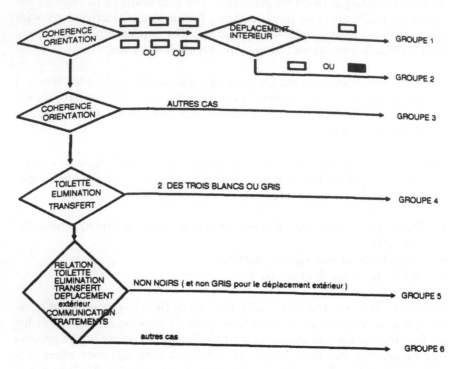

Figure 9.3 Provisional algorithm for AGGIR. Source: Arnaud *et al.* 1993, 97.

J.-M. Vetel declared in the *Revue de Gériatrie* that the 'time for AGGIR has come' – a bit of wordplay in French, since 'AGGIR' is close to *'agir'*, meaning to act. Six resource utilization groups were defined (Groupes Iso-Ressources, GIR), corresponding to six levels of dependency. They were tested on a large scale (10,000 individuals) in coordination with some local-level health coverage offices (branches of the national Social Security program). All this 'paves the way for funding care for the elderly according to their dependency level'.

The geriatricians thus seem to have successfully constructed an instrument closely resembling those they had rejected shortly before, but for a practical reason this time: to promote dependency risk as something different from simple sickness or long-term care, making it something that deserves special funding in times of budgetary austerity. But meanwhile they were joined by other actors, to which we turn now.

The state and other public actors

Once again, the story starts in the United States, where there was a growing preoccupation with public deficits in the 1970s. The election of Ronald

Reagan in 1980 opened a period of retrenchment for the welfare state (Pierson 1994). In the healthcare sector, an instrument named Diagnosis-Related Groups (DRGs) was introduced to limit costs. Created by Yale University management professor Robert Fetter and Alain Enthoven, a researcher at the Rand Corporation, the instrument theoretically allowed comparison of healthcare providers' efficiency. DRGs were used like products on a standard market: an expenditure level was defined for each DRG, and providers were given the corresponding lump-sum payment for each patient's DRG, even if expenses were ultimately higher. This shift to such a Prospective Payment System (PPS) was intended to boost productivity and cut costs, but its incentives induced lower quality of care and patient selection (Newhouse 1996).

Where the elderly are concerned, the risk of patient selection is particularly high, since their costs are higher than those of younger people, all other things being equal. Some even see the PPS as an instance of the divide-and-conquer and obfuscation techniques identified by Pierson. It divides health providers, who are incited to act counter to their professional ethics, from elderly consumers, who can only suffer lower quality care or be denied access; it obfuscates because budget cuts targeting the ageing population are hidden in the everyday operation of the new payment system (Preston *et al.* 1997).

In France, the PPS is imported through the PMSI (see above). The programme started in 1982, headed by the high-ranking official Jean de Kervasdoué (who earned his MBA and Ph.D. in the US). Some of its administrators asserted that it was only a way to better know hospital costs, not a way of fixing prices. This probably reduced physician opposition and made implementation of the information system possible. Regardless, some 20 years later, in 2003, a new administration turned the information system into a full-fledged payment system (Benamouzig 2005, Pierru 2007, Belorgey 2010, Juven 2014). It was first implemented in acute care, where it is easier to identify DRGs. The desire to also implement it in geriatrics (non-acute care), seen in the 1993 texts mentioned earlier, is therefore directly rooted in this history of the transformation of the payment system.

More specifically concerning public geriatric and elder policy, some official documents reveal the presence of the same preoccupations and mind-set. For instance, in 1990 the Ministry of Social Affairs published a document on dependency indicators. Written by General Director of Hospitals Gérard Vincent, it begins, 'In the current context of cost containment, the search for indicators contributing to optimal resource allocation for the socio-medical system is a priority'. In 1991, two official reports from M.P. Boulard and high-ranking civil servant P. Schopflin both express the aspiration that the State have an instrument for dependency assessment to understand and contain costs in the sector and establish a payment system. Geriatricians themselves, as we have seen, are influenced by the same preoccupations, including developing indicators, behaving strategically under financial austerity and working towards resource optimization.

Another great transformation impacting public policy for the elderly, and nearly all policy domains at the time, was the 'new public management' movement. Initially launched by conservative governments in the US and the UK, it was continued, albeit with some changes, by their moderate successors and imported by most Organisation for Economic Co-operation and Development (OECD) countries (Hood 1991, Osborne and Gaebler 1992, Pollitt & Bouckaert 2011). The movement aimed to introduce private business management methods into public administration in order to cut costs with tools including project management methods and benchmarking. It also had a significant impact on public policy in France (Bezes 2009), where the new form of management was mainly implemented by consulting firms (including the international 'big four') working to change professional practices in the public healthcare sector and more broadly at the State level (Belorgey 2010, Henry & Pierru 2012).

This taste of 'new public management' happens to have been introduced by one of the three main developers of the AGGIR scale, J-M Ducoudray, who we encountered earlier with J.-M. Vetel and R. Leroux. Unlike the two geriatricians, Ducoudray started out as a hospital director (thus a civil servant) with 'another view of gerontological questions', as Vetel put it in Leroux's obituary, adding that Leroux had had a 'strong sense of social justice'. J.-M. Ducoudray's writing indeed reveals a much more State-centred approach, more informed by general constraints than clinical knowledge of the human body. For instance, in 1993, immediately after Vetel's introductory article in the special journal issue, he published a text on project management that appears to be a translation of 'new public management' ideas into the journal's house style: a way to acclimate French gerontologists to the idea. He also developed connections between the group and Senator Jean-Pierre Fourcade (of the right-leaning UMP party), President of the Social Affairs Commission, who would pass the amendment creating the first dependency allowance.

We can actually best understand State intervention by looking at the final stages of the scale's development, especially its publication in an official decree. In March 1994, the Ministry of Social Affairs informally presented the scale to a group of experts on the sector, of whom some were quite critical. Despite this opposition, J.-P. Fourcade inserted an amendment into a law passed in July of that year, thus instituting the Experimental Dependency Allowance in 12 French administrative departments. J-P Fourcade and the French Senate in general are known for being particularly attentive to departmental issues, and this allowance might just have eased financial strain in these departments by limiting the elderly's access to the previous, more generous allowance that was later slated to be phased out. Benefits in those

12 departments were henceforth calculated using the AGGIR scale. Three years later, in 1997, another law was passed that transformed the experiment into national law in the form of the Specific Dependency Allowance.[4] The AGGIR scale was sanctioned and translated into a decree for the application of the law (Décret n° 97–427), validating all the geriatricians' work. The text states that the SNGC remains the sole proprietor of the classificatory algorithm, which can be summed up as follows:

1   Ten variables are given to assess the level of dependency (see Table 9.1). The first and second (mental coherence and orientation in time and space) correspond to Géronte's hat, resolving the lack of mental elements in Katz's ADL. The next six are Katz's ADL (with 'walking inside' as an extension of 'going to toilets'), which had also received much criticism. The last two, although present in Géronte and influential in the 1993 PCA, surprisingly receive no value. They had been among Lawton's IADL.
2   Each of these variables must be coded with the now-usual three Géronte ratings: A for full autonomy, C for full dependency, B for an intermediate situation.
3   An elderly person receives a certain number of 'points' as a result of the coding, which in turn determine which of the 13 'ranks' he or she will be given. The assignation of a rank process, i.e. the algorithm, is iterative. The more serious disabilities, such as a 'C' for mental coherence, are worth many points and lead to immediate classification in rank 1 (the maximum level of dependency). Below a given threshold (when someone is sufficiently autonomous), coding results lead to the next iteration, which in turn leads to lower ranks, and so on. The method used may thus be labelled as binary iterative, i.e. potentially quite close to the pattern of the rejected 1993 blueprint (see above).
4   The 13 ranks are then grouped in six GIR, the five found in the 1993 version plus one more (see Table 9.2). The scale is therefore clearly the result of cooperation between the State and favourable geriatricians.

Eventually the Pensions and Healthcare branches of the Social Security administration, also invested in the cost-containment movement, fostered the scale's development through their infrastructure and publications. Thus, ultimately numerous public actors contributed to the emergence of the risk of dependency.

The opponents and their critiques

We will first meet the opponents, and then proceed to summarize their criticisms, which are often similar. The opponents come from three main fields,

Table 9.1 Points of dependency in the AGGIR scale (first iteration)

Variables / Coding	A	B	C
Coherence	0	0	2000
Orientation	0	0	1200
Bathing	0	16	40
Dressing	0	16	40
Feeding	0	20	60
Continence	0	16	100
Transfer	0	120	800
Walking inside	0	32	200
Walking outside	0	0	0
Communication	0	0	0

Source: Décret 97–427, table by the author.

Table 9.2 From ranks to GIR

Ranks	GIR
1	1
2, 3, 4, 5, 6, 7	2
8, 9	3
10, 11	4
12	5
13	6

Source: Décret 97–427.

the first being the scientific world. Other kinds of physician are prominent here, like public health professors Alain Colvez and Jean-Claude Henrard who had developed their own dependency measurement tool (Ennuyer 2002: 111–119). As for geriatricians, they are far from united. The SNGC had only been created in 1980 and did not represent all relevant professionals; there was also the French Gerontology Society (Société Française de Gérontologie, SFG), and another instrument for dependency assessment, the Kuntzmann scale. Numerous geriatricians also voiced their criticism through the 1993 issue of the *Revue de Gériatrie* discussed earlier in this chapter. Critique was also expressed by other State-affiliated organizations, including the national school for hospital directors and CREDOC, an observatory of social consumption trends.

The second kind of sceptic was found among experts and grassroots activists. One particularly interesting case is that of Frédéric Bevernage, because he is a geriatrician and director of one of the new computerized hospital departments presented earlier. He believed AGGIR was 'a road to hell paved with good intentions' (1998). Another is Bernard Ennuyer, whose work is quoted abundantly in this chapter because he is a leading specialist of the field, a sociologist and the director of a homecare association. A third is a high-level civil servant at the Ministry of Social Affairs who did not want his name to be published.

The third field of opposition is more political, since it encompasses political actors like Ministry for Elderly in the socialist government (2001–2002) Paulette Guinchard and the Economic, Social, and Environmental Council (Conseil Economique, Social et Environnemental; CESE), the third national assembly (after those of Parliament) that mainly represents unions and civic associations.

Criticism was along two lines. The first signalled that the scale would not accurately express the needs of the elderly, leaving them with huge uncovered charges after receiving the allowance ('*reste à charge*', a remainder to be paid) or inflicting the same on their (institutional) caregivers. The second critique was that this was mainly due to the scale's bias for nursing homes over home care, which we will address later. The first critique actually comes from four flaws in the instrument.

First, dependency levels for determining allowances are only an average: people are sorted into six dependency-level categories, but there are significant variations within each category. The algorithm sorts for practical budget allocation reasons, but reduces the number of dependency levels and financial needs relative to the actual situations. As a matter of fact, all PPSs are criticized on this count, although most of the aforementioned critics seem unaware of that and arrive at their position by their own paths.

Second, there is a discrepancy between geriatric and managerial indicators. To take but one example, the managerial approach uses the average length of stay as an indicator of performance, shorter averages indicating higher performance. But from a geriatric approach longer care increases the likelihood of an elderly person leaving the ward in better health, thus further forestalling the need to return. Saint-Jean and his team (1993) concluded in this respect that 'the validity of this instrument [*the PMSI*] remains to be proven, especially in geriatrics, and its use for financial allocations may impoverish departments caring for elderly patients'. This flaw is also a discrepancy between medical and cost perspectives.

Third, Katz's ADL do not account for mental disorders and their behavioural consequences. The developers of AGGIR had already observed this oversight, and eventually added this dimension as AGGIR's first two variables.

Fourth, the last two AGGIR variables, walking outside and communication, were not assessed at all, and so the instrument fails to take account of these kinds of potential disability. This is despite their definition as IADL by Lawton and Brody, making them factors in dependency.

A subsidiary controversy arose later concerning the reproducibility of the scale given the variety of people using it in evaluations nationwide (Colvez *et al.* 2005, David 2006). Assessments are not all done in the same way, so a given person could have different results from different evaluators. Scale proponents explained this as evaluator error – due to divergent professional backgrounds, for instance. Opponents suggested instead that it came from a flaw in the instrument, which is poorly reproducible.

If the first criticism of the scale was of its poor ability to measure the elderly's real dependency levels, the second line of criticism added that this was in fair part due to its bias to nursing home care as opposed to homecare. Katz's ADL, Lawton and Brody's IADL, Exton-Smith's scale, Leroux's Géronte and Vetel's AGGIR were indeed all conceived from the outset in long-term care hospitals or nursing homes. There is a good reason for that: these authors are all physicians in such institutions themselves, which gave them access to a good sample of the elderly. Vetel responded to this criticism by explaining that AGGIR was tested on a range of patients in many places before its official recognition (see above). But opponents insisted that this validation came too late to prevent the structural flaw, which they anticipated would lead to three problems. First, IADLs (housekeeping, personal accounting, etc.) are performed by staff in institutional settings, but by the elderly themselves in home settings. As a result AGGIR would not accurately depict home situations. Second, the instrument is silent about help from families, for the same reason and with the same consequences. An elderly person living at home alone is not in the same situation as one surrounded by a caring family, and public assistance should vary accordingly. Third, the scale is also blind to peoples' living environments and the 'technical assistance' (as opposed to the 'human' kind) that the elderly may require at home. For instance, an aged woman who heats her house with wood and has to fetch the wood outside is, of course, much more dependent on other people for everyday life than one with modern conveniences, and should receive financial assistance accordingly.

Surprisingly, the available official documents are usually silent on these issues. They only describe how to fill out the scale. With time, much of the discussion has moved to the meaning of the three adverbs already found in Géronte: 'completely, usually, correctly', to which a fourth, 'spontaneously', was added in 2008. The link between the scale and the dependency level is only described as resulting from 'a complex algorithm that requires computer calculations', as a 2008 decree puts it. The weights of the coded variables are only found in the 1997 decree. Despite all these problems, then, the most important part of the instrument is now taken for granted. The black box we have been exploring thus far is now closed. The first 'taken for granted' effect is making people behave in accordance with this new risk and believe in it (Desrosières 1993), therein making it an essential component in the emergence of dependency as new social risk.

Let's consider this effect in the regular application of the scale.

The paradoxically comforting action of the street-level bureaucrats

Michael Lipsky (1980) described the dilemma of street-level bureaucrats, faced with the allocation of public resources that are usually insufficient for meeting the needs of their clientele. In this setting, they are the people responsible for using the AGGIR scale to evaluate elderly dependency levels since it became legally required. Most of them are nurses and social workers. The formal logic of the framework is as follows: three-way coding of each item in the scale → automatic rendering of a dependency level, the GIR → automatic attribution or refusal of a given level of public benefits, valuated in euros → determination of the number of hours of professional aid available to the elderly person (known as an 'Assistance Plan'). However, ethnographic observation of the work of the people conducting such evaluations in the home setting shows that the reverse order prevails instead (see Table 9.3).

As we can see, the agent starts from the elderly person's living situation and needs, which are not well represented on the scale. She asks not only about personal care needs but also about 'environmental aids' like housekeeping and cooking. She is supposed to code those IADLs into the scale, but as we saw earlier, they are not included in the algorithm's calculations of benefits.[5] The elderly woman is generally reluctant to receive public assistance and behaves modestly throughout the visit. The agent must especially press her to accept help with personal care, but once she agrees, she can get the help that she actually needs but is lacking in the scale: housekeeping aid. In so doing, the agent defends the interests of the elderly woman against the State. At the same time, she tries to change how the woman lives in a way she thinks better for her. She thus develops a patronising attitude (the carpet question), making her own diagnostic of the situation and defining what is to be done in consequence in the Assistance Plan. She then makes her diagnostic fit the legal framework.

This is not isolated behaviour. The Scientific Committee for Adaptation of Autonomy Evaluation Tools, founded by law in 2001 (by a left-leaning government) also wants evaluation to start with the Assistance Plan, and the AGGIR scale applied afterwards in order to determine the sum of benefits to be allocated. The Committee shares many of the critical views we have seen of the scale. It implicitly recognizes that the scale does not accurately evaluate what should be done for the elderly. An analogous conclusion was drawn by Ministry experts in a working group of the Caisse Nationale de Solidarité pour l'Autonomie (CNSA), a hybrid national agency for disabled and dependent persons created in 2004 (Graz 2006).

Street-level bureaucrats contribute to this tendency as well, by willingly overestimating the extent of dependency in filling out the scale when they think that the sum allocated to each GIR at the national level is inadequate for responding to the needs of some flesh-and-blood people.[6] This is a very well-known practice in the healthcare policy sector, where the same

Table 9.3 Example of an evaluation

Discussion (extracts)	Comments
Agent: Can you still cook?	The agent evaluates an IADL: cooking
Elderly woman: No, I eat ready-to-eat meals after heating them up in the microwave.	
Agent: You have trouble staying standing ...	
Woman: Yes (...). My kitchen isn't big, but with my cane I can't carry things (...).	
You must have a little cart.	
I have one	
Do you use it?	
Yes, I can push it, pull it ...	
You should be careful it doesn't tip. Some are specially designed to avoid that (...). You can find them in those shops I was speaking about, too (...). If I can give you some advice, even if the tiles are cold... You've never fallen?	The agent checks a well-known cause of problems: the carpets. She insists, even against the will of the woman
I know my carpets.	
Carpets still cause falls.	
I know them. I know where I have to lift my foot. They've been here for 37 years. It would be a pity [*to remove them*] (...).	
So, how long would you need someone in your home?	The agent does not evaluate with the scale, asking the elderly woman's needs directly
Let me explain (...). You can have the allowance if you need personal care. You have difficulties bathing and dressing, so you need it...	She recaps the difficulties in two ADL, which should be coded 'B' in the scale, leading to a GIR #4, and therefore to an allowance.
Living environment aids [*like housekeeping, as opposed to personal care*], the maximum is 2 times 2 hours a week.	The old woman is rather embarrassed at the prospect of receiving personal care, but she would accept someone for housekeeping. The agent negotiates the former, the presence of which allows her to give the latter. She starts from the woman's real need and tries to meet it within the legal framework.
If it were possible ...	
Would you like someone to help you with bathing, even partially, for the feet, for a shampoo from time to time?	
[*mumbling*] I've never had help, I don't want to abuse...	
So, the maximum I give for housekeeping is twice 2 hours a week.	The agent embodies the State: 'I give'

Direct observation, French middle-size town suburb, April 2011.

problems emerged decades before and were dubbed 'upcoding'. Street-level bureaucrats' dilemma in responding to citizens' needs while being dealt insufficient resources is thus temporarily solved, either by discarding the scale to define the real needs of the elderly, and/or by upcoding the situation in the scale in order to obtain sufficient funding for a given person. Of course, these solutions are not final. But what matters most for our purposes is that in so doing, everyone contributes to making the new dependency risk more substantial, however dissatisfied they are by the notion. However critical they may be of AGGIR, they breathe life into dependency by qualifying the elderly for benefits and labelling their needs as 'dependency'. Since situations of dependency command the attribution of benefits, the elderly and agents have a common interest in dependency really existing.

Back to medical indicators?

The actions of two groups, however, may lead the new risk of dependency to fade back into the older category of sickness. The first group is composed of private insurers, which have gone through a three-phase search for new markets and stricter criteria for defining their contracts. As usual, the story starts in the United States. The literature on the economics of insurance is rather pessimistic (e.g. Pauly 1990, Cutler 1993). It seeks to explain why people do not purchase insurance against the risk of long-term care (which will later be termed 'dependency' in Europe). The rare companies daring to offer contracts covering real expenses went bankrupt from the high variability of costs. Since then, only partial insurance contracts have been available, meeting a limited demand. It was also rather slow to take off in France. The financial press explains it by the elderly's distrust of such contracts, due, for instance, to their unclear definitions of 'dependency'.

In this context, the 1997 development of an official, State-authorized definition of the situation of dependency gave insurers arguments to soothe this distrust. In the following years, the AGGIR scale rose to prominence in newspapers, especially the financial press, which presented AGGIR-based contracts (see Figure 9.4 and Table 9.4). In 2011 and 2014, legislation was presented that lead to a certain amount of discussion. President Nicolas Sarkozy spearheaded a 'national debate on dependency' (2011), which fuelled the new risk's development in the press. The President strongly implied that part or all of this risk would be handled by private insurers, due to public budgetary constraints. One can see the traces of this debate in the graph.

But insurers found the definition of the new risk was still not clear enough. They worked within the aforementioned CNSA Committee to simplify the definition, stating, 'the AGGIR algorithm and weighting of variables are unclear for lay people. [*They*] prefer an eligibility threshold based on a given number of non-realized ADL, rather than the belonging to a GIR'. They agreed that ADLs take insufficient consideration of mental disorders, and

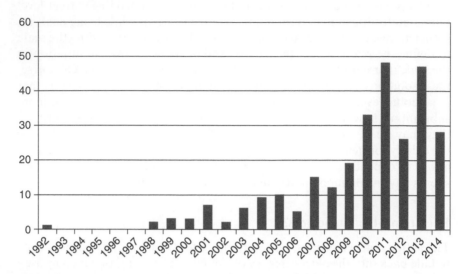

Figure 9.4 Number of media articles containing 'AGGIR' (per year). Data source: Personal search on Factiva 2015, Personal search on Factiva, accessed 10 February 2015.

wanted to replace AGGIR with the Mini-Mental State Examination, a genuinely medical test, for that purpose. They insisted that dependency is nearly always the consequence of a health problem. This position is purely pragmatic: insurers need the most precise definition of the risk possible in order to set the best premium and increase their share of the market. It is thus worth noting that, after benefitting from the new risk's emergence facilitating the development of a new market parallel to health insurance, they demanded that it be at least partially merged back into risk of illness, for the pure sake of accurate accounting and clarified communication.

If insurers are the first group to make the new notion of dependency fade back into the old category of sickness, the second group to do so is paradoxically comprised of geriatricians, who appear unsure of whether the risks

Table 9.4 Number of media articles containing 'AGGIR' (per media sector)

Sector	N	%
Financial	99	42
Regional	86	36
National	28	12
Social	16	7
Other	8	3
Total	237	100

Data source: Personal search on Factiva, accessed 10 February 2015.

facing the elderly are of a medical or dependency order. They had always insisted both were concerned. Geriatrician authors in the 1993 *Revue de Gériatrie* had also discussed using the Resources Utilizations Groups (RUG) proposed by the American team of Fries (1989), and they used the exact translation in French to name their GIR. Fries *et al.*'s model is far-reaching, as it uses not only ADL but also behavioural and even many medical elements, such as an elderly person's clinical situation, special therapies (i.e. physical therapy), and main diagnoses. Geriatricians discarded the tool in 1993, but changed their minds in the 2010s. They created a new instrument called 'Pathos', a new transposition of the PMSI for geriatrics, which was initially required by the health insurance branch of Social Security. It calculates elder care costs on the basis of the medical situation. Another instrument, 'Socios', is intended to account for the social situation. Consequently, AGGIR is only one of many instruments used today, and the connection between an older person's medical indicators and living situation has been renewed. The 'old' risks are still alive and well.

Concluding remarks

Two kinds of conclusions may be drawn, one on the invention of dependency and another, more theoretical, on the relationship between theory and action.

We now know that dependency did not exist as a social risk until it was invented by Katz and those who followed, or more precisely prior to the promulgation of legal instruments claiming to measure it. Dependencies may have existed between the elderly and others, but not in the sense that they were perceived as 'risks' (that must be measured and compensated for when they occur) or social phenomena (recognized at a collective level). For dependency to become a new social risk according to the welfare state's definition, i.e. an accident of life to be addressed at the macro-level, many people had to intervene: some geriatricians gave it a formal structure and assessment, some politicians and branches of Social Security advocated for it, and other geriatricians and some grassroots activists and politicians fruitlessly fought its institutionalization, State and local governments eventually institutionalized it. Once the 'assessment' instrument – in France, the AGGIR scale – became law, it was used to invent dependency as an accident of life that should be compensated by the welfare state. Street-level bureaucrats then brought dependency into genuine existence by claiming and obtaining compensation for elderly people on the grounds of dependency, in so doing silencing some of the opposition. Private insurers, looking for new markets and policies inspiring greater trust, also gave dependency life – in the press, in people's minds, and through payments when the risk became reality. The new risk of dependency remains frail, however, since it is repeatedly pulled back into basic medical risk. Use of the alternative term 'long-term care' instead of 'dependency' illustrates that the latter remains closely associated with sickness, even when it is not acute.

From a more theoretical point of view, we have already distinguished between medical and cost perspectives, but there is actually a third perspective between them, known as the 'clinical experience perspective' in the sociology of applied knowledge (Freidson 1988 [1970]; Becker *et al.* 2008 [1961]). Aiming for action rather than knowledge, participants such as physicians prefer actions that are successful, have little chance of success, or may even be based solely on their own experiences to an intellectually rigorous but inactive approach. In this they resemble some other actors, such as politicians and businessmen, who are prompt to scoff at 'armchair intellectuals'. J.-M. Vetel obviously shared this perspective, as we saw earlier in his declaration that the 'time to AGGIR [*to act*] has come', as do other proponents of the scale. There are therefore three perspectives that shed light on the emergence of dependency: medical (common to opponents, in the name of the elderly), cost (common to proponents), and clinical experience (explaining some participants' abandonment of the first to embrace the second). Blurring the boundaries between science and action, they are likely to be found in case studies in other countries as well.

Notes

1 In this, it shares Carnap's view that 'it was not until thermometers were invented that the concept of temperature could be given a precise meaning' (1966, p. 68). For analogous approaches in ageing issues, see Katz (1992, 2002).
2 Fifteen days of observation, from October 2010 to June 2011, in an average-size town and its suburbs.
3 For a similar approach, see Blaug (1964). The selected articles come from the literature and the overview of the two French leading journals presented below.
4 In 2001 the left-leaning government transformed it into a less restrictive Personalized Autonomy Allowance, but the scale used to evaluate the dependency is the same – only the resulting allowances are modified.
5 Except for a very brief assessment of 'walking outside' in the algorithm's last iteration.
6 Email from a social worker, 2011.

References

Arnaud C., Ducoudray Jean-Marc, Leroux Robert, Martin J. & Jean-Marie Vetel (1993), 'PMSI en gériatrie; lexique de l'évaluation en gérontologie; les groupes iso-ressources de charges en soins gérontologiques', *Gérontologie et société*, 64, pp. 78–108.
Arnold June & Arthur Norman Exton-Smith (1962), 'The Geriatric Department and the Community Value of Hospital Treatment in the Elderly', *The Lancet* 280 (7255), pp. 551–553.
Becker Howard (1985), *Outsiders. Etudes de sociologie de la déviance.* Paris, Métailié [1963].
Becker Howard, Strauss Anselm, Everett Hughes & Blanche Geer (2008), *Boys in White.* New Brunswick, Transaction Books [1961].

Belorgey Nicolas (2010), *L'hôpital sous pression: enquête sur le 'nouveau management public'*. Textes à l'appui – Enquêtes de terrain. Paris, La Découverte.

Benamouzig Daniel (2005), *La santé au miroir de l'économie*. Sociologies. Paris, PUF.

Bevernage Frédéric (1998), 'La grille AGGIR, un enfer pavé de bonnes intentions'. www.bevernage.com/geronto/aggir.htm, accessed 6 February 2017.

Bezes Philippe (2009), *Réinventer l'État*. Le lien social. Paris, PUF.

Blaug Mark (1964), *Economic Theory in Retrospect*. London, Heinemann.

Carnap Rudolf (1966), *Philosophical Foundations of Physics. An Introduction to the Philosophy of Science*. New York, Basic Books.

Colvez Alain, Royer Véronique, Berthié-Mourgaud Stéphanie & Cécile Pociello (2005), 'Étude de la fiabilite de l'instrument aggir: reproductibilité (test/re-test) entre évaluateurs, dispersion des temps d'aide requise entre groupes iso-ressources'. Montpellier, Pôle d'Etude et de Formation en Gérontologie du Languedoc-Roussilon, pour la DGAS.

Cutler David M. (1993), 'Why doesn't the market fully insure long-term care?' National Bureau of Economic Research. www.nber.org/papers/w4301, accessed 6 February 2017.

David Albert (2006), *Aide méthodologique à l'analyse et à l'amélioration de l'outil AGGIR*. Paris, Armines.

Desrosières Alain (1993), *La politique des grands nombres. Histoire de la raison statistique*. Textes à l'appui. Anthropologie des sciences et des techniques. Paris, La Découverte.

Durkheim Emile (2007), *De la division du travail social*. Paris, PUF [1893].

Elias Norbert (1991), *La société des individus*. Éd. Agora. Paris, Pocket [1987].

Ennuyer Bernard (2002), *Les malentendus de la dépendance: de l'incapacité au lien social*. Action sociale. Paris, Dunod.

Freidson Eliot (1988), *Profession of Medicine. A Study of the Sociology of Applied Knowledge*. Chicago, University of Chicago Press [1970].

Fries Brant, Don P. Schneider, William J. Foley & Mary Dowling (1989), 'Case-Mix Classification of Medicare Residents in Skilled Nursing Facilities: Resource Utilization Groups (RUG-T18)', *Medical Care* 27 (9), pp. 843–858.

Frinault Thomas (2005), 'La dépendance ou la consécration française d'une approche ségrégative du handicap', *Politix* 72 (4), pp. 11–31.

Frinault Thomas (2009), *La dépendance: un nouveau défi pour l'action publique*. Rennes, PUR.

Graz Jean-Christophe (2006), 'Les hybrides de la mondialisation', *Revue française de science politique*, 56 (5), pp. 765–787.

Gusfield Joseph R. (1986), *Symbolic Crusade: Status Politics and the American Temperance Movement*. Urbana, University of Illinois press [1966].

Henry Odile & Frédéric Pierru (2012), 'Les consultants et la réforme des services publics', *Actes de la recherche en sciences sociales,* 193 (3), pp. 4–15.

Hood Christopher (1991), 'A Public Management for all Seasons?', *Public Administration* 69 (1), pp. 3–19.

Juven Pierre-André (2014), 'Une santé qui compte ? Coûts et tarifs dans la politique hospitalière française', Thèse de doctorat, Mines-ParisTech.

Katz Stephen (1992), 'Alarmist Demography: Power, Knowledge, and the Elderly Population', *Journal of Aging Studies*, 6 (3), pp. 203–225.

Katz Stephen (2002), *Disciplining Old Age: The Formation of Gerontological Knowledge*. Charlottesville, University of Virginia Press.

Katz Sidney, Moskowitz Roland W., Jackson Beverly A. & Marjorie W. Jaffe (1963), 'Studies of Illness in the Aged: The index of ADL: A Standardized Measure of Biological and Psychosocial Function', *Journal of the American Medical Association*, 185 (12), pp. 94–99.

Lardy, B. 1993. 'Définition et objectifs du PMSI'. *Revue de gériatrie*, 18 (8): 479–482.

Lawton Powell M. & Elaine M. Brody (1969), 'Assessment of Older People: Self-Maintaining and Instrumental Activities of Daily Living', *The Gerontologist*, 9 (3), pp. 179–186.

Leroux, Robert, G. Attalli, M. Godon & G. Viau. 1981. 'Naissance de Géronte au congrès de gériatrie du Mans'. Symbiose - Revue des professions de santé 20.

Lipsky Michael (1980), *Street-Level Bureaucracy. Dilemma of the Individual in the Public Service*. New York, Russel Sage Foundation.

Manciet Gerard, Corompt, A.C., Decamps Arnaud, Galley Pierre, Dedieu Catherine, Simonetti, M. & Jean Marc Daubos (1993), 'Relation entre les niveaux de soins requis et la dépendance des personnes âgées en unité de long séjour'. *Revue de gériatrie*, 18 (8): 511–516.

Newhouse Joseph P. (1996), 'Reimbursing Health Plans and Health Providers: Efficiency in Production Versus Selection', *Journal of Economic Literature*, 34 (3), pp. 1236–1263.

Osborne David & Ted Gaebler (1992), *Reinventing Government: How the Entrepreneurial Spirit Is Transforming the Public Sector*. Reading (Mass.) Amsterdam Paris, Addison-Wesley, A. W. Patrick.

Pauly Mark V. (1990), 'The Rational Nonpurchase of Long-Term-Care Insurance', *Journal of Political Economy*, 98 (1), pp. 153–168.

Pierru Frédéric (2007), *Hippocrate malade de ses réformes*. Raisons d'agir. Paris, Editions du croquant.

Pierson Paul (1994), *Dismantling the Welfare State? Reagan, Thatcher, and the Politics of Retrenchment*. Cambridge, Cambridge University Press.

Pollitt Christopher and Bouckaert Geert (2011), *Public Management Reform: A Comparative Analysis - New Public Management, Governance, and the Neo-Weberian State*. 3rd Edition. Oxford and New York, Oxford University Press.

Preston Alistair M., Wai-Fong Chua & Dean Neu (1997), 'The Diagnosis-Related Group-Prospective Payment System and the Problem of the Government of Rationing Health Care to the Elderly', *Accounting, Organizations and Society* 22 (2), pp. 147–164.

Saint-Jean Olivier, Denis Mayeux, Josian Holstein, Robert Moulias & Membres du groupe PMSI Gériatrie (1993), 'Programme national de recherche sur le PMSI en gériatrie', *La revue de gériatrie*, 18 (8), pp. 495–500.

Vetel Jean-Marie (1993), 'Informatique en gériatrie: bouée de sauvetage ou boulet?' *Revue de gériatrie*, 18 (8), p. 447.

Part IV

Experiencing, playing, shifting boundaries

10 Discerning ageing in relation to the law?

Debates on the legal framework of freedom of movement of the elderly in France between 2004 and 2015

Lucie Lechevalier Hurard and Benoît Eyraud

Introduction

In France, an independent administrative body, the General Controller of Deprivation of Liberty Sites (CGLPL), monitors the enforcement of the fundamental rights of persons deprived of freedom as a result of a judicial or administrative decision.[1] The scope of CGLPL's control covers prisons, custody centres and detention centres where foreigners awaiting deportation are held (the administration does not recognize their right to remain on the territory). It also concerns psychiatric hospitals, insofar as certain hospital statutes specific to these institutions allow (under certain conditions) dispensing with the person's consent.

In May 2012, the CGLPL proposed extending the scope of its control to establishments for the dependent elderly. Although retirement home admission and residence are not subject to a judicial or administrative decision, the proposal was justified by the view that 'many elderly or very elderly people are not allowed outside their accommodation since, lacking sufficient capacity, there is too great a risk of them physically distancing themselves' (CGLPL, 2013, pp. 213–214). Although the proposal was ultimately rejected during parliamentary debates, it nonetheless illustrated the problem of the *de facto* existence of restrictions on the freedom of movement for seniors living in establishments.

In a context where professionals of such establishments seek to completely detach themselves from the unflattering image of the total institution (Loffeier, 2015), contrasting it to the domestic character of their institutions (Mallon, 2004), many have publically expressed outrage at this proposal and pushed for a clarification of the legal guidelines that frame their daily work. An article published by a geriatric psychiatrist, entitled, 'Freedom of movement in nursing homes: are we on the wrong side of the law?' (Hazif-Thomas, 2014) reflects the concern of professionals in the face of the legal framework they perceive as insufficiently clear and that consequently offers too little protection, both for themselves and for seniors they treat. This concern is considerably heightened in an environment where such practices may also be subject to allegations of 'mistreatment' (Dujarier, 2002; Hugonot, 2007; Molinier, 2009; Beaulieu & Crevier 2010; Lechevalier Hurard, 2013)

In this chapter, we intend to revisit these recent issues by analysing the different stages of the freedom of movement of the elderly debate as it has occurred in the French gerontological world over a 10-year period. We are particularly interested in regulatory actors[2] in this domain and the questions they ask themselves: How can we frame the restriction on freedom of movement practices like those in nursing homes (Lechevalier Hurard, 2013)? Should there be specific legislation for seniors whose state of health appears to especially diminish their faculties? Do these impairments justify the development of specific legal statutes?

After (1) re-evaluating how the debate on the existing legal framework has gradually emerged, we will (2) outline how regulatory actors of the gerontological sector initially failed to agree on whether to legislate restrictions on the freedom of movement of certain seniors, especially considering the risk of discrimination that such a text potentially represented. They therefore turned towards defining forms of 'soft law' (based on best practice recommendations) (Conseil d'Etat, 2013) since such 'laws' made it possible to differentiate between several types of populations without institutionalizing them. (3) Incentives to write possible restrictions on the freedom of movement into law were nevertheless maintained during the following period. We observe that it led to the passage of a law in 2015, which specifically established enacting these restrictions under certain conditions, while still upholding the refusal to identify distinctions among the elderly.

Retracing the evolution of how legal figures and responses were questioned, and considering their contributions to the stages of debate, allows us, beyond the notion of freedom of movement, to highlight a broader issue: the framings of age. In practice, since for a large part of the sector's actors certain seniors quite automatically fall into the category of 'normal' ageing persons, they are associated with the fundamental rights of ordinary adults. On the other hand, in 'pathological' ageing, which justifies special measures restricting these rights, is it not essential then to set legal limits and define legal boundaries (that no one seems prepared to undertake)?

Empirical data

The proposed analysis is based on empirical data of varying natures. A legal analysis was first based on a collected set of French and international laws that currently govern the care of the vulnerable elderly and their freedom of movement. It was supplemented by an assessment on a national scale of French case law on the subject, as well as by a body of eleven best practice guidelines of professional care practices of the elderly (those either suffering from Alzheimer's disease or generally living in geriatric institutions). The jurisprudence analysed, like good practice recommendations, span over a decade, between 2000 and 2015. The different public action procedures were documented by a series of interviews of involved parties, through observations conducted by two bodies of the National Committee of Positive Treatment and Rights (CNBD) as well as through analyses of summary documents of ensuing debates, made public during the processes.

A gradual and increasingly debated legal context

The debate on opportunities of a specific legal framework for restrictions of the freedom of movement of the elderly begins slowly emerging from the 1990s. If restrictions of these liberties are regulated by a set of laws applicable to the general adult population, it is the development and institutionalization of closed units in the early 2000s that leads gerontology regulatory actors to acutely problematize the issue of a framework of the restrictions for some elderly residents who live in institutions.

The legal framework of the freedom of movement in the care of vulnerable seniors

In France, as in most countries of civil law systems or common law, care practices and support are historically regulated by general legal principles, which are not specific to the age of the persons, provided they are adults.[3] The common law generally prohibits restrictions on the freedom of movement not agreed to by the person. This general principle carries no age limit. Legally, an adult individual of any age remains entitled to exercise his rights and free to make decisions regarding his person (Cornu, 1961, p. 9; Gridel, 2001, p. 4). These principles are also asserted by advocates of an international convention on the rights of the elderly.[4]

Admittedly, institutions may take measures restricting freedom to satisfy 'security' standards, provided they obtain the person's consent. This requirement of consent was accentuated during the legislative cycle of the 2000s, during which several laws were passed in order to reinforce patients' and service users' rights.[5] In terms of care, barring exceptions, no medical procedure or treatment can be performed or given without the free and informed consent of the person, and this consent may be revoked at any moment.[6] The regulations applicable to health and medico-social institutions established the principle of prior consent of treatment and ensuing constraints, which is problematic if the capacity to consent of the residents is undetermined.

In this particular case, two clauses allow for derogation from the general law. First, the initiation of a measure of legal protection: a guardian may be vested with power to decide personal matters, subject to judicial guardianship rules.[7] In fact, of the 800,000 guardianships existing in 2012, many cases concerned the elderly (Eyraud, 2013). Under certain conditions,[8] the guardian could oblige a person to leave his home or to sign a residence contract with a hospital or a nursing home. Furthermore, there is a measure of care without consent. In this context, the person may be subject to mandatory hospitalization and the limitations of movement associated with it, but the hospitalization should take place in a psychiatric ward. Historically, many elderly persons with impaired cognitive abilities have been hospitalized in psychiatric units (Chapireau, 2007). Although specialized services of Geriatric Psychiatry have evolved today, they still do not accept all seniors with impaired cognitive abilities.

These two provisions do not cover all the cases where seniors with impaired cognitive abilities, residing in health or medico-social sector institutions, are subject to restrictive freedom measures.

Are the existence of closed units legally justifiable?

A number of institutions for the elderly are equipped with closed units. This practice was encouraged by the development of specific units at the local level from the 1980s. Often used for persons whose cognitive abilities are impaired, they are referred to as 'Alzheimer units' or 'protected units'; even 'security' units (Lechevalier Hurard, 2015).

Gradually, the legal framework of these practices was questioned by professionals in a context of increasing concern for the rights of the elderly. In the late 1980s, the Gerontology National Foundation established a 'Dependent elderly charter' in which 'freedom of movement' of the elderly was reaffirmed, soon followed by the 'Charter of the European Federation of Establishment Directors'. In the process, gerontological and geriatric sector professionals created the Francophone Association for Human Rights of the Elderly. If social rights topics took centre stage as the main event, issues of obtaining consent and restrictions on the freedom of movement were also mentioned in various texts during the association's various conferences held throughout the 1990s. Ploton and Souillard were preoccupied with the few cases valuing the point of view of seniors in the measurement of consent in institutions (Ploton & Souillard, 1991). In the late 1990s and early 2000s, the question of elderly rights was becoming increasingly a subject of public debate. Assuredly, the case will demonstrate that judges will recognize the restrictive measures of the freedom of movement of residents with impaired cognition in certain circumstances (Lacour, 2012; Véron, 2017). However, this judicial response does not appear fully satisfactory to industry figures, including facility directors who wish to avoid legal litigations.[9]

After the legal measures of the early 2000s, which strengthened the obligation to respect the rights of persons by consensus of their consent, the modalities of application of the law in establishments and medico-social services were discussed. In this context, the issue of specific legislation to regulate reductive practices of movement in institutions was actively addressed.

Turning towards soft law: allowing for legal non-establishment of new categories of ageing

The idea of introducing new legal provisions was broached and opened up a debate on the consequences of a specification of legal rules for some of the elderly. Discussions took place primarily in the form of consensus conferences, a classic tool of public health professionals (Got, 2005) since its emergence in the late 1970s in the United States. In 2004, the scientific and professional community gathered to discuss Freedom of Movement.

Debating a relevant legal framework

Organized by a federation of public hospitals (FHF) according to the methodology promoted by the independent agency responsible for regulating the health sector,[10] this consensus conference led to the production of a written summary of recommended practices in this field. Its aim was to specify the 'medical' conditions in which the freedom of movement could be 'exceptionally limited', including without the person's consent, despite the fact that the 2002 laws made consent mandatory (FHF, 2004, p. 8). Although the problem was not limited to the elderly, the specific issue pertaining to them was mentioned:

> The situation of the vulnerable elderly today, often deprived of their freedom to exercise their consent, must be subject to consideration on a solely individual basis. For, if the disabled can now benefit from protection thanks to the strength of their associations, the same cannot be said for the elderly who are not associated with any advocacy group and are therefore all the more vulnerable.
>
> (FHF, 2004, p. 10)

The conclusive element of these problems was one of the central issues of the consensus conference. In terms of the rule of consent under fundamental rights, some members of the jury felt that exceptions should be laid out in a legislative text. Others feared that such legislation would lead to 'separating those suffering with cognitive disorders' and were concerned about the potential stigma of a discriminatory system. No satisfactory agreement being found, the issue was temporarily shelved. Mentioning these seemingly irreconcilable positions, the recommendation of the conference text suggested that 'thorough reflection be given to this subject' (FHF 2004, p. 18). To fill the void left by this period of suspension of the decision on the transformation of the legal framework, the jury then proposed to 'improve the practices of respect for the will of the people, despite difficulties of expression' through best practice guidelines issued by public regulatory bodies such as the High Authority of Health and the National Assessment of Social and

Medico-social Council.[11] Indeed, as a result of this consensus conference, at least a dozen best practice guidelines were published, with a national vocation and using professional management practices with the elderly living in institutions and those suffering from Alzheimer's disease. These are texts designed to regulate professional practices. They involve especially independent agencies of the state who regulate the intake system in health and social care (Castel & Robolet, 2009; Benamouzig, 2010).

Two corpus of recommendations for two separate populations

Analysis of this corpus of good practice guidelines nevertheless shows that, in the set of texts, the authors make a distinction between the two populations of elderly residents in institutions. The first group includes ordinary residents; the other group, 'Alzheimer's patients', who receive separate treatment, are candidates for the restriction of freedom of movement.

In the first group of guidelines of best practices we studied, laws establishing the rights of patients and users, as well as major national and international texts on the fundamental rights of persons[12] are reiterated. In this context of legal condemnation of practices restricting freedoms, only medical prescriptions are presented as able to define the conditions under which an exception could be made to the rule of consent. Certain conditions for using contention are nevertheless specified. Since it represents 'an infringement on the inalienable right of freedom of movement' (FHF, 2004, p. 21) and a 'risky act' (HAS and Forap, 2012, p. 20), it must be used for a limited time, and fall within a specifically dictated monitoring procedure (ANESM, 2009, p. 22). The recommendations in the guidelines therefore contribute to strictly defining this action.

Alongside this detailed framework of the use of restraints, the regulatory authority for the medical-social sector, ANESM, issues a recommendation on 'positive treatment' that puts at the heart of its definition, 'respect for the person and his history, his dignity and his uniqueness' and 'giving value to users' opinions' (ANESM, 2008, p. 15). Through this broad definition, the ANESM goes beyond compliance with the consent of the person receiving care. It therefore excludes all practices that would, in one manner or another, go against the choice of the person.

If the guidelines extend the scope of the prohibition of non-consensual practices, a second set of texts, specifically dedicated to the care of Alzheimer's disease, provides a regulatory framework in which certain restrictive practices of freedom can be used as in exceptional cases. This delineation appears in the unequal treatment of the issue of rights by recommendations for the general population of elderly and those that relate directly to the care of Alzheimer's disease. In the first subset of guidelines, references to fundamental rights and freedoms is a structuring factor, since all the guidelines follow from the legal and moral regulatory framework. From the second subset of texts, this reference is essentially absent.

Persons suffering from cognitive impairment are characterized by the risk of danger they pose. This risk exists for persons in care, primarily for themselves, physically, but also indirectly, in terms of legal liability for those involved in ensuring their safety. In fact, nursing home managers have more to fear in the courts being questioned on liability for infringement of their safety obligations than for violation of the freedom of movement of residents. The effective litigation indeed deals mainly with compliance with the obligation of residents' safety, unlike the psychiatric field, where there are rulings on violations of freedom of movement.

The lexical field of danger and risk tends to define a particular segment of the population in the recommendations. 'Dangerous behaviour' (ANAES, 2000b, p. 10; DGS, DGAS and SFGG, 2007, p. 34) for the person or those in his inner circle, or 'at risk' (ANAES, 2000b, p. 15; FHF, 2004, p. 18; ANESM, 2009, p. 13; HAS, 2008, p. 67) in the guidelines, justify exceptions to the respect for rule of freedom of movement and justify consent that can give rise to restrictive measures partially in the name of 'security' and 'protection'. Unlike strictly regulated medically qualified practices such as contention, their definition is not explicitly defined, and their degree of acceptance fluctuates. Practices referred to as the 'control' and 'mastery' or 'limitation', according to certain texts, can be deemed medically binding practices, and, similarly regulated by supporting restriction (ANESM, 2009, p. 22). In other texts, their use in certain circumstances and with populations whose behaviour is considered dangerous seems justified (ANAES, 2003, p. 21; Anaes, 2000b, p. 30; FHF, 2004, p. 14).

In spite of the absence of legal provisions that place Alzheimer's in a legal category opening the possibility of a specific and particular law (Aïdan, 2007), the contours of a certain population group are being defined in the best practice guidelines. Using recommendations reiterates the legal principle of prohibition of restrictive practices of freedom while establishing exceptions and allowing the development of differentiated practices between two types of populations (the elderly without cognitive alteration and the elderly with cognitive alteration), without these categories being institutionalized in the law.

Yet the nature of these texts is not directly legal and thus they are not enforceable in the same ways laws or administrative regulations are. Conceived as a transitional mode of regulation, the best practice guidelines did not resolve the issue of specific legal rules for elderly with cognitive impairments.

New legislation on ageing ... lacking specifics

Beyond the spread of best practice recommendations resulting from the 2004 consensus conference, the question of a specific legal status authorizing the restriction of the freedom of movement of seniors in certain circumstances remains unresolved. Political commitment to finding a legal resolution to the problem has been strongly reaffirmed in several political proposals in recent years.

A specific status for Alzheimer's elderly?

The question of a legal status of vulnerable seniors was first addressed in the framework of public action dedicated to Alzheimer's disease.[13] The third 2008–2012 Alzheimer's Plan took form by launching its measure 39 that called for reflecting on the legal status of the persons with Alzheimer's disease in institutions:

> The goal is to end the legal uncertainty linked to the difficulty of understanding consent of the person with Alzheimer's disease and to clarify the role of different persons in relation to the patient, be they persons of trust, a guardian, or a caregiver.

The manifestation of this measure gave rise to legal recommendations made by the services of the Ministry in a preliminary draft law in 2009. The reform considered creating, in the medico-social sector, placement in retirement homes without a form of consent by giving the Director the power to restrict freedom of movement of persons staying at his/her establishment on the basis of two medical certificates; one of which from the coordinating physician of the institution after possible consultation with the institution's staff.

Certain regulatory actors who published tribunes in the national press made harsh criticisms. They accused the provisions of stigmatizing people and seeking to protect society (Causse *et al.*, 2009). Due to a lack of consensus, the measure was ultimately abandoned. Erema, an ethics organization set up within the framework of policies dedicated to the disease, was responsible for advancing the lively discussion. Their resulting viewpoint, however, in 2012, only raised further questions, without responses. 'It is worth asking whether Alzheimer's justifies a special adaptation of existing texts or the development of specific legal protection adapted to the particularities of the disease' (Erema, 2012, p. 14). The Alzheimer Plan 2008–2012 had expired, thus no specific status was established.[14]

The 'society's adaptation to ageing' law reaffirms the principles of common law

The arrival of a new majority government in 2012 saw a reform of the measure, with the proposition of a general law on 'the adaptation of the society to ageing', containing provisions on users' rights and their protections. Preliminary reports (Aquino, 2013; Broussy, 2013; Pinville, 2013) evoke neither the Alzheimer's Plan, nor discussion of a specific status, but the need to act: '[Residential facilities for seniors] in the future, will be establishments specializing in dependence or in Alzheimer's disease' (Broussy, 2013, p. 68). But they demonstrate a strong will to legally reaffirm the fundamental rights of the elderly, while creating the possibility of limiting the freedom of movement of residents in institutions under certain conditions.

Political commitment of the new majority to get involved in the issue of rights and freedoms of the elderly and their legal framework was also reflected in the creation of a new body: the National Committee for Positive Treatment and the Rights of the Elderly and Disabled Persons (*Comité National pour la Bientraitance et les Droits des personnes âgées et des personnes handicapées* (CNBD).[15] One of its subcommittees was responsible for discussing the issue of rights. Within the committee, the working group[16] on the freedom of movement sought to draft a 'charter of best practices of using a geo-location system in gerontology for the benefit of persons with impaired intellectual functions', and to discuss new legislative provisions. The proposal of a geo-location charter led to a text where the older audiences, to whom geo-location techniques could be applied, remained unspecified. The authorization of certain restrictions on the freedom of movement in the text is only at the price of the reaffirmation of the principle of consent and maintains relative silence on all uncertain situations where the validity of consent is not guaranteed.

Further discussions, this time of a legislative nature, encouraged the participants to discuss the medical and judicial guarantees that must be applied to the measures of restriction. The written text before the issue and argued in front of the CNBD, stipulated that restrictions on the freedom of movement could be authorized on medical advice.

This provision is criticized by a magistrate,[17] on the grounds that the Constitution gives the judge the mandate to be the guarantor of individual liberty, and therefore it is up to the judge, not the doctor, to control restrictions of freedom.

Upon considering this case, when the president of the commission, David Causse,[18] repeatedly states the risk of placing such measures under the control of a judge, he does so more due to the lack of resources of the Ministry of Justice than as a critique of a judicialization of freedom of movement. This provision will be removed from the text submitted to the State Council, since the Office of the Ministry of Justice has clearly confirmed this legal hurdle.

A lack of agreement involves the monitoring to be established on the restrictions of freedom of movement.

Ultimately, the law on the adaptation of the society to ageing adopted on 28 December 2015, reaffirms the concern of 'inscribing the freedom of movement among the rights and freedoms guaranteed to persons received in social and medico-social institutions'. Article 27 nevertheless provides for a limitation of freedoms for the persons accommodated in nursing homes, but only if the restrictions are specified in an annex to the residence contract, *signed by the accommodated person*. They must be in accordance with the state of the person and the objectives of his care, after a collective procedure carried out at the initiative of the coordinating physician of the establishment or the patient's personal GP.

Through the use of an appendix in the residence contract as leverage, the primacy of consent is reiterated, leaving aside all other situations where its validity is not guaranteed. It is as if the person suffering from Alzheimer's disease has a reduced capacity to consent. Thus although a person's rights are reiterated, the question of her actual capacity to act is circumvented.

In short, after the proposals for specific legislation for certain members of the elderly population, the legislature opted for a new legislation that merely reaffirms the general principles of law. Since the resolution employs a technique of avoidance (the existing legal framework is not changed but merely restated), we can comprehend the frustration of those involved in the process, who attempted to address a problem they wished to resolve.

Conclusion

After observing that the grounds of legal rules in institutions for the elderly authorize the restriction on the freedom of movement only through the accordance of the said person consent, we emphasized the difficulties in solving the issue of a legal framework specific to seniors with cognitive difficulties.

Beyond the single issue of the freedom of movement, the challenge that regulatory actors of the gerontological sector face seems to lie in the reluctance to legally establish a distinction between 'regular' ageing, where the reference to common law or even universal rights is applied, and 'diminished' or 'pathological' ageing, for which specific provisions would be implemented.

This conflict is evident, both in the guides to good practices – which do not distinguish between 'general' recommendations and recommendations for ageing persons who present a danger – and in the legislature's hesitancy to establish a law on 'ageing' or for those who suffer cognitive impairment.

Moreover, the differential treatment as a source of conflict between the soft laws and the legislation gives us a glimpse into the ambiguous relationship between those involved in the gerontology sector and the law. Proclaimed by those who hold high expectations and perceive it as a means of bringing public attention to a social problem, the laws also serve as powerful vehicles for institutionalizing categories of the ageing. Such rules risk reinforcing forms of discrimination and sustaining the stigma experienced by the elderly. In conclusion, those involved in the gerontology sector may have recourse to the law, but only with a great ambivalence; they are unaware of what an appropriate law would be.

Notes

1 This contribution took place under the auspices of the research project 'Specialz', funded by the Fondation Mederic Alzheimer and Fondation Plan Alzheimer.

2 The term 'regulating actors' includes all those whose activities contribute to regulating professional practices of the gerontology sector on various levels: administrative agencies (ANAES, National Health Authority, ANESM) conciliatory systems set up through ministerial initiatives (CNBD), professional associations of general interest (National Foundation of Gerontology), federations of professional institutions and services (FEHAP) or individual professionals who, due to the institutional positions they occupy, are successively led to actively intervene in the evolution of the rules governing professional practices.

3 Whether dealing with the protection of adults, end-of-life arrangements, or care decisions where a person's ability to express his views is in question, French law, like laws in other Western countries, do not create distinctions based on age. The elderly are thus legally treated like all other adults. For example, in England, the Mental Capacity Act addresses the issue from the perspective of the lack of capacity. This law applies to all persons over 16 years of age whose mental capacity to take care of and undertake decisions are temporarily or permanently altered. When the person is considered incapable, it provides the possibility of decisions that lead to a tightly regulated deprivation of liberty (Bartlett, 2005, 2014, 2015). In Quebec, the focus is more on care without consent; whether or not they apply to the area of mental health (Bernheim, 2012, 2015). Many European countries also have legal systems of protection of majors, which again are aimed at the entire population, regardless of age (Sénat français, 2005; Dayton, 2014).

4 Various convention proposals have been made that all concern prohibiting any legal or de facto discrimination related to age. Read more on this topic: (FIAPPA, 2012; Dabbs Sciubba, 2014; HelpAge International).

5 In particular, Law No. 2002–2 of 2 January 2002 renewing social action, JO 3 January 2002, p. 124 and Law No. 2002–303 of 4 March 2002 on patients' rights, JO 5 March 2002, p. 4118.

6 Article L. 1111–4 of the Public Health Code.

7 Article 459 of the Civil Code.

8 The termination of a property lease agreement or a sale must be done with the permission of the guardianship court, and with a detailed medical certificate. The protected person has a free choice of residence, knowing nevertheless that the judge will rule in case of conflict.

9 The studies of directors undergoing training are very enlightening to this concern in the sector in this regard.

10 A reference to the ANAES era, which later became the National Health Authority.

11 In French, the 'Haute Autorité de Santé' and the 'Conseil national de l'évaluation sociale et médico-sociale'.

12 The recommendation by ANESM (2008) on positive treatment cites for example the Universal Declaration of Human Rights of 10 December 1948, the Declaration of the Rights of Disabled Persons of 9 December 1975, the Charter of Rights and Freedoms of the Elderly Dependent person written in 1988 by the National Foundation of Gerontology, or the Charter of Fundamental Rights of the European Union of 2000.

13 In the early 2000s, the issue of Alzheimer's was taken up by the State Councilor Jean-François Girard, who advocated the 'medicalization of the diagnosis and the de-medicalization of care'. This was the beginning of public actions specifically focused on Alzheimer's disease that resulted in three successive public health plans between 2001 and 2012: The Kouchner Plan, in 2001, the Douste-Blazy Plan in 2004 and the Alzheimer Plan from 2008–2012. In 2014, a fourth plan continued the advancement and was extended to include all neurodegenerative diseases.

14 The neurodegenerative diseases 2015–2020 plan does not address this issue.

15 The National Committee for positive treatment and rights was created in January 2013 by the Prime Minister. It is defined as an 'instance of exchanges between representatives of the elderly and disabled, industry professionals, administration and the two ministers', and is composed of sixty representatives.
16 The group is composed of about twenty people, representing institutions federations, doctors, associations of older people, but no representatives of people with Alzheimer's disease.
17 Commission of October 18; discussions with magistrate Anne Caron d'Eglise.
18 Then deputy director of an important federation of institutions (the FEHAP), David Causse is notably the former main organizer of the 2004 consensus conference.

References

Aïdan Géraldine (2007), *Pour une phénoménologie juridique de la maladie d'alzheimer*. Paris, Association France Alzheimer.
Aquino Jean-Pierre (2013), *Anticiper pour une autonomie préservée: un enjeu de société*. Paris, Comité avancée en âge, prévention et qualité de vie.
Bartlett Peter (2005), *Blackstone's Guide to the Mental Capacity Act 2005*. Oxford, Oxford University Press.
Bartlett Peter (2014), 'Reforming The Deprivation Of Liberty Safeguards (Dols): What Is It Exactly That We Want?', *Web Journal of Current Legal Issues*, 20(3).
Bartlett Peter (2015), 'Décisions de la cour européenne en matière de liberté d'aller et venir et droit des établissements sanitaires et sociaux: le cas anglais', *Revue de droit sanitaire et social*, (6), pp. 995–1006.
Beaulieu Marie & Marie Crevier (2010), 'Contrer la maltraitance et promouvoir la bientraitance des personnes aînées', *Gérontologie et société*, 133(2), pp. 69–87.
Benamouzig Daniel (2010), 'L'évaluation des aspects sociaux en santé. La formation d'une expertise sociologique à la haute autorité de santé', *Revue Française des Affaires Sociales*, 1(1–2), pp. 187–211.
Bernheim Emmanuelle (2012), 'Le refus de soins psychiatriques est-il possible au Québec ? Discussion à la lumière du cas de l'autorisation de soins', *McGill Law Journal*, 57(3), pp. 553–596.
Bernheim Emmanuelle (2015), 'La judiciarisation des soins sans consentement. De la force idéalisée du droit à sa mise en œuvre pratique. L'exemple du Québec', *Revue de droit sanitaire et social*, (6), pp. 1007–1015.
Broussy Luc (2013), *L'adaptation de la société au vieillissement de sa population. France: année zéro!* Paris, Rapport pour la Ministre déléguée aux Personnes âgées et à l'Autonomie.
Castel Patrick & Magali Robelet (2009), 'Comment rationaliser sans standardiser la médecine? Production et usages des recommandations de pratiques cliniques', *Journal de gestion et d'économie médicales*, 27(3), pp. 98–115.
Causse David, Delaunay Michèle, Guinchard Paulette & Denis Jacquat (2009), 'Alzheimer, une maladie à "confiner"?', *Libération*, www.liberation.fr/societe/2009/09/04/alzheimer-une-maladie-a-confiner_579323, accessed 8 February 2017.
CGLPL (2013), *Rapport d'activité 2012*. Paris, Contrôleur général des lieux de privation de liberté.
Chapireau François (2007), 'Le recours à l'hospitalisation psychiatrique au XXème siècle', *L'Information Psychiatrique*, 83(7), pp. 563–570.
Conseil d'État (2013), *Etude annuelle 2013: le droit souple*. Paris, La documentation française.

Cornu Gérard (1961), 'L'âge civil'. In *Mélanges en l'honneur de Paul Roubier*. Paris, Dalloz.

Dabbs Sciubba Jennifer (2014), 'Explaining Campaign Timing and Support for a UN Convention on the Right of Older People', *The International Journal of Human Rights*, 18(4–5), pp. 462–478.

Dayton Kimberley (2014), *Comparative Perspectives on Adult Guardianship*. Durnham, North Carolina, Carolina Academic Press.

Dujarier Marie-Anne (2002), 'Comprendre l'inacceptable: le cas de la maltraitance en gériatrie', *Revue internationale de psychosociologie*, 8(19), pp. 111–124.

Eyraud Benoît (2013), *Protéger et rendre capable: la considération civile et sociale des personnes très vulnérables*. Toulouse, Erès.

FIAPPA (2012), *Comment obtenir le vote du projet de convention internationale relative aux droits des personnes âgées?*, www.fiapa.net/wp-content/uploads/2013/07/Comment-obtenir-le-vote-du-projet-de-convention-internationale-relative-aux-droits-des-personnes-âgées.pdf, accessed 8 February 2017.

Got Claude (2005), *L'expertise En Santé Publique*. Paris, Presses Universitaires de France.

Gridel Jean-Pierre (2001), 'La Sénescence Mentale et Le Droit', *La Gazette du Palais*.

Hazif-Thomas Cyril (2014), 'Liberté d'aller et venir en Ehpad: sommes-nous des hors la loi ?', *NPG Neurologie, Psychiatrie, Gériatrie*, 14(83), pp. 275–284.

HelpAge International Ageism, Discrimination and Denial of Rights in Older Age Continue to Be Tolerated across the World... *HelpAge International*. available at www.helpage.org/what-we-do/rights/towards-a-convention-on-the-rights-of-older-people/ [accessed 15 June 2016].

Hugonot Robert (2007), *Violences invisibles: reconnaître les situations de maltraitance envers les personnes âgées*. Paris, Dunod.

Lacour Clémence (2012), 'La liberté d'aller et venir en établissement d'hébergement pour personnes âgées dépendantes'. In Gzil Fabrice & Emmanuel Hirsch (eds.), *Alzheimer, éthique et société*. Toulouse, Erès, pp. 365–376.

Lechevalier Hurard Lucie (2013), 'Faire face aux comportements perturbants: le travail de contrainte en milieu hospitalier gériatrique', *Sociologie du Travail*, 55(3), pp. 279–301.

Lechevalier Hurard Lucie (2015), 'Être présent auprès des absents: ethnographie de la spécialisation des pratiques professionnelles autour de la maladie d'alzheimer en établissements d'hébergement pour personnes âgées', *Thèse de doctorat*, Université Paris 13 Nord.

Loffeier Iris (2015), *Panser des jambes de bois ? La vieillesse, catégorie d'existence et de travail en maison de retraite*. Paris, Presses Universitaires de France.

Mallon Isabelle (2004), *Vivre en maison de retraite: le dernier chez-soi*. Rennes, Presses Universitaires de Rennes.

Molinier Pascale (2009), 'Vulnérabilité et dépendance: de la maltraitance en régime hospitalier'. In Jouan Marlène & Sandra Laugier (eds.), *Comment penser l'autonomie? Entre compétences et dépendances*. Paris, Presses Universitaires de France, pp. 433–458.

Pinville Martine (2013), *Relever le défi politique de l'avancée en âge: perspectives internationales*. Paris, Rapport remis au Premier Ministre.

Ploton Louis & Françoise Souillard (1991), 'Quand l'acceptation passive, pour ne pas dire la résignation, tient lieu de consentement'. In Saussure (de) Christian (ed.), *L'homme très âgé, quelles libertés ?* Genève, Actes du 3ème Congrès francophone des droits de l'homme âgé.

Sénat français (2005), *La protection juridique des majeurs*. Paris.

Véron Paul (2017), 'L'apport jurisprudentiel dans la régulation de la liberté d'aller et venir des personnes âgées en institution', *Médecine & Droit*, (à paraître).

Annex: assessment of best practice recommendations

Anaes (2000a), *Recommandations pratiques pour le diagnostic de la maladie d'alzheimer*. Paris, Evaluation of professional practices in health establishments, ANAES.

Anaes (2000b), *Limiter les risques de la contention physique de la personne âgée*. Paris, Evaluation of professional practices in health establishments, ANAES.

Anaes (2003), *Prise en charge non médicamenteuse de la maladie d'alzheimer et des troubles apparentés*. Paris, Evaluation of professional practices in health establishments, ANAES.

FHF (2004), *Liberté d'aller et venir dans les établissements sanitaires et médico-sociaux et obligation de soins et de sécurité*. Consensus conference, Paris, Fédération Hospitalière de France (French Hospital Federation).

SFGG, Vellas Bruno, Gathier Serge, Allain Hervé, Aquino Jean-Pierre, Berrut Gilles, Berthel Marc, Blanchard François, Camus Vincent, Dartigues Jean-François, Dubois Bruno, Forette Françoise, Franco Alain, Gonthier Régis, Grand Alain, Hervy Marie-Pierre, Jeandel Claude, Joël Marie-Pierre, Jouanny Pierre, Lebert Florence, Michot Patricia, Montastruc Jean-Louis, Nouhrashémi Fati, Ousset Jean-Pierre, Pariente Jérémy, Rigaud Anne-Sophie, Robert Philippe, Ruault Geneviève, Strubel Denise, Touchon Jacques, Verny Marc & Jean-Marie Vetel (2005), 'Consensus sur la démence de type Alzheimer au stade sévère', *Revue de Gériatrie*, 30(9), pp. 627–640.

Benoit Michel, Arbus Christophe, Blanchard François, Camus Vincent, Cerase Valérie, Clement Jean-Pierre, Fremont Patrick, Guerin Olivier, Hazif-Thomas Cyril & François Jeanblanc (2006), 'Concertation professionnelle sur le traitement de l'agitation, de l'agressivité, de l'opposition et des troubles psychotiques dans les démences', *La revue de gériatrie*, 31(9), pp.689–696.

DGS, France Alzheimer and AFDHA (2007), *Alzheime: l'éthique en questions*. Recommendations, Paris, Direction générale de la santé, France Alzheimer, Association francophone des droits de l'homme âgé (French Health Authority, France Alzheimer, Francophone Association for Human Rights of the Elderly).

DGS, DGAS and SFGG (2007), *Les bonnes pratiques de soins en établissements d'hébergement pour personnes âgées*. Recommendations, Paris, Direction générale de la santé, Direction générale de l'action sociale, Société française de gérontologie et de gériatrie, (French Health Authority, General Commission of Social Action, French Society of Gerontology and Geriatrics).

HAS (2008), *Diagnostic et prise en charge de la maladie d'alzheimer et des maladies apparentées*. Recommendations, Paris, Haute Autorité de Santé (French Health Authority).

ANESM (2008), *La Bientraitance: définitions et repères pour la mise en œuvre*. Recommendations, Paris, Agence nationale de l'évaluation et de la qualité des établissements et services sociaux et médico-sociaux National Agency of Assessment of Social and Medico-social Services.

ANESM (2009), *L'accompagnement des personnes atteintes d'une maladie d'Alzheimer ou apparentée en établissement médico-social*. Recommendations, Paris, Agence nationale de l'évaluation et de la qualité des établissements et services sociaux et médico-sociaux (National Agency of Assessment of Social and Medico-social Services).

HAS (2009), *Maladie d'Alzheimer et maladies apparentées: prise en charge des troubles du comportement perturbateurs*. Recommendations, Paris, Haute Autorité de Santé (French Health Authority).

HAS (2011), *Maladie d'Alzheimer et maladies apparentées: diagnostic et prise en charge*. Recommendations, Paris, Haute Autorité de Santé French Health Authority).

HAS and Forap (2012), *Le Déploiement de la bientraitance*. Recommendations, Paris, Haute Autorité de Santé et Fédération des organismes régionaux et territoriaux pour l'amélioration des pratiques et des organisations en santé (French Health Authority and Federation of Regional and territorial agencies for the Improvement of Health practices and organizations).

Erema (2012), *Alzheimer, éthique, science et société*. Paris, Espace national de réflexion éthique sur la maladie d'Alzheimer (National Center of the Ethical Considerations of Alzheimer's Disease).

11 Different initial training, different professional practices?

Latitude and interprofessionality in dependency assessment

Jingyue Xing and Solène Billaud

The French State has established a succession of diverse political arrangements to meet the growing care needs of dependent older people over the past two decades (Le Bihan, 2005). The 'Personalized Autonomy Allowance' (Allocation Personnalisée d'Autonomie, hereafter APA), established in 2001, is the only programme specifically dedicated to this purpose. The APA is a subsidy mandated by the French State and administered by the governments of lower-level administrative departments called General Councils (Conseils Généraux). The central State's role in the APA programme is limited to the law establishing eligibility criteria and benefits, annual decrees setting the various legal parameters of the programme, and a certain degree of co-funding. Each departmental General Council has a key role in structuring and implementing the APA programme.

The APA programme is open to people living in institutions or at home. The programme's objective is defining what they determine to be the 'needs' of people aged 60 years or over that have difficulty performing everyday activities, and providing grants to help defray the cost of corresponding care services. For beneficiaries living at home, the APA essentially helps to pay for services such as household chores, grocery shopping, meal preparation and personal hygiene. According to the research agency Directorate for Research, Studies, Evaluation and Statistics, Direction de la recherche, des études, de l'évaluation et des statistiques (DREES), affiliated with the French Ministry of Social Affairs and Health, there were nearly 1.2 million APA beneficiaries as of 31 December 2011 (DREES, 2012).

One of the most important eligibility criteria for the APA is that the applicant be designated as 'dependent'. Departmental governments created new divisions to handle this task, commonly referred to as 'medico-social service teams': When an individual still living at home applies for APA benefits, the General Council sends team members to visit the applicant to assess the degree of their dependency using a national 'degree of autonomy' scale, an assessment instrument called AGGIR (Autonomie Gérontologie Groupe Iso-Ressources).[1]

The law leaves General Councils considerable flexibility in the composition and operation of medico-social service teams. First, by merely indicating that they must include 'at least one doctor and one social worker', the law gives no firm definition of a 'medico-social service team' and says nothing of its organization. Moreover, the term 'social worker' is a relatively broad label (Ion & Ravon, 2005) that may correspond to a variety of specializations, such as social service assistant, specialized counsellor, or social economy and family advisor. Finally, the law does not specify which specific initial training members of such teams should receive:[2] between administrative departments and even within the same medico-social team, the people conducting home visits may have been trained quite differently. In the departments where this research was conducted, most medico-social service personnel held degrees in paramedical professions (nursing) or social work. There are considerable differences in the content of these two courses of study, particularly in the place given to the teaching of clinical skills and diagnostic, therapeutic and social sciences. Moreover, medico-social service team members generally receive little specific on-the-job training for using the AGGIR scale to assess applicants' degrees of dependency and establish 'personalized care plans'. Finally, the nature of their task is such that visiting caseworkers often work alone and spend most of their time visiting APA applicants, which logically does not favour the harmonization of assessment practices. So, we may ask, do their professional practices differ according to their initial training?

The first section presents a brief literature review on conceptual understandings of interprofessionality. We will then explain our research methods, which are based on an ethnographic approach. In the third section, we will turn to analysis of the professional practices of medico-social caseworkers and present our research findings. The chapter ends with some interpretations of these results.

The legal framework of the APA programme and the role of medico-social teams

The APA programme eligibility criteria are as follows: (i) age 60 years or older, (ii) has resided legally in France for at least three months, and (iii) has been assessed as 'dependent' (detailed definition follows).

The Social Action and Families Code (Code de la Famille et de l'Aide Sociale, CFAS) details the APA application procedure for people living at home in over twenty articles. When an individual residing at home applies for APA benefits, the General Council sends medical and/or social work personnel to visit the applicant. The CFAS requires that 'the APA application [*be*] processed by a medico-social team that includes at least one doctor and one social worker'.[3] This

(Continued)

medico-social work team assesses the degree of dependency using AGGIR, a national 'degree of autonomy' scale established by a group of doctors. This scale is based on seventeen measures indicating mobility, memory, coherence, communication, continence and ability to successfully undertake the basic essential activities of daily living, such as personal hygiene, dressing, meal preparation and eating. The AGGIR assessment instrument is used to assign one of six levels of dependency to individuals. Those assessed at 'moderately dependent' (GIR4) through 'extremely dependent' (GIR1) are eligible for APA benefits. Individuals rated GIR5 ('mildly dependent') and GIR6 ('not dependent') are ineligible.

Once an individual has been designated as eligible for APA benefits, a medico-social caseworker establishes a 'personalized care plan' tailored to meet his or her everyday needs.[4] The total monthly cost of the care plan cannot exceed a pre-determined ceiling, set annually by national authorities for each degree of dependency. For an individual categorized as GIR1, for example, the total cost of his or her personalized home care plan can in theory add up to 1,304.84 euros per month, whereas the maximum amount available for an individual at GIR4 is 559.22 euros per month.

Literature review

Many French sociologists have studied the internal heterogeneity of professions – how they may be 'segmented' and 'fragmented'[5] – and a number of them were particularly inspired by symbolic interactionism (Bûcher and Strauss, 1961; Strauss *et al.*, 1964; Freidson, 1986). Most of these studies addressed only one occupation where members had followed relatively similar initial training. But people working in many occupations, especially in some of the jobs referred to as *'petits métiers'*,[6] may have initial training in a variety of fields.

The term 'interprofessionality' has often been used to study the encounter of multiple professional backgrounds in the same system. In the United States, 'interprofessionality' is studied under the sociology of professions, and is often framed as competition or confrontation among professions sharing the same workplace (Abbott, 1998; 2003), which is to say in terms of how the various professions defend their 'territory' from each other. In the French context, the term is mainly employed in analysis of collaborative efforts among professionals from different backgrounds in the fields of healthcare or the medico-social care of vulnerable populations (Aubert *et al.*, 2005; Castel, 2005; Couturier *et al.*, 2009). In such cases, there is a pre-established division of labour among members of each profession, each playing a different role according to their particular skills and abilities.

The 'competition' among professions is mostly a game of power (Sirota, 2005).

This study sets itself apart in this regard, as we are interested neither in competitive or confrontational relationships between two professions as is the case in some American studies (Abbott, 1998; 2003; Hartley, 2002; Salhani and Coulter, 2009), nor in collaborations between workers from different professions as found in some French studies in healthcare or medico-social care settings (Aubert *et al.*, 2005; Castel, 2005). We use the term 'interprofessionality' to explore whether workers initially trained in paramedical or social work possess different professional practices when holding the same job.

Our study's focus is relatively close to the issues addressed in professional socialization studies. Indeed, initial training can be seen as a form of secondary socialization, 'post-process to incorporate an individual already socialized to new sectors of the objective world of his society' (Darmon, 2006). Other forms of secondary socialization also exist, notably professional socialization in apprenticeship for a new occupation (Linhart, 1978) or in daily professional practice (Dubois, 2003). We could turn our question another way: does socialization through initial training play a more important role than forms of secondary socialization? Medico-social service teams composed partly of people trained as nurses and partly of people trained as social workers that all perform the same job are rich settings for addressing this question.[7]

Methods

Our analysis is based on ethnographic research conducted between 2010 and 2012 in seven French administrative departments as part of a collective research programme on the territorial dimensions of public policy for dependent older people (Gramain *et al.*, 2012). The analysis presented here is based on findings from four of these departments, where we could study professional practices during home visits to aged people more deeply. These departments are designated by the letters A, B, C and D.

A purposive sample

The material was collected using purposive rather than statistically representative sampling in order to assemble a set of contrasting cases that could be compared case by case to reveal common processes (Glaser & Strauss, 1967; Paillet & Serre, 2014).

We chose the four departments for the diversity of social interventions they offered to dependent older people, based on four main indicators: average per capita expenditure on social assistance, number of APA beneficiaries at the time of its implementation, proportion of APA expenditures relative to social assistance expenditures, and the proportion of beneficiaries residing in institutions (Jeger, 2005; Mansuy, 2011; Guenguant & Gilbert, 2012).

Table 11.1 General characteristics of four departments investigated

	A	B	C	D	Mainland France
Environment					
Percentage of people over 75 years in the population (2012) (*)	**8.75%–10.4%**	**8.75%–10.4%**	<8.75%	<8.75%	9.2%
Median living standards in 2012 (in euro / year)	<18,500	>20,150	>20,150	<18,500	19,786
Social assistance expenditure					
Average expenditure per capita on social assistance in euros (2012) (*)	**>570**	501–570	**<460**	**>570**	516
Percentage of APA spending in social assistance, 2012 (*)	>21.2%	16%–18.6%	<16%	<16%	16.5%
Beneficiaries of the APA					
Number of beneficiaries of APA, per 1000 citizens aged 75 or more, at the time of its establishment in 2003 (**)	**>185**	160–180	**<155**	160–180	170
Proportion of beneficiaries residing at home, 2012 (*)	**>63%**	58%–63%	**<52%**	58%–63%	59%

(*) Source: INSEE departmental social indicators.
(**) Source: Jeger, 2005.

An ethnographic survey

We conducted over sixty interviews with people at different hierarchical levels in these four departments (the vertical dimension): directors of General Council senior services, medico-social team managers, supervising doctors and the medico-social caseworkers that assess APA applicants in their homes. We made a particular effort to interview a variety of these visiting caseworkers, differentiated by age, initial training (nursing, social work, social economy and family advising, etc.) and professional career path (horizontal dimension). In an ethnographic perspective (Beaud & Weber, 2003), we had the opportunity to accompany them on home visits and observe their interactions with applicants and their families during over twenty assessments in three of the departments (A, B and D).[8]

Table 11.2 Number and recruitment of visiting caseworkers in the four departments investigated

Department	A	B	C	D
Number of caseworkers	65	40	23	35
Represented initial training	Social workers ('Assistant social'); Social economy and family advisors; nurses	Social workers; Social economy and family advisors; nurses	Social workers; Social economy and family advisors; specialized counsellors; administrative officers	Nurses (sometimes working in pairs with social workers of the healthcare insurance service)

Source: field survey.

Sociological literature has clearly demonstrated that professional practices frequently involve tacit knowledge that is only partially explained in interviews (Giddens, 1984); this may be unconscious because it is difficult to verbalize, or more deliberate when a sensitive issue is concerned. Observing home visits was therefore crucial to concretely understanding the work of conducting home visits (Champy, 2009).

Results

Do assessment practices differ according to the initial training of people conducting home visits, or do they converge? The answer differs depending on whether it is department heads and medico-social team managers describing home-visit practices, or the people who conduct the visits describing their own work.

The doctors' and hierarchical superiors' perspective: Differentiated home-visit practices

As mentioned above, the training for a nursing degree is substantively quite different from that for social work or social economy and family advising. According to doctors, team managers and department heads, initial training differences of caseworkers conducting home visits correspond to different professional practices in nurses and social workers, breaking down along three lines: assessment practices, generosity of allocated allowance and relationships with hierarchy.

Although everyone conducting home visits in all four departments uses the AGGIR scale, their managers and supervising doctors maintain that the occupation they initially trained for influences how they use the instrument and thus the degree of dependency resulting from their assessment: nurses apply the AGGIR scale 'more rigorously' (manager, department A),[9] with 'a medical eye' (supervising doctors, departments A and B), which is seen as being closer to what is expected from instrument users (Xing, 2015). In the managers and supervising doctors' opinion, social workers tend to give greater weight to applicants' social situations (isolation, for example) and adjust the scale's results accordingly. Although such social factors do appear on the AGGIR form, they do not enter into calculation of the degree of dependency that determines eligibility and the aid ceiling.

> Well, they [visiting caseworkers] certainly have different training, it's true that we can see the difference between a social worker and a nurse … A social worker – even if a person is assessed at GIR5 [thus ineligible for APA benefits] – would try to say, 'But she's isolated, she's alone,' etc. Here she'll do pure social work and will give us the spiel for two hours … Well sure, but this person isn't eligible for the APA, she doesn't fall under the APA framework, she can't be considered as an APA beneficiary. Here, we certainly see the social work approach.
>
> (A supervising doctor in department B)[10]

Social workers are also perceived as more 'generous' in granting public assistance. According to a department head working for General Council A, social workers 'often prescribe more hours of home care services. This is actually one of our concerns'.[11] Although he lacks precise statistics, he believes that social workers are more prone to establishing a personalized care plan equal to the legally determined ceiling for each degree of dependency.

Finally, in interviews managers and supervising doctors present nurses as being more respectful of administrative orders and causing 'fewer problems for management' (medico-social team manager, department A).[12] In contrast, social workers are often described as pushing the limits of hierarchical instructions and being more difficult to control in terms of professional practices.

Caseworkers conducting home visits: similar discourse and practices despite different initial training

Our observations of home visits and interviews with medico-social caseworkers give a more nuanced picture, in fact revealing similarities in the home-visit practices of workers from both professional backgrounds.

Finding latitude in the AGGIR scale

When it came to using the AGGIR scale as an assessment instrument, we observed that regardless of initial training, no one applied it literally.

Observations of home visits begin most often with fairly general questions about the applicant's situation and family configuration, any help they might already be receiving from family or other institutions, why they applied to the APA programme, and the older person's particular expectations. Caseworkers begin to fill out the AGGIR scale during this discussion. The scale may not yet be complete, but they have already drafted an applicant profile and often have an idea of how dependent he or she is and the benefits that should be accorded.

An excerpt from our field notes:

GÉRALDINE: [nurse, department D] and Catherine [social worker, health coverage service of department D] visit an APA applicant at her home:

GÉRALDINE: asks the lady the first question: your date of birth?

APPLICANT: [she gives the correct answer]

GÉRALDINE: How old are you?

APPLICANT: 64. No, 84, I didn't think about it.

GÉRALDINE: How many children do you have?

APPLICANT: Five.

GÉRALDINE: Where are they?

APPLICANT: [responds precisely for her three daughters and two sons, naming them by their first names].

GÉRALDINE: and Catherine simultaneously fill out the AGGIR scale on paper.

GÉRALDINE: asks applicant's son-in-law why they are submitting an application for APA.

He says it's because she lives in a nursing home three weeks per month, and they would like a small public subsidy.

GÉRALDINE: Because we cannot accept your application, given the degree of your mother-in-law's dependency. (Géraldine has not yet fully filled out the scale but she already knows it will be a rejection.)[13]

Although the law sets a benefits cap for each degree of dependency, caseworkers conducting home visits find latitude in the personalized care plan by 'tweaking' AGGIR scale coding; in other words, they play on the 'translation' process converting an applicant's situation into administrative coding. For example, a visiting nurse for General Council A explained in an interview: 'Yes, I know that some variables are more important than others – transfer, for example. I know very well that the GIR level [*degree of dependency*] will be higher if I tick this or that box'.[14] A social worker of General Council B told us: 'Sometimes I cheat – if it is really necessary – between GIR4 and GIR3'.[15] For most visiting caseworkers we interviewed, the AGGIR scale is just a working tool. This translation 'game' converting applicants' situations into AGGIR coding in order to make coding results come as close as possible to the benefit level that caseworkers deem appropriate is not the excusive purview of social workers; it is frequently found in nurses' practices as well.

Whatever their initial training, caseworkers conducting home visits make conscious use of the assessment instrument. When they tick boxes on the AGGIR worksheet, they are not really leaving it up to the instrument; quite to the contrary, they use it to better represent their perceptions of applicants' assistance needs by assessing their overall situations. In their assessment practices, visiting nurses and social workers have, to use Giddens' term, a form of professional 'reflexivity' when faced with each applicant's particular situation, and do not merely mechanically implement administrative directives or tools (1984).

Following implicit principles

The APA-assessment coding game reflects the rationale of the street-level bureaucrat, as described by Lipsky (1980): whatever their initial training, when establishing a personalized care plan visiting caseworkers tend to take account of the applicants' social environment, family life and sometimes the kinds of pathologies they suffer from, in addition to their degree of dependence strictly speaking. In other words, beyond the law and administrative instructions, caseworkers have developed tacit principles guiding their professional practices for assessment and establishing care plans. These principles concern applicant hygiene, social risk prevention and social accompaniment, as well as family wellbeing.

The principle of maintaining or improving hygiene seemed to be rather central in visiting caseworkers' decisions. There is a sanitary aspect – 'its good/bad for a person's health' – and a moral and normalizing aspect – 'dependent older people should accept grooming help'. Visiting caseworkers from both training backgrounds attach greater importance to bodily hygiene than environmental hygiene, which leads to an increase in personal assistance activities (grooming, dressing, meals) relative to housework. For example, a social worker for General Council B explained:

> When people only ask for housework, sometimes I'll just give them two hours. I am very clear. In contrast, when I see someone between GIR4 and GIR3, where there is a real need and the family has already gotten them some help, and I really see their difficulties, waiting for nursing and professional care services… Well, I am not ashamed to, quote, 'tweak my assessment' and say, 'well, alright…'[16]

Two visiting caseworkers trained as nurses, interviewed in different departments, agree on priorities: 'the APA programme is not for household chores, but for personal care',[17] and 'for us, the priority of the APA programme is grooming or dressing help, … our priority is the person'.[18]

Not always appreciated by APA applicants, grooming aid is subject to negotiation. According to visiting caseworkers, its acceptance justifies some generosity in coding the AGGIR scale. During a visit to a 'rather independent' first-time applicant, a nurse caseworker for General Council D justified her GIR4 assessment, which makes him eligible for APA benefits, by saying, 'He's a "low" GIR4; what played [*in favour of GIR4*] is that this man has accepted grooming help. It [*the coding*] is subjective'.[19]

The second commonly recurring principle concerns social risk prevention and social accompaniment. Visiting caseworkers do not just make a one-time assessment, 'at a given point in time' as stipulated by law. All those interviewed consider it more appropriate to take a short-term and even a medium-term view, taking into account probable developments in applicants' health conditions in the succeeding months: if they anticipate that applicants will worsen, they prefer to assess the degree of the applicant's dependency more 'broadly' and 'generously'. For example, a nurse visitor said,

> To a person with Alzheimer's disease, who still manages for the moment, I prefer to give access to the APA programme, since [*otherwise*] he will need to submit his application again later. It is a very complex process for a person like him, and the wait is very long.[20]

Beyond a preventive view of awarding public aid, visiting caseworkers are also sensitive to the isolation experienced by some applicants, and try to line up APA-funded home care services to keep applicants living at home for as long as possible. For example, in a rural area in department A, a 90-year-old applicant living alone in an apartment on top of a hill was assessed GIR4 despite his nearly total independence in daily life. In the debriefing after the visit, the caseworker (a social worker) for General Council A explained:

> Despite everything, he still needs help. He lives alone, and if we remove the home care aid, he couldn't stay at home. He is 90 years old, so ... so I am not going to do something stupid. But if I had to be really strict, he would not have gotten a subsidy from the APA programme.[21]

A nurse caseworker in the same department also raised this concern during an interview: 'Staying at home without family ... As they become more and more dependent, when there is no family, it is difficult, or even impossible [*to stay at home*]'.[22]

This principle of social prevention and accompaniment also reflects case-workers' workload-reduction considerations. As stated explicitly in some debriefings, rejecting the applications of people who are borderline GIR4 (slightly dependent)/GIR5 (almost independent) benefits neither caseworkers nor beneficiaries in the long run, because these applicants would have to re-submit their application and go through the same process a few months later, as soon as their conditions worsen slightly. The caseworkers would then have to conduct another home visit to reassess their dependency, meaning that one person's application would be treated twice in a short period of time, creating a heavier workload and unnecessarily complicating the application process.

The third principle that emerges concerns family wellbeing. We found that the family caregivers' health, especially mental health, is an implicit assessment criteria common to visiting caseworkers from both training backgrounds.[23] In their daily practice, caseworkers not only consider potential APA home care services in relation to the individual applicant, but to the family as well. The conceptual framework applied in establishing a personalized care plan is not in fact individual, as dictated by law, but rather collective, insofar as visiting caseworkers take account of each applicant's whole family and his or her environmental constraints.

Excerpt from our field notes:

> Catherine is talking to the applicant's wife, while Géraldine talks to me privately: 'I remember her, I came here two years ago … She tends to depression. She cried during the visit.' The applicant's wife told Mrs C that she does not sleep well because she sleeps next to her husband, who wakes up at night.
>
> [Catherine and Géraldine ask her questions about how her husband's home care is organized, his health, and how dependent he is]
>
> GÉRALDINE: Does he go out?
>
> Without waiting for the wife to answer, Géraldine turns to Catherine, saying, 'If I give him a C [on the AGGIR scale] for "transfer", that will make [GIR] 4'. And that is what she did right away on her AGGIR worksheet. She turns to me: 'Actually, it's possible to know what the GIR will be ahead of time.'
>
> In the debriefing after the visit, both caseworkers expressed their concern about the mental health of the family caregiver [the wife]: 'She will not hold out for much longer. She will wear herself out. Especially if he does not sleep through the night. She is depressed'.[24]

This principle sometimes leads visiting caseworkers to extend professional care services under the APA programme to relieve 'tired' or 'exhausted' family caregivers, or prompt them to grant assistance to a relatively independent person that is socially or geographically isolated.

Finding latitude in instructions from above

In addition to strategic use of the AGGIR scale and the implicit assessment principles shared by all interviewed visiting caseworkers, we also observed that those from different professional backgrounds had analogous practices in response to hierarchical constraints.

French local authorities' financial situation has deteriorated sharply since 2009 (Broussy, 2012). As a result, all four General Councils concerned by this study had established administrative directives in an attempt to reduce APA programme expenditures. One approach was to limit the maximum number of subsidized hours of home assistance accorded to GIR4 (less dependent) beneficiaries; another approach was to encourage these beneficiaries to choose direct employment, meaning they employ individual caregivers themselves, which is more economical than going through a home services organization. There is no guarantee, however, that caseworkers will respect these rules when they establish personalized care plans. We observed two types of response to hierarchical directives among visiting caseworkers, which do not differ according to initial training (as their hierarchical superiors believe), but instead depend on the type of instructions.

When instructions are formulated in quantified and personalized (the target is set at the individual level) terms, hierarchical superiors can readily verify their evaluation, so caseworkers will comply literally. For example, department B has capped the personalized care plans of GIR4 beneficiaries at 20 hours, instead of the 27-hour maximum prescribed by law. General Council caseworkers 'must' obey this requirement because their practices are 'visible' to hierarchical superiors. But it does not prevent them from developing other strategies to subvert administrative orders, notably through AGGIR scale coding and shifting the ratings of applicants assessed at GIR4 to GIR3 when they conclude that more aid is necessary.

When administrative instructions are expressed as either a qualitative goal or a more general quantified goal, formulated at the level of the service rather than the individual, caseworkers' practices can more easily diverge from the instructions. For example, departments A and D ask visiting caseworkers to steer more GIR4 beneficiaries towards direct employment. In department A, the objective was to get 15 per cent of 'new applicants' rated GIR4 to choose direct employment, while previously only 6 per cent had chosen that option. A nurse caseworker we interviewed told us that the direct employment model 'is not very appropriate for the dependent elderly'.[25] She would only recommend direct employment if the applicant and his or her family asked for it specifically, and if 'the applicant is very well supported by the family'. All visiting caseworkers, regardless of their initial training, resist administrative instructions they consider inappropriate. Contrary to their hierarchical superiors' opinion, nurse caseworkers subvert hierarchical orders just as often as social workers, in order to fulfil what they consider their 'real mission'; they are mainly guided by the three implicit principles discussed above. We emphasize that both those with nursing training and those with social work training tend to act in a social work spirit, not only by transgressing hierarchically imposed rules, but also by aiming to do their work 'well'.

This brings us to a key point already analysed by other researchers, namely the resistance of street-level bureaucrats to administrative instructions (Lipsky, 1980; Spire, 2005, 2008; Serre, 2009; Dubois, 2013). In this case, the physical working conditions contribute to the caseworkers' room for manoeuvre: because home visits take place off-site, they are not monitored by hierarchical superiors, providing caseworkers with an additional resource for resistance. Another important factor is that the conversion of applicant situations into AGGIR coding remains elusive and invisible to their administrative superiors.

Discussion

Regardless of their different initial training backgrounds in nursing or social work, visiting caseworkers' professional practices are truly marked by a spirit of social assistance. How to understand the observed similarity of practices? We offer two lines of thought in response.

The particular profile of nurse caseworkers

We will now turn to examining nurse caseworkers' career paths and professional socialization in particular detail. We observed a great similarity among them: the six we studied had all worked for a long time in the social services division of a local-level administration; three of them had worked in a General Council's Mother and Child Welfare Service. Moreover, none had worked in a hospital or clinic in the preceding 15 years.

The nurse caseworkers' professional socialization mainly took place in departmental administrations, specifically in services responsible for allocating assistance to vulnerable social groups (children or seniors). Their primary task was assessing and helping people's living situations rather than providing physical care, so they were more concerned with social, educational and hygienic issues than with medical ones. These nurses were also used to working with social workers and the administration, thus marking their professional ethos with a spirit of social work.

In sum, we observe a distinct nurse profile: the 'social' nurse. This would explain the similarity of nurses and social workers' professional practices. In a way, our study shows that 'continuing' professional socialization can play a more important role in professional ethos and practices than 'initial' professional socialization.

Administrative organization of the APA division and caseworker working conditions

The administrative organization of General Council APA divisions also deserves further exploration, especially the relationship between doctors and visiting caseworkers. In all four departments in this study, supervising doctors do not re-evaluate caseworkers' decisions (except when an applicant contests their assessment), as seen in the following field notes from a home-visit debriefing in department A:

RESEARCHER: Will this case be discussed again?
CAROLE [social worker, department A]: No, no, I take responsibility.
RESEARCHER: It won't be discussed again?

CAROLE: The risk is that, if a General Council supervising doctor checks up on it, and he asks me 'Ms Carole, when did you actually visit this man?' 'I met him on November 3'. 'So you found this man dependent?'... [To us]: You see, that's the risk.

RESEARCHER: And the supervising doctors, do they often make checks?

CAROLE: No, not often. But this is what we said, Magalie [a nurse caseworker colleague] and I – it's our conscience, our professional conscience. Of course this is public money etc., but if we take away this assistance, the applicant will no longer be able to stay at home.[26]

The organizational form of these General Councils' APA implementation divisions leads to specific working conditions for visiting caseworkers: even though supervising doctors are theoretically their supervisors, they do not impose that role in their everyday work. Caseworkers have significant flexibility in applying the AGGIR scale, converting an applicant's situation into administrative coding, and developing personalized care plans – a situation closely resembling the working conditions of social workers described by sociologists such as Delphine Serre (2009) but bearing little resemblance to hospital nurses' working conditions.

Conclusion

The ways in which departmental administrations interpret national guidelines for establishing medico-social teams for APA assessments and personalized care plans leads to the hiring of visiting caseworkers with diverse initial training backgrounds.

A priori, two caseworker profiles can be identified. Some come from paramedical professions and thus, according to interviewed superiors and supervising doctors, their assessment practices take a rather medical approach. The rest come from social work professions and tend, according to their superiors, to be too generous in their everyday practices and regard instructions from the their higher-ups with greater flexibility.

Upon observation of caseworker practices during home visits, we found instead that those trained as nurses and as social workers tend to have convergent assessment practices, share a few implicit principles guiding their daily work, and take similar liberties regarding the tools and instructions the administration imposes on them to standardize and monitor their work. Regardless of their initial training, all the caseworkers we studied have the professional ethos of street-level bureaucrats and subscribe to the moral position of social work.

This similarity in practices seems especially related to the career paths of nurse caseworkers. Indeed, most of them have had a 'social nurse' career, working more in contact with administrators and social workers than with doctors. Hiring this specific type of nurse consequently contributes to the

convergence of professional practices among caseworkers in the APA programme. Additionally, the working conditions we observed in the analysed
departments, particularly their working off-site and without fear of checks
by supervising doctors, also help reinforce the implicit principles of work
and the space for flexibility that all caseworkers create to redefine the content and rules of their 'social assistance mission' in their own terms.

Study of the professional practices of street-level bureaucrats, who in this
case had very different initial training but do the same job, has thus allowed
us to demonstrate that strongly convergent practices and common principles of action can develop under certain conditions. It is interesting to note
that this convergence occurred in favour of the spirit of social work rather
than medical wellness. Our study also suggests that professional socialization through the everyday implementation of a task has a stronger effect
than professional socialization through initial training. This result seems
particularly interesting in the French context, where public operations are
increasingly entrusted to street-level bureaucrats from different professions.

Notes

1 For a detailed presentation of the AGGIR scale, see http://vosdroits.service-
  public.fr/particuliers/ F1229.xhtml, accessed 6 February 2017; for a more
  detailed analysis of the scale, see Belorgey's chapter in this volume.
2 We define 'initial training' as an individual's formal education before first entering the labour market.
3 Article R232-7 of The Code of Social Action and Families.
4 According to law a committee must validate caseworkers' recommendations
  before assistance is granted, but in practice they are almost always accepted
  without discussion, except when contested by an applicant.
5 In France, sociologists have studied various professional practices by professional generation Rayou & Van Zanten, 2004), workplace (Baszanger, 1981; Van
  Zanten, 2003), gender (Paillet & Serre, 2014) and career path (Zalio, 2007).
6 French research on the sociology of professions covers work of all levels and
  statuses, including skilled and semi-skilled occupations such as as nursing aux-
  iliary, letter carrie and construction worker (Champy, 2009).
7 Some French researchers have worked on the implementation of the APA programme, but they have mainly focused on the role of what we will call 'supervising
  doctors' in assessment or the relationship between these doctors and medico-
  social team members conducting the home assessment visits (see Mulet, 2014 for
  an example). These 'supervising doctors' are physicians working as governmental
  bureaucrats that supervise casework and may also conduct medical visits.
8 The fourth department, C, did not authorize researchers to accompany caseworkers on home visits.
9 Interview with the head of Senior and Disabled Services, General Council A, 26
  November 2010.
10 Interview with two supervising doctors working for General Council B, 29
  November 2011.
11 Interview with the head of Senior and Disabled Services, General Council A, 26
  November 2010.

12 Interview with the head of Senior and Disabled Services, General Council A, 26 November 2010; interview with the medico-social team manager, General Council A, 18 January 2011.
13 Excerpt from our field notes from home visits in department D, 23 March 2009.
14 Interview with a visiting caseworker trained as a nurse, General Council A, 8 March 2011.
15 Interview with two visiting caseworkers (one nurse, one social worker), General Council B, 29 November 2011. The maximum amount allowed for an individual increases with the level of GIR: 559.22 euros per month for GIR4 and 838.83 euros for GIR3.
16 Interview with two visiting caseworkers (one nurse, one social worker) General Council B, 29 November 2011.
17 Ibid.
18 Excerpt from our field notes from home visits in department D, 23 March 2009.
19 Ibid.
20 Interview with a nurse caseworker, General Council A, 8 March 2011.
21 Excerpt from our field notes from home visits in department A, 24 November 2009.
22 Interview with a nurse caseworker, General Council A, 8 March 2011.
23 Family caregivers are also a hot topic in research on older people and it is garnering increasing political attention. For more on the subject, see Barylak *et al.*, 2006; Villez *et al.*, 2008; Loïc & Weber, 2009; Bloch, 2012.
24 Excerpt from our field notes from home visits in department D, 23 March 2009.
25 Interview with a nurse caseworker, General Council A, 8 March 2011.
26 Extract from our field notes from home visits in department A, 9 March 2011.

References

Abbott Andrew (1998), *The system of professions: An essay on the division of expert labor.* Chicago, University of Chicago Press.
Abbott Andrew (2003), 'Écologies liées: à propos du système des professions'. In Menger Pierre-Michel (ed.), *Les professions et leurs sociologies. Modèles théoriques, catégorisations, évolutions.* Paris, Edition de la MSH, pp. 25–50.
Aubert Martine, Manière Dominique, Mourcy France & Sabrine Outata (eds.) (2005), *Interprofessionnalité en gerontologie.* Toulouse, Érès.
Barylak Lucy, Guberman Nancy, Fancey Pamela & Janice Keefe (2006), 'Examining the Use of a Caregiver Assessment Tool – Barriers, Outcomes and Policy Implications', *Final report*, contract 4500116739 with Health Canada.
Baszanger Isabelle (1981), 'Socialisation professionnelle et contrôle social: le cas des étudiants en médecine, futures généraliste', *Revue française de sociologie*, Vol. 22, no. 2, pp. 223–245.
Beaud Stéphane & Florence Weber (2003), *Guide de l'enquête de terrain.* Paris, La Découverte, coll. 'Guides repères'.
Bloch Marie-Aline (2012), 'Les aidants et l'émergence d'un nouveau champ de recherche interdisciplinaire', *Vie sociale*, Vol. 4, no. 4, pp. 11–29.
Broussy Luc (2012), 'Les finances des Conseils généraux face au défi de la dépendance', *Revue politique et parlementaire*, 5 April, pp. 77–82.
Bûcher Rue & Anselm Strauss (1961), 'Professions in process', *American Journal of Sociology*, Vol. 4, no. 66, pp. 325–334.

Castel Patrick (2005), 'Le médecin, son patient et ses pairs: une nouvelle approche de la relation thérapeutique', *Revue française de sociologie*, Vol. 46, no. 3, pp. 443–467.

Champy, Florent (2009), *La sociologie des professions*. Paris, PUF, coll. 'Quadrige Manuels'.

Couturier Yves, Trouvé Hélène, Gagnon Dominique, Etheridge Francis, Carrier Sébastien & Dominique Somme (2009), 'Réceptivité d'un modèle québécois d'in-tégration des services aux personnes âgées en perte d'autonomie en France', *Lien social et Politiques*, no. 62, pp. 163–174.

Darmon Muriel (2006), *La socialisation*. Paris, Armand Colin, coll. '128'.

Direction de la Recherche, des Études, de l'Évaluation et des Statistiques (DREES) (2012), 'APA – Résultats de l'enquête trimestrielle', Technical Report, no. 1.

Dubois Vincent (2003), *La vie au guichet*. Paris, Economica, coll. 'Études poli-tiques' » [1999].

Dubois Vincent (2013), 'Le rôle des street-level bureaucrats dans la conduite de l'ac-tion publique en France'. In Eymeri-Douzans Jean Michel & Bouckaert Geert (eds.), *La France et ses administrations. Un état des savoirs*. Bruxelles: Brylant-De Boeck, pp. 169–176.

Freidson Eliot (1986), *Professional powers. A study of the institutionalization of for-mal knowledge*. Chicago, Chicago University Press.

Giddens Anthony (1984), *The constitution of society. Outline of the theory of structur-ation*. Cambridge and Oxford, Polity Press/Basil Blackwell.

Glaser Barney & Anselm Strauss (1967), *The discovery of grounded theory: Strategies for qualitative research*. Chicago, Aldine Publishing.

Gramain Agnès, Billaud Solène, Bourreau-Dubois Cécile, Lim Helen, Weber Flor-ence & Jingyue Xing (2012), *La prise en charge de la dépendance des personnes âgées: les dimensions territoriales de l'action publique*, Rapport final, convention MiRe/DREES, BETA (Univertié Lorraine), CMH (ENS/EHESS/CNRS).

Guenguant Alain & Guy Gilbert (2012), *Une contribution à l'évaluation des poli-tiques décentralisées et des dispositifs nationaux de péréquation*, Rapport DREES, Paris.

Hartley Heather (2002), 'The system of alignments challenging physician profes-sional dominance: An elaborated theory of countervailing powers', *Sociology of Health & Illness*, Vol. 24, no. 2, pp. 178–207.

Ion Jacques & Bertrand Ravon (2005), *Les travailleurs sociaux*. Paris, La Décou-verte, coll. 'Repères' [1984].

Jeger François (2005), 'L'Allocation personnalisée d'autonomie: une analyse des dis-parités départementales en 2003', *Etudes et résultats*, Vol. 1, no. 372.

Le Bihan Blanche (2015), 'Quinze années d'observation des politiques de prise en charge des personnes âgées en perte d'autonomie en Europe'. In Viriot Duran-dal Jean-Philippe, Raymond Émilie, Moulaert Thibauld & Michèle Charpentier (eds.), *Droits de vieillir et citoyenneté des aînés. Pour une perspective internationale*. Montréal, Presses Universitaires du Québec, pp. 45–56.

Linhart Robert (1978), *L'Établi*. Paris, Minuit.

Lipsky Michael (1980), *Street-level bureaucracy: Dilemmas of the individual in public services*. New York, Russell Sage Foundation.

Mansuy Michèle (2011), 'Intervention sociale en faveur des personnes âgées dépendantes : regard croisés entre la France et la Loire-Atlantique', *Revue française des affaires sociales*, Vol. 65, no. 4, pp. 56–87.

Mulet Pascal (2014), 'Évaluer la dépendance: jeux et enjeux autour de la codification'. In Weber Florence, Trabut Loïc & Solène Billaud, *Le salaire de la confiance. L'aide à domicile aujourd'hui.* Paris, Éditions Rue d'Ulm, pp. 195–215.

Paillet Anne & Delphine Serre (2014), 'Les rouages du genre. La différenciation des pratiques de travail chez les juges des enfants', *Sociologie du travail*, Vol. 56, no. 3, pp. 342–364.

Rayou Patrick & Agnès Van Zanten (2004), *Enquêter sur les nouveaux enseignants. Changeront-ils l'école?* Paris, Bayard.

Salhani Daniel & Ian Coulter (2009), 'The politics of interprofessional working and the struggle for professional autonomy in nursing', *Social Science & Medicine*, Vol. 68, no. 7, pp. 1221–1228.

Serre Delphine (2009), *Les coulisses de l'État social. Enquête sur les signalements d'enfant en danger.* Paris, Raison d'agir.

Sirota André (2005), 'Le renoncement narcissique auquel le travail en équipe oblige est-il possible?'. In Aubert Martine, Manière Dominique, Mourey France & Sabrina Outata (eds.), *Interprofessionnalité en gérontologie.* Toulouse, Érès, coll. 'Pratiques gérontologiques'.

Spire Alexis (2005), *Étrangers à la carte. L'administration de l'immigration en France (1945–1975).* Paris, Grasset.

Spire Alexis (2008), *Accueillir ou reconduire. Enquête sur les guichets de l'immigration.* Paris, Raisons d'agir.

Strauss Anselm, Schatzman Leonard, Bucher Rue, Ehrlich Danuta & Melvin Sabshin (1964), *Psychiatrists ideologies and institutions.* New York, The Free Press of Glencoe.

Trabut Loïc & Florence Weber (2009), 'Comment rendre visible le travail des aidants ?', *Idées économiques et sociales*, Vol. 4, no. 158, pp. 13–22.

Van Zanten Agnès (2003), 'Les cultures professionnelles dans les établissements d'enseignement. Collégialité, division du travail et encadremen'. In Menger Pierre-Michel (ed.), *Les professions et leurs sociologies. Modèles théoriques, catégorisations, évolutions.* Paris, Edition de la MSH, pp. 161–181.

Villez Marion, Ngatcha-Ribert Laëtitia & Paul Ariel Kenigsberg (Coord.) (2008), *Analyse et revue de littérature française et internationale sur l'offre de répit aux aidants de personnes atteintes de la maladie d'Alzheimer ou de maladies apparentées*, Paris, Fondation Médéric Alzheimer.

Xing Jingyue (2015), 'L'expertise médicale, un acteur décisif dans les réformes des financements publics des établissements d'hébergement pour personnes âgées dépendantes', 6th Congrès des Associations Francophones de Science Politique (Cospof), Lausanne, Suisse, 5–7 February.

Zalio Pierre-Paul (2007), 'Les entrepreneurs enquêtés par les récits de carrières: de l'étude des mondes patronaux à celle de la grammaire de l'activité entrepreneuriale', *Sociétés contemporaines*, Vol. 68, no. 4, pp. 59–82.

12 Shaping old age

Innovation partnerships, senior centres and billiards tables as active ageing technologies

Aske Juul Lassen

Over the past decade, active ageing has been positioned as a solution to the challenges of global ageing (Moulaert & Paris, 2013). While the scientific, economic, and even moral arguments for being more active later in life have been many (e.g. EC, 1999; WHO, 1999; Walker, 2002; Collinet & Delalandre, this volume), there are difficulties facing the adoption of active ageing into everyday practices. Although older Europeans in general lead more active lives today than in previous generations, many pursue activities that do not correspond to active ageing policy ideals (Clarke & Warren, 2007; Venn & Arber, 2010; Lassen, 2014a; Lassen, 2014b). This chapter explores how active ageing policy becomes part of everyday practices, using the proposed concept of *active ageing technologies*. I use the concept of technology to mediate between policy and everyday practice, inspired by readings of Foucault and Science and Technology Studies (STS) literature. The technologies explored in this chapter are embedded with knowledge and meaning. By operationalising this embedded knowledge, the technologies inform practice in specific ways. Looking at these phenomena as technologies thus implies that they can bridge the practices in which they participate and carry intention from one practice to another. But as the cases will show, everyday practices not only absorb technologies developed elsewhere, they also transform them.

I develop the concept of active ageing technologies through three cases selected from ethnographic fieldwork I conducted in Denmark for my dissertation research (Lassen 2014a). The first case is a Danish public–private innovation partnership (PPIP) working to develop innovative technologies facilitating social and physical activity in the older population. I was a participant in the PPIP, and through ethnographic descriptions of the workshops, I describe how the PPIP itself can be seen as a technology that shapes old age. I analyse the PPIP as an active ageing technology that aims to promote activities and independent living for older people. The second form of technology is the senior centre, analysed here through two centres where I conducted ethnographic fieldwork. Supported by the local municipalities, these senior centres are manifestations of active ageing policies, facilitating participation, independence, and active later lives through the spatial and temporal organisation of activities in their communities. As such, the centres are active ageing technologies, as they anchor a politically established ideal of old age while also providing a space where everyday practices can appropriate and adapt active ageing. The third technology is the billiards table. While a billiards table might not be obvious as an active ageing technology, it does facilitate activity. Billiards tables do not exactly fit into the active ageing discourse, but they enable players to alter active ageing to fit their pre-existing practices. It allows players to stay active for several hours a day thanks to its rhythmic pace and mild level of physical activity.

Active ageing has been subject to some academic scrutiny in recent years. Active ageing policies in the European Union (EU) and the World Health Organization (WHO), and their relationships to previous qualifications of the ageing process, have received some attention (Boudiny & Mortelmans, 2011; Moulaert & Paris, 2013; Lassen and Moreira, 2014). However, more research is needed on the concrete initiatives trying to implant active ageing in people's everyday practices. While the EU does this quantitatively through the active ageing index (European Centre Vienna, 2012), the integration of active ageing in practice is qualitatively and ethnographically understudied. By focusing on active ageing technologies, I wish to emphasise the ways active ageing policies take hold in everyday practices. In so doing, this chapter shifts the focus from themes developed in my previous publications – the epistemologies and models behind active ageing policies (Lassen & Moreira, 2014) and the expressions of active ageing in everyday practices (Lassen, 2014b; Lassen, 2015) – to how active ageing becomes part of everyday practices. In the terminology of this book, active ageing policies are the frame, but this frame is transformed when it becomes fixed in everyday practices. Everyday practices generate their own active ageing technologies – such as billiards tables – and change those offered by active ageing policies – such as PPIPs and senior centres. At the same time, technologies are not passive messengers that see an undisturbed and pure ideal of active ageing through from policy to practice; rather, active ageing is transformed when the technologies transport knowledge and meaning. The move from policy to practice consequently involves a tangle of mediations and transformations that create local versions of active ageing.

Active ageing in the EU and the WHO – a brief background

In the late 1990s the EU and the WHO established active ageing as the basis for their ageing policies. Through occasions such as the United Nations (UN) naming 1999 the 'International Year of Older Persons', its 2002 'Second World Assembly on Aging: Building a Society for All Ages' and the EU's declaration of 2012 as the 'European Year for Active Ageing and Solidarity between Generations', both organisations have promoted active ageing as the solution to the challenges of ageing populations.

Active ageing policies draw on findings and theories from a wide range of disciplines that together generate the idea that various forms of activity possess rejuvenating qualities. The image of older people as passive, dependent and frail is becoming obsolete, considered a mistake inherent to the provisions of twentieth-century welfare states. As social gerontologist Alan Walker, one of the scholarly contributors to EU active ageing policies, has stated about the link between older people and the welfare state:

> [I]t raised their living standards substantially in most Western European countries, but on the other hand, it contributed to their social construction as dependent in economic terms and encouraged popular ageist stereotypes of old age as a period of both poverty and frailty (Walker, 1980; Townsend, 1981, 1986; Binstock, 1991).
>
> (Walker, 2009, p. 77)

In this regard, active ageing in the EU can be seen as a policy response to the social construction of old age, and a detachment from the fatalistic view of demography as destiny (Nordheim, 2000). In the EU, active ageing is being developed as a new mindset on ageing to make people realise the advantages of a longer working life. Changing cultural expectations of ageing and prolonging working lives go hand in hand. Mandatory retirement and early retirement patterns are products of twentieth-century industrial society and welfare states. Working conditions have changed and people are living longer. Currently people in most EU member states live 20 to 24 years after retirement (EU 2012, p. 14). The EU's vision of active ageing connects the potential of future sustainable economies to a higher quality of life for older people, who have until now been victims of pacifying and disempowering mandatory retirement. Walker states that this is a rare occasion for policy that is both morally correct and economically sound (Walker, 2002, p. 1). This policy is leading to pension reforms, healthcare reforms, labour market reforms, age management strategies and local initiatives to support more active later lives.

In the WHO, active ageing is based on the connection between activity and functional capacity (WHO, 1999). Until the 1990s opinions differed on the benefits of physical activity in old age, but when an increasing body of research built consensus on the benefits of physical activity, the WHO assembled a range of scholars to establish the 'Heidelberg Guidelines for Promoting Physical Activity among Older Persons' (WHO, 1996). This growing consensus moreover coincided with a drastic decline in global fertility and mortality rates over the latter half of the twentieth century. This made it even more necessary to foster population health over the entire life course, and lifestyle interventions had to be developed to ensure a high quality of life in the years continuously being added to lifespans. It was time to 'explode the myths of ageing' (WHO, 1999) and show how a healthy lifestyle could lead to a good and long later life, during which new interests could be pursued and participation in society could continue. Active ageing thus gained ground internationally as the best possible solution to challenges arising from ageing populations. In 2002, the WHO launched a policy framework on active ageing that explicitly aimed to influence ageing policies globally (WHO, 2002).

In 2007, the WHO used its active ageing policies as a springboard for its Age-Friendly Cities initiative (WHO, 2007). It was intended to disseminate some of active ageing's conceptions of older people as resources and the need for urban infrastructure and community-building to include health intervention, security and participation for lifelong quality of life. The idea was that activity and enablement could be facilitated through the proper community and urban assets. Focus groups were formed to develop a checklist of essential features for an age-friendly city. This checklist was and is used in a wide range of cities worldwide to join the network of age-friendly cities. With the move from lifestyle interventions to infrastructure, the WHO widened its focus to include other aspects of life quality, such as social participation, transportation, civic participation and employment (WHO, 2007). The WHO 2002 policy framework was recently reviewed and updated, with a new focus on lifelong resilience, 'defined as having access to the reserves needed to adapt to, endure, or grow from, the challenges encountered in life' (International Longevity Centre, Brazil, 2015, p. 40). Such thinking holds that the active person is resilient, and active ageing policies should support this resilience through, for example, cultural safety (p. 51), better sleep (p. 57), the physical environment (p. 61), the social environment (p. 63) and inter-sectorial action (p. 80). Active ageing is thus positioned as a collective goal to which civil society, the media, academia, the private sector, individuals and governments should all contribute. Furthermore, the focus on resilience means that the updated active ageing policy framework represents an even clearer departure from twentieth-century ageing policies that tended to focus on individual and societal adaptation to old age. The introduction of resilience negates the decline to which society and individuals would have to adapt.

The concept of technology

The three case studies developed in this chapter - PPIP, senior centres and billiards tables – are different in many respects. In a Foucauldian reading, the billiards table could be defined as *techne* – a form of 'practical rationality governed by a conscious goal' (Foucault, 1984, p. 255), whereas the other two are more abstract condensations of knowledge. These could be seen as institutions and regulatory decisions forming part of an apparatus (*dispositif*) that strategically responds to an urgent need (Foucault, 1977), i.e. the need to discipline the growing ranks of older people in order to create active older citizens. But in this chapter I use the concept of technology to refer to *techne*, institutions, and regulatory decisions that shape old age in a specific way. In so doing, I use a conception of technology inspired by the field of STS.

STS has explored how technologies are socially constructed (Bijker *et al.*, 1987) and the ways in which the social is co-produced by a variety of actors, which shed light on the material, technological, and scientific composition of the social (Latour, 1987). Technologies are not passive objects, but mediate and intervene in the practices in which they participate (e.g. Latour, 1991; Oudshoorn & Pinch, 2003). The active ageing technologies in this chapter are thus material and immaterial strategic devices that mediate between active ageing policies and everyday practices, shaping old age in a specific way.

Active ageing technologies combine old age and technologies differently than they are usually paired. Technology is often framed as a possible solution to the predicament of ageing populations, through new and innovative ways of providing care and accessibility. Aged people themselves are often considered to be passive recipients of these assistive technologies imposed on them. Several scholars have argued against this passive approach to technologies (e.g. Peine *et al.*, 2014). In this chapter, ageing people are regarded as co-producers of technologies, because they negotiate and transform them in their practices. Blaschke *et al.* describe how the EU considers information and communication technologies (ICTs) to be economically necessary to maintaining a satisfactory level of care for aging members of the population but as yet there is little certainty as to whether this is actually so, or which kinds of ICTs are best suited (2009). Technologies have been proposed to solve the ageing challenge by assisting ageing people who are frail (see Dorsten *et al.*, 2009) and prolonging people's ability to age in place (see Cook, 2006).

As described earlier, political and normative regimes of activity are another way of meeting the challenges that ageing populations present to welfare states. Activity and technology thus represent different proposed solutions to the same problem. Activities predominantly foster prevention; technologies predominantly provide assistance. Each solution shapes a different vision of 'good old age'. In general terms, older people either become passive recipients of care and technologies or active and empowered citizens. While this empowerment is indeed a way to facilitate a more positive and optimistic view of old age, it can also become a forced form of empowerment that leaves little room for those who do not wish to be empowered. In this regard, disempowerment and dependence become forms of disobedience and dissent.

I introduce the concept of active ageing technologies to argue that this distinction between pacifying assistive technologies and empowering regimes of activity is not congruent with how many older people appropriate technologies into their everyday practices. The technologies at hand activate ageing people, instead of catering to their increasing care needs. In this regard, technologies are strategic material and non-material condensations of knowledge that contain ideals of 'the good life' that are transformed through everyday practices. Consequently, the active ageing technologies described in this chapter are not necessarily tangible objects with an enduring presence. The PPIP is only present temporarily during workshops, but its very specific conception of 'good old age' transcends these timeframes. Senior centres have a physical presence, but they are first and foremost hubs gathering and organising various kinds of activity. The billiards table is a tangible object, but one that is connected to a range of practices, traditions and inherited forms of knowledge. All three technologies are characterised by the fact that they are all embedded with the knowledge that a 'good old age' is an active old age.

The case of a Danish public–private innovation partnership

Lev Vel (Live Well) was a PPIP that aimed to develop technologies facilitating more active later lives.[1] With my colleagues Julie Bønnelycke and Lene Otto, I have previously described how the partnership developed active ageing technologies (Lassen *et al.*, 2015). I wish to focus here on how the partnership itself can be seen as an active ageing technology. It is a non-tangible technology that forms a specific 'old age' through the development of new objects. This foundation for an ideal old age is a strategic technology, due to how it distributes and translates condensed knowledge across sectors and practices.

Lev Vel was the initiative of a diverse partnership of universities, private companies, and public organisations with the support of The Capital Region and The Danish Council for Technology and Innovation for a 3-year period starting in 2010. Initially, *Lev Vel* was divided into three 18-month sub-projects. Some of these were extended, and new sub-projects were also initiated after the completion of the initial projects. As part of my doctoral work, I participated in the sub-project called *Mødestedet* (The Meeting Place), whose goal was to develop technologies that would promote physical, mental and social fitness among older people.

The private partners in *Mødestedet* were a medical device business incubator, a fitness centre, a robotics manufacturer and an insurance company. In addition, three municipalities, three private organisations, five universities/university colleges and a municipal senior centre participated. As an ethnologist, I was part of the project in order to provide background knowledge about older people and old age and to conduct ethnographic fieldwork intended to provide insight in the user-driven innovation process.

Lev Vel aimed for a type of 'good old age' that was a form of active ageing mediated by technology. We therefore had to look among prospective users for kinds of practices and problems that could somehow be solved with technology. We disseminated knowledge of the needs of active ageing at levels from the political to the vernacular, by, as the research proposal put it, 'developing innovative solutions, which enable independent older people to maintain their desired life space and functional capacity for as long as possible'.

We then tried to reverse the flow of knowledge, by developing the insights provided by the ethnographic study of everyday practices and using them in the innovation partnership to create prototypes. In so doing, the PPIP functioned as a mediating technology between the centrally established goals for innovation and the targets of the intervention, who were given a voice by the project's user-centred approach. What is important here is the distribution and transfer of knowledge between different practices: from research policy to innovation partnership to everyday practices and back. It is this knowledge transferral that consolidates the partnership as a strategic technology. It attempts to fix active ageing into everyday practices, but also aims to adapt active ageing by taking account of the everyday practices in which it intervenes.

As described above, active ageing transforms many of the meanings associated with old age and reshapes the ideal of what 'good old age' is. Independence is a key notion in this reconceptualisation. Its opposite, dependency, was closely tied to the meaning of old age throughout the twentieth century (e.g. Townsend, 1981), but the dependency of old age is now cast as being part of an out-dated conception of the life course. The ageing people of today are often described as increasingly independent, and are said to be able to maintain this independence into very old age through an active lifestyle (e.g. WHO, 1999). The objective of active ageing then becomes facilitating this lifestyle by promoting good health and societal reorganisation, accomplished through a range of strategies including pension reform, healthcare reform, and, in this case, PPIPs. The PPIP is an active ageing technology in how it attempts to instil the ideal of active ageing into older people, by assembling a variety of different organisations and people and facilitating a synergetic knowledge transfer between them that leads to new technology-mediated behaviours. PPIP's aim was to shape a specific, independent and active old age, and it tried to reach that goal in a variety of ways.

First, the PPIP was intended to develop innovations through mutually beneficial strategic cooperation between public and private partners. Improved efficiency, quality and coercion were key words in the framing of the project. This should align the diverse sectors to facilitate independent living. The partners would participate in the creation of 'living laboratories' in hospitals and municipalities with the aim of forming consensus on the applicability of specific innovations to everyday practices – both those of older people and those of staff handling the innovations. The goal was to synchronise the public sector and private companies with an ageing society, and to adjust their services to a new life course. Second, this reorganisation of specific institutions catering to an ageing society would be based on insights on aged people generated through ethnography and co-design. As such, the PPIP attempted to create a user-driven innovation process that would ideally improve services and benefit everyone involved, supporting older people in various ways of living independently. Third, the specific prototypes developed in *Mødestedet* would all facilitate particular activity types that would support older people in an active lifestyle, thereby ideally improving their functional capacities and independent living. The prototypes emerging from *Mødestedet* were an online exercise-oriented senior community, interactive modular tiles used for rehabilitation after a fall, an interactive yoga mat and interactive Nordic walking sticks. The PPIP thus supported independent living by bringing institutions into alignment on this view of old age, based on user-driven insights and the development of prototypes that ageing people could use to extend their independence later into old age.

Two Danish senior centres

As part of my doctoral research, I conducted participant-observation at two senior centres in the Copenhagen area. Both centres were associated with the PPIP through programme participants. One, Wiedergården, was a partner in the PPIP, and the other, The Cordial Club was in a PPIP partner municipality. Senior centres in Denmark are local centres where retirees from the municipality can attend various activities during the week. They are often located in nursing home facilities and are used by residents and non-residents alike, although this was not the case for the two senior centres I studied, which, instead of being connected to nursing homes, are independent organisations that are largely organised and run by the users themselves. Regardless, the diversity of senior centre types all represent variations of an active ageing technology that is increasingly widespread in Denmark: local centres for organising activities. They offer a wide range of pursuits and provide a place for older people to participate in the community, arrange their own activities, and spend time during the day chitchatting, participating in activities, and simply hanging out.

Wiedergården is located in an affluent part of the capital area. Most users are well off and have a high level of education. In early 2011, there were 1100 weekly users. The centre was 20 years old and was created after the municipality called a public meeting to ask older citizens to express their wishes. The municipality agreed to create the centre on condition that the citizens organise it themselves and establish user councils. The only paid staff at the centre is the day manager and cafeteria employees (only the manager was employed by the municipality, as the cafeteria was a private company). The municipality funds the centre, but the town council was discussing a monthly user-fee of approximately 100 dkr. (about 15 euros) at the time of fieldwork. The offered activities ranged from classic diversions for older people such as billiards, decoupage, bridge and weaving to physical activities often associated with younger people such as ping-pong, Zumba, a fitness centre and Pilates. I followed a Pilates class, the fitness centre, a computing class and the metalworking shop. I usually participated in the activity and then hung around to talk afterwards, which meant that I also talked to users attending other activities.

The Cordial Club has a different socio-economic profile than Wiedergården. The Cordial Club has 110 members who are primarily from working-class backgrounds. The members pay an annual fee of 115 kroners (app. 17 euros), which covers club expenses: memberships in various senior advocacy organisations, basic equipment, and backup when excursions and parties run over budget. They have free use of the facilities from 10:00 to 16:00, 4 days a week, so long as the club is run as an association with a member list, board, chairman and treasurer. The club started as a billiards club for the workers at a local telephone factory. When many of the members retired, they organised as an association for retirees, and expanded club offerings in order to include their wives. The members run the club themselves, and organise activities such as a billiards tournament, a darts tournament, weekly dice and card games, bingo, parties and excursions. A group of around 20 people run the club and go there all 4 days a week. Most of them play billiards, but others play cards and dice, make lunch to sell to members, or just hang around and talk. I mainly participated in billiards, but also in dice, cards, bingo and darts, and I often hung around and chitchatted, drank coffee or had lunch.

While the two centres differ in many ways, they are both active ageing technologies because they facilitate active ageing among the users and shape a specific old age enabled by the regulation of local authorities. The senior centres structure the everyday lives of its users around activities and facilitate an active old age, while also allowing for the older people's own interpretations of what constitutes a good activity (billiards, darts, etc.). Municipalities' decision to fund senior centres determine the general conditions for a specific kind of old age, but it is largely up to older users to decide how to use the centres and the kinds of activities they will organise. This kind of active ageing technology thus does not stress the kind of activity older people should engage in, but seeks to empower them to choose their activities for themselves. This leads to a negotiation and transformation of active ageing by the aged users of the centres, who adapt active ageing to their existing practices, and thereby appropriate active ageing.

One example of such a negotiation and adjustment is how a group of older men at Wiedergården created a metalworking shop, which I followed for 2 months. They collected a multitude of machines and tools from former workplaces and contacts into an outbuilding, where they meet twice a week to repair and build various accessories for their gardens, boats or houses. They share the space with a group of woodworkers, who use the facilities the other two days of the week. While few of the users had actually worked as woodworkers or metalworkers, many had been labourers in related occupations, and they identify as metalworkers or woodworkers and differentiate sharply between the two. They spend much of their time in the workshop drinking beer or coffee and talking, often about their working lives, hobby projects, politics and women. The metalworking group also talks a lot about how they differ from the woodworkers, who are not seen as real labourers, as

well as how they differ from the health- and fitness-oriented users of Wiedergården. One day, the woodworkers' organiser, Hans, came into the workshop to arrange the pick-up of a bag of cement with Bent, a metalworker:

BENT: I want a case of beer for it, and you're picking it up yourself. And why
are you woodworkers not cleaning up after yourselves? It's two cases of
beer now.

HANS: Ok, ok. By the way, why are none of you sorry old guys joining the
line dance group?

BENT: Why on earth would we do that?

OVE [ANOTHER METALWORKER]: I thought you claimed to be a labourer.

HANS: You guys don't know what you're missing. Your wife is there, Bent
[drawing her figure sensually in the air], she's really swinging it. You are
missing out on 43 lovely old birds, swinging …

BENT: Are you calling my wife an old bird? Why are you standing there
jerking off? You should watch out for your heart, old man. Next time
we might not find you in time [referring to a time when Hans had a heart
attack and was found on the pavement between the main building and
the outbuilding]. And why the hell would you lie down on the pavement?
Please lie down inside, in the heat, next time. I won't stand there freez-
ing, next time. I'll let you lie there.

HANS: Aahhh, they sewed me up real good and gave me a new vein from
my leg. I'm good as new. You guys should keep better watch over your
wives. Us woodworkers are known to be ladies' men, and while you
stand here with your ten thumbs and useless metal, we might just steal
them.

There are many such conversations in the workshop. After Hans left, they
spent the next hour slandering the woodworkers, in the same tough but joking tone as in the conversation above. Despite the joking, there is a subtle
conflict over the proper use of the room and metalworkers form themselves
as a group with the woodworkers as their opposite. Furthermore, Ove's re-
mark implying Hans is not a real labourer reveals another demarcation in
the group. The metalworkers find all the focus on health and physical activity to be excessive and feminine. They often say that disease is part of
growing old, and find that the demand for active ageing is a hopeless and
irrational battle. At the same time, they all state that it is important for them
to keep going and engage in activities, and they see the workshop as a way
to maintain their skills, continue their interests, engage in their community
and fill their day with a meaningful pastime. In this regard, they negotiate
and adapt active ageing, by embracing the parts of it that highlight community engagement, participation and contribution, and by denouncing its
health-oriented aspects. In a previous article I have described how a group
of billiards players negotiate and recompose active ageing in a similar manner (Lassen, 2014b). The senior centres are active ageing technologies that

older users can customise while embracing different aspects of active age-ing. Active ageing is often negotiated and adapted in local versions, and the user-managed senior centres seem to be a technology that allows for this type of adjustment.

The billiards table

In previous work I have analysed how a billiards group at The Cordial Club engages in a culturally specific form of practice that reconstitutes active age-ing (Lassen, 2014b). Billiards is a popular and widespread activity at many Danish senior centres, and can be seen as an alternative active ageing activ-ity. At The Cordial Club, billiards facilitates togetherness and mild physical activity for a group of men who would be neither able nor willing to engage in other types of activity. Some of them play for 6 hours a day, 4 days a week, and are only able to do so due to the rhythm of billiards, where breaks and conversation are intrinsic to the game. This active ageing activity plays out according to the previously outlined premises of The Cordial Club. As de-scribed earlier, the senior centres are active ageing technologies in that they allow users to adjust active ageing to their practices; in the process users negotiate and stretch the meaning of active ageing. The billiards table will be the next to be described as an active ageing technology, although darts and dice also seem to possess many of the same qualities.

Most of the billiards players at The Cordial Club have played billiards their whole lives and take great pride in it. Family histories, a working-class affiliation and male togetherness are embedded in the table. In this regard, the billiards table is not just a table. Many of the players tell their life story through the table, by focusing on different periods of their lives and how play frequency, locations and company have changed over the life course. The billiards table is thus an active ageing technology that allows players to connect the current phase of their lives to their life courses. Players adopt different strategies in order to keep playing into very old age, such as taking more breaks and changing their play strategy. One example is more frequent use of a bridge,[2] a support for the cue allowing players to take otherwise nearly impossible shots if their arms are not long enough or they cannot make the necessary stretch. Players often tease others using a bridge, but at the same time it is a widely accepted tool allowing players to make difficult shots despite the stiff limbs that often come with old age.

As an active ageing technology, the billiards table permits players to adapt active ageing to their pre-existing practices. Many players stress that they play because of their personal histories and fondness for the game. They em-phasise the beauty of the game, their group and how they look out for each other. Like the metalworkers, many of the billiards players denounce what they call the 'health regime', to which they feel subjected. However, at the same time they inscribe billiards into active ageing by stating that the game keeps them going, the community is good for them, the social aspects of the game are themselves healthy, it is not good to just sit at home, and all these attributes postpone old age, dependency and death. Many say that they would be in their graves already if it were not for the game and the group. But it is a form of active ageing that apparently pays no heed to health advice, physical activity or possible contributions to society: they say they just like to play billiards and enjoy the company. But they play on the premises of a senior centre, and they seem to incorporate many of the ideas behind active ageing despite explicitly disavowing it. The billiards table is an active ageing technology in how it allows players to engage in an activity of their own choosing that they enjoy, but that is subsequently inscribed into active ageing in various ways. The billiards table is ambiguously both associating the players with, and dissociating them from, active ageing.

While billiards is perhaps not an ideal active ageing activity it still involves some movement, which is often described by the players as an asset of the game. They sometimes experience exhaustion and soreness after 6 hours of playing, and one of the women, Lissie, declares that 'as long as I can stand I won't sit there and play cards'. This is why billiards is perceived as a physical activity and accepted as such by many of the players, although this is not why they play. Nonetheless, billiards is not immune to the discourse of active ageing and is constantly associated with it and in negotiation with it. The table facilitates active lives, and is a condensation of knowledge about how to live actively as an old person. The condensed knowledge here is manifest in the players' knowledge, playing skills, functional capacities, life histories, and even craftsmanship that went into creating the game and the table (which one of the players actually helped build in his youth). This knowledge is in negotiation with the ideal of active ageing, however, when they describe billiards as something that helps them keep going and is a form of physical activity adapted to aged players' capacities.

While active ageing is a powerful idealisation of old age, it is mixed with a range of other discourses about and conceptions of old age, such as the right to freely enjoy retirement after a long working life or that old age is a period of natural decline and disengagement. Everyday life is not the object of a single external ideology that intrudes and intervenes. Rather, it is constantly entangled with and penetrated by numerous, diverse, and often contradictory discourses and ideals. Everyday practices are neither pure associations with nor dissociations from active ageing, but are in constant, messy negotiation with contradictory ideals of old age. The billiards players declare that active ageing is not for them, but with the next breath connect billiards to active ageing. They describe how billiards was better accepted as a good activity in the good old days, but then go on to praise the municipality that provides them with facilities. Hoards of older people are playing billiards at a time when people their age are expected to use Stairmasters instead of Zimmer frames (walkers), and are expected to engage in their communities and society instead of being passively served by the public sector. Defence of the billiards table negotiates and twists active ageing, but is not enough to escape it.

It nevertheless does generate new versions of active ageing and 'good old age' that might prove to be more robust and widely accepted by ageing people than narrower, ready-made strategic technologies for active ageing.

Concluding remarks

As the case studies have shown, everyday practices are not simply absorbing technologies developed elsewhere. Everyday practices generate their own active ageing technologies – such as billiards tables – and change the ones that are offered to them, such as PPIPs and senior centres. Treating such phenomena as technologies implies that they can act as bridges between various practices involving these phenomena and carry intention and meaning from one practice to another. It also implies, by extension, that policies do affect everyday practices through technologies, but that everyday practices also affect policies through technologies in return. Technologies are not just passive messengers that carry an ideal of active ageing through from policy to practice; rather, the technologies mediate between the practices and shape them in relation to each other. There is a form of mutual synchronisation work taking place, wherein the political and everyday practice continuously negotiate what 'good old age' is through technology. As such, the technologies participate in forming the world – both as carriers of specific ideals of 'good old age' and as entities that can contain ambiguous and contrasting ideologies – that then tinkers and fiddles with active ageing so that it can be integrated into everyday life. The senior centres and the billiards table are examples of such technologies that allow older people to negotiate and appropriate active ageing when everyday life is penetrated by so many expectations of just how one should go about ageing actively.

While the WHO and the EU continuously engage in shaping old age through policies for active ageing, more qualitative and ethnographic research is needed on how these policies are transformed locally. While active ageing has to some extend been scrutinised discursively (e.g. Katz, 2001; Moulaert & Biggs, 2013), the ways local municipalities employ active ageing and the ways older people practice active ageing have been understudied. In Denmark, the active ageing framework has led to initiatives such as rehabilitation programmes (attempting to regain functional capacity to forestall homecare) and co-creation projects (bridging the divide between municipalities and civil society by engaging NGOs and volunteers in the development and implementation of local policies), which are currently being studied by ethnographers researching the intersections between local forms of governance and older persons. While this will shed light on the local versions of active ageing in Denmark, there is need for more worldwide scrutiny of the different ways in which active ageing is locally situated and shapes old age to provide greater understanding of the complex ways that old age is being transformed, defined, and experienced in the first decades of the twenty-first century.

Notes

1 Website: http://lvvl.dk/forside/0/2 (in Danish), accessed 31 January 2017.
2 In Danish, a bridge is informally called a 'bedstemorkø', which translates literally to 'grandma-cue'.

References

Bijker Wiebe, Hughes Thomas & Pinch Trevor (eds.) (1987), *The social construction of technological systems: New directions in the sociology and history of technology.* Cambridge MA/London, UK, MIT Press.

Blaschke Christina, Freddolino Paul & Erin Mullen (2009), 'Ageing and technology: A review of the research literature', *British Journal of Social Work*, Vol. 39, pp. 641–656.

Boudiny Kim & Dimitri Mortelmanns (2011), 'A critical perspective: Towards a broader perspective of "active ageing"', *Electronic Journal of Applied Psychology*, Vol. 7, no. 1, pp. 8–14.

Clarke Amanda & Lorna Warren (2007), 'Hopes, fears and expectations about the future: What do older people's stories tell us about active ageing?', *Ageing & Society*, Vol. 27, pp. 465–488.

Cook Diane (2006), 'Health monitoring and assistance to support aging in place', *Journal of Universal Computer Science*, Vol. 12, no. 1, pp. 15–29.

Dorsten Aimee-Marie, Sifford Susan, Bharucha Ashok, Mecca Laurel Person & Howard Wactlar (2009), 'Ethical perspectives on emerging assistive technologies: Insights from focus groups with stakeholders in long-term care facilities', *Journal of Empirical Research on Human Research Ethics*, Vol. 4, pp. 25–36.

European Centre Vienna (2012), *Active ageing index 2012 for 27 EU Member States.* Vienna, European Centre for Social Welfare Policy and Research.

European Commission (1999), *Towards a Europe for all ages. Promoting prosperity and intergenerational solidarity.* Brussels, European Commission.

European Union (2012), *Pension adequacy in the European Union 2010–2050.* Brussels, European Commission.

Foucault Michel (1977), 'The confession of the flesh'. In Gordon Colin (ed.), *Power/knowledge: Selected interviews and other writings, 1972–1977 by Michel Foucault.* New York, Pantheon Books, pp. 194–228 [1977].

Foucault Michel (1984), 'Space, knowledge and power'. In Rabinow Paul, *The Foucault Reader.* New York, Pantheon Books, pp. 239–256.

International Longevity Centre Brazil (2015), *Active ageing: A policy framework in response to the longevity revolution.* Rio de Janeiro, International Longevity Centre Brazil.

Katz Stephen (2001), 'Busy bodies: Activity, aging, and the management of everyday life', *Journal of Aging Studies*, Vol. 14, no. 2, pp. 135–152.

Lassen Aske Juul (2014a), *Active ageing and the unmaking of old age – The Knowledge productions, everyday practices and policies of the good late life*, PhD diss., University of Copenhagen.

Lassen Aske Juul (2014b), 'Billiards, rhythms, collectives – billiards at a Danish activity centre as a culturally specific form of active ageing', *Ethnologia Europaea*, Vol. 44, no. 1, pp. 57–74.

Lassen Aske Juul (2015), 'Keeping disease at arm's length: How older Danish people distance disease through active ageing', *Ageing & Society*, Vol. 35, no. 7, pp. 1364–1383.

Lassen Aske Juul, Bønnelycke Julie & Lene Otto (2015), 'Innovating for "active ageing" in a public-private innovation partnership: Creating doable problems and alignment', *Technological Forecasting & Social Change*, Vol. 93, pp. 10–18.

Lassen Aske Juul & Tiago Moreira (2014), 'Unmaking old age – political and cognitive formats of active ageing', *Journal of Aging Studies*, Vol. 30, no. 1, pp. 33–46.

Latour Bruno (1987), *Science in action: How to follow scientists and engineers through society*. Cambridge MA, Harvard University Press.

Latour Bruno (1991), 'Technology is society made durable'. In John Law (edLo.), *A sociology of monsters: Essays on power, technology and domination*. London and New York, Routledge, pp. 103–131.

Moulaert Thibauld & Simon Biggs (2013), 'International and European policy on work and retirement: Reinventing critical perspectives on active ageing and mature subjectivity', *Human Relations*, Vol. 66, no. 1, pp. 23–43.

Moulaert Thibauld & Mario Paris (2013), 'Social policy on ageing: The case of "active ageing" as a theatrical metaphor', *International Journal of Social Science Studies*, Vol. 1, no. 2, pp. 113–123.

Nordheim Fritz von (2000), 'Active ageing: Facing the challenges of demographic change', *Eurohealth*, Vol. 6, no. 3, pp. 1–2.

Oudshoorn Nelly & Trevor Pinch (eds.) (2005), *How users matter: The co-construction of users and technology*. Cambridge MA, London, MIT Press.

Peine Alexander, Rollwagen Ingo & Louis Neven (2014), 'The rise of the "innosumer" – rethinking older technology users', *Technological Forecasting & Social Change*, Vol. 82, pp. 199–214.

Townsend Peter (1981), 'The structured dependency of the elderly: A creation of social policy in the twentieth century', *Ageing & Society*, Vol. 1, no. 1, pp. 5–28.

Venn Susan & Arber Sara (2010), 'Day-time sleep and active ageing in later life', *Ageing & Society*, Vol. 31, no. 2, pp. 197–216.

Walker Alan (2002), 'A strategy for active ageing', *International Social Security Review*, Vol. 55, no. 1, pp. 121–139.

Walker Alan (2009), 'Commentary: The emergence and application of active aging in Europe', *Journal of Aging & Social Policy*, Vol. 21, no. 1, pp. 75–93.

World Health Organization (1996), *The Heidelberg Guidelines for promoting physical activity among older persons*. Geneva, World Health Organization.

World Health Organization (1999), *Ageing Exploding the Myths*. Geneva, World Health Organization.

World Health Organization (2002), *Active ageing: A policy framework*. Geneva, World Health Organization.

World Health Organization (2007), *Global age-friendly cities: A guide*. Geneva, World Health Organization.

List of contributors

Editors biographies

Loffeier, Iris is a permanent research fellow in sociology at HESAV (Haute École de Santé Vaud), in Lausanne, Switzerland. For three years, she was a postdoctoral researcher in the FRAMAG research programme led by Benoît Majerus at the University of Luxembourg. She was, for two years, research and teaching assistant at the University of Western Brittany (UBO, Brest, France). She received the *Le Monde* award for academic research for her doctoral thesis in sociology – which she completed at Aix-Marseille Université, France and was subsequently published under the title *Panser des jambes de bois? La vieillesse, catégorie d'existence et de travail en maison de retraite* (Presses Universitaires de France, 2015).

Majerus, Benoît is Associate Professor for European History at the University of Luxembourg. He has widely published on the history of psychiatry in the twentieth century, most recently 'Making Sense of the "Chemical Revolution". Patients' Voices on the Introduction of Neuroleptics in the 1950s', *Medical History*, 2016, Vol. 60, no. 1, p. 54–66 and 'The Straitjacket, the Bed, and the Pill: Material Culture and Madness', G. Eghigian (dir.), *The Routledge History of Madness and Mental Health* (Routledge, 2017).

Moulaert, Thibauld is Associate Professor at the Université de Grenoble-Alpes, France. After a postdoctoral Fellowship in sociology at the National Fund for Scientific Research, Université Catholique de Louvain, including a Visiting Research at King's College London, UK in 2010, he worked as scientific coordinator for REAICTIS (Réseau d'Étude International sur l'Âge, la Citoyenneté et l'Intégration Socio-économique) on older people volunteering and on older people citizenship and environments. His first book *Governing the End of the Career at a Distance. Outplacement and Active Ageing in Employment* (Peter Lang, 2012) received a prize for publication from the Fondation Universitaire.

Contributors biographies

Belorgey, Nicolas is a permanent Researcher at the Centre National de la Recherche Scientifique (CNRS), France. He is posted at Societies, Actors and Government in Europe, a joint laboratory from the CNRS and the University of Strasbourg. He is invested mainly in sociology, and has also degrees and publications in economics and political science. His publications include: *L'hôpital sous pression: enquête sur le 'nouveau management public'* (La Découverte, 2010); 'Reducing the Wait Time at the Emergency Room: The Effects of a Public Service Reform', *Actes de la recherche en sciences sociales*, 2011.

Billaud, Solène is a sociologist specialised in sociology of health and ageing and an Assistant Professor at Université Grenoble-Alpes in France. She works on the professional and family long-term care of dependent older people. More generally, she is interested in the dynamics of the daily help to people with health problems, in public grants of care services and in public policy for dependent older people.

Collinet, Cécile is Professor at the university Paris-Est Marne-La-Vallée, France. She is Assistant Director of a research team focused on sociology and history of sport. She works on public policies and especially on health policies and prevention of ageing. She leads a research program called 'The governance of wellbeing in France'.

Delalandre, Matthieu is a Senior Lecturer at the Université Paris-Est Marne-La-Vallée, France. His research focuses on issues related to the production and the diffusion of scientific knowledge in the field of sport and physical activity. He is particularly interested in scientific controversies and in scientific knowledge reception and use.

Eyraud, Benoît is a Senior Lecturer in sociology at the University Lyon 2 (France) and researcher at the Max Weber Centre. He is leading with Livia Velpry the Collectif Constrast, a French multidisciplinary research group composed of sociologists, philosophers and legal experts. https://contrastcollectif.wordpress.com/.

Keller, Richard C. is Professor of Medical History at the University of Wisconsin-Madison (USA), where he is also Associate Dean of the International Division. He is the author of *Fatal Isolation: The Devastating Paris Heat Wave of 2003* (Chicago University Press, 2015) and *Colonial Madness: Psychiatry in French North Africa* (Chicago University Press, 2007), and is co-editor of *Unconscious Dominions: Psychoanalysis, Colonial Trauma, and Global Sovereignties* (Duke, 2011), *Enregistrer les morts, identifier les surmortalités. Une comparaison Angleterre, Etats-Unis et France* (Presses de l'EHESP, 2010), and a special issue of *South Atlantic Quarterly*, 'Life after Biopolitics' (2016).

Kramer, Nicole is a postdoctoral researcher at Frankfurt University, in Germany. Her recent research deals with gender history, the history of old age and the twentieth-century welfare state in Europe. Among her recent publications are 'Volksgenossinnen on the German Home Front: An Insight into Wartime Nazi Society', in B. Gotto and M. Steber (eds), *Visions of Community in Nazi Germany. Social Engineering and Private Lives* (Oxford University Press, 2014); 'Welfare, Mobilization, and the Nazi society', in L. Raphael (ed.), *Welfare and Poverty in Modern German History* (Berghahn Book, 2016).

Lambelet, Alexandre is Associate Professor in the School of Social Work (EESP) at the University of Applied Sciences & Arts Western Switzerland (HES-SO), Lausanne.

Lassen, Aske Juul, PhD, is a postdoc at the Copenhagen Centre for Health Research in the Humanities (core.ku.dk), SAXO-Institute, University of Copenhagen, Denmark. He is an ethnologist who specialises in ageing, humanistic health research, everyday practices, co-creation, cultural analysis, public engagement and ethnography. He is currently engaged in the two cross-disciplinary research endeavours Centre for Healthy Ageing (ceha.ku.dk) and Counteracting Age-Related Loss of Skeletal Muscle Mass (calm.ku.dk).

Lechevalier Hurard, Lucie holds a PhD in sociology (University Paris 13). She is a post-doctoral researcher at CNRS and the Max Weber Centre in Lyon (France), and a member of Collectif Contrast (http://contrastcollectif.wordpress.com/).

Messerschmidt, Reinhard, MA, studied Sociology, Philosophy and Political Sciences. Afterwards, he was a scholarship holder of the European Doctoral School of Demography at the Institut national d'études démographiques (INED) in Paris. Furthermore, he held a doctoral scholarship at the a.r.t.e.s. Graduate School for the Humanities Cologne, where he started his discourse analytical research on demographic change. From 2012 to 2014 he worked as a research scientist at GESIS – Leibniz Institute for the Social Sciences in the BMBF-funded digital humanities project eTraces. Since 2015, he has been a research scientist at the Cologne Center for eHumanities at the University of Cologne, Germany.

Nilsson, Magnus earned his PhD from the National Institute for the Study of Ageing and Later Life, Linköping University, Sweden. He currently holds a position as Assistant Professor in Social Work at the University of Gothenburg, Sweden. His research has engaged with different ageing-related themes, for example ageing in rural areas, ageing and masculinity, representations of old age and ageing in public discourse and the process of marketization of elder care in Sweden.

Pérez-Caramés, Antía is Senior Lecturer in Sociology at the University of A Coruna, where she received her PhD in 2010 with a thesis on the process of demographic ageing and gender relations in care work for dependent people in Galicia (Spain). She is a member of the Research Group on the Sociology of International Migrations, based at the same university. Her research focuses on demography and migration studies. She is mainly interested in the analysis of care work and gender relations, the political production of population ageing, and several aspects of the phenomenon of international migrations in Spain.

Pfaller, Larissa (Dr. phil.), is Research Associate at the Institute of Sociology at the Friedrich-Alexander-University of Erlangen Nürnberg (FAU) in Germany. She is especially interested in cultural sociology and qualitative social research, and recently published her PhD thesis on the topic of anti-ageing medicine.

Schweda, Mark (PD Dr. phil.) is Senior Researcher at the Department for Medical Ethics and History of Medicine at the University Medical Center Göttingen. He has a background in philosophy and German language and literature. His research focuses on philosophical, bioethical, and sociocultural aspects of ageing and the life course as well as on questions of political philosophy. Among his recent publications is the edited volume *Popularizing Dementia. Public Expressions and Representations of Forgetfulness* (Bielefeld, 2015) (together with Aagje Swinnen).

Xing, Jingyue is a PhD student in the Department of Sociology at the École Normale Supérieure of Paris, France. Her research interests are in political sociology, sociology of organizations, sociology of health and of ageing. She studies the pricing practices of local and central authorities relative to the rates for nursing homes and homes for the disabled. More broadly, she analyses the State reform and its impact on the daily work of low-level functionaries, and the relations between authorities and public service producers.

Index

active ageing 34, 45–56. *See also* ageing; as everyday practices 222–34
active ageing technologies 222, 226
Activities of Daily Living (ADL) 167, 175, 177, 181
Adams, Vincanne 64
adult disability dependency ratio (ADDR) 26–27
AFSSA 53, 54
Age Friendly Cities initiative 225
ageing. *See also* older adults; older people: active (*See* active ageing); attitudes of French towards 112–16; banal nationalism and 86–90; defining boundaries for 11–12; dependency in 228; disciplines exploring 3; as epitome of disaster 152–3; exercise improving wellbeing of 45–56; expert knowledge and 131–2, 144; gender and 11, 131–44; health and exercise in 45–49; historiography of 5–6; international perspective of 2; medicalisation of 3, 60, 71; moral economy of 10, 79–92; nationalism and 90–92; physical activity of 45–56, 222–36; political economy perspective of 6; preventive policies on 45–56; 'problem of,' 116–18; as a region of knowledge 1–2; as a risk factor for diseases 60, 62; science and policy 9, 19–40; social production of 5; society's adaptation to 197–8; structuring research on 6–7; study of social dimensions of 3–4; sub-categories of 7; threatening vitality of the population 112
ageing well 46; individual responsibility for 54–55
Ageing Well Plan 54
ageism 120–1

Agence Française de Sécurité Sanitaire des Aliments (AFSSA) 53, 54
age of subject impacting effects of physical activity on wellbeing 50
AGGIR scale 11, 166, 172–81, 204, 206; conducting evaluations using scale 179–81; criticism of 176–8; latitude in applying 210–12; strategic use of 210–14
alarmist demography 2, 11, 19, 35–36, 38, 152, 155–7, 159
Alliance nationale pour l'accroissement de la population française 113
Allocation Personnalisée d'Autonomie (APA) 204–17
Alzheimer Plan 2008–2012, 196
Alzheimer's patients: legal status of in institutions 196; restriction of movement and 194–5
Alzheimer units 192
American Academy of Anti-Ageing Medicine (A4M) 60, 62
American College of Sports Medicine (ACSM) 48
ANESM 194
anti-ageing medicine 60–73; abductive argument 67; attitudes towards 65–71; avant-garde perspective of 67; extending lifespan 63; future perspective of 60–61, 63–64, 71; limiting aesthetic signs 63; pharmaceutical interventions in 63; varieties of evidence in 68–69
anti-immigrant sentiments 37, 83–86, 91
anti-Islam sentiments 82–83
anxiety impacted by exercise 51
APA programme: administrative organization of 216–17; dependency as eligibility criteria 204; initial